Opioids in Medicine

Opioids in Medicine

A Comprehensive Review on the Mode
of Action and the Use of Analgesics
in Different Clinical Pain States

By

Enno Freye
Heinrich-Heine-University, Düsseldorf, Germany

In collaboration with

Joseph Victor Levy
University of the Pacific, Webster Street, San Francisco/California, USA

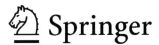 Springer

Library of Congress Control Number: 2008920685

ISBN 978-1-4020-5946-9 (HB)
ISBN 978-1-4020-5947-6 (e-book)

Published by Springer,
P.O. Box 17, 3300 AA Dordrecht, The Netherlands.

www.springer.com

Printed on acid-free paper

Contents

Part II   Mechanism of Action of Opioids and Clinical Effects

Part III   Opioids, an Integrative Part in Perioperative Medicine

Part V   Detection of Illicit Use of Opioids in Primary Care

Introduction

The book centers on the treatment of pain using the appropriate opioid and a suitable co-medication whenever necessary. While many physicians or health care providers either subscribe or advocate analgesics in response to a painful situation, their basic knowledge when and how to apply them frequently is scarce. And often there is a lack of sufficient knowledge on their potential side-effects, their mode of action, their possible interactions with other agents such as ß-blockers, Ca^{2+}-antagonists, ACE inhibitors and/or benzodiazepines. In addition, not all analgesics are equivalent or equally proficient at alleviating certain painful ailments. Although there have been many of articles and books written on the subject of effective pain treatment, very few have centered on the rational use of opioids. In fact opiophobia is still around with some caregivers who consider an opioid not to be the first-line drug in severe pain. On the contrary, the myth is still around that an opioid is potentially dangerous even when used in serious painful situations, and although the WHO has stated that opioids are elementary in therapeutic strategy taking into account that they are used by mouth, by the ladder, at fixed time intervals and advocating a time consistent release formulation, they are not available in every country. This book is a basis for those people who have decided to use opioids for pain relief in a meaningful way, not putting too much emphasis on academic discussion and controversies but rather to give the potential user something practical at hand for safer use.

Considering chronic pain to be an intruder in someones life, the book will:
- Give practical defense strategies using active and passive tactics,
- advocate the types of opioids (weapons) to use,
- give a strategy how to gain the edge over pain,
- build a plan to suit the situation when it comes,
- prepare you for uncommon side-effects,
- provide you with basic building blocks of tactics in pain therapy,
- make sure that the odds are in favor of your patient.

While any ailment that is accompanied by pain in principle has the tactical advantage, this book is also meant for the significant majority of therapists who want to build up their first line of defense beforehand. Not wanting to be left alone with the sole information given in the prescription information, or avoiding the cumbersome task of searching through the vast number of articles and textbooks related to opioid use, this book covers viable information in a compact and comprehensive format, which otherwise can not be found easily.

While there is no absolute prescription for every situation that will cover every case, the approach is to lay out the basics for the therapist before pain becomes a "self-inflicting disease".

Düsseldorf, January 2008   Enno Freye, MD, PhD

Part I

Rational for the Use of Opioids in Nociceptive Transmission

The Nociceptive System, an Elementary Part of the Body's Protective Scheme

Pain is an unpleasant sensory and emotional experience associated with real or potential tissue damage. Described in terms of such damage, it is an integral part of our existence. In its acute state, pain is localized and transient and displays a direct stimulus-response relationship. Because pain serves to protect us by warning of contact with potentially damaging thermal, mechanical, or chemical factors, a relatively high threshold stimulus is required. Pain when it is persistent and chronic becomes the primary reason for seeking medical attention. In its pathological state, either during inflammation or neuropathy (injury or disease to the nervous system, including dystrophy and deafferentiation pain) pain outlasts its biological usefulness and has become the target of extensive research. This is because over one-third of the world's population suffers from persistent or recurrent pain. In the United States alone some 100 million people suffer from moderate to severe pain during any given year. In addition, approximately $100 billion per year is spent on health care, compensation, and litigation related to chronic pain [1]. Only 50% of the individuals who seek treatment for intractable pain are satisfied with the treatment options they are offered. Evaluation of the mechanism of pain is complicated by the fact that the clinical diagnosis of pain is often imprecise, reflecting the emotional state of the sufferer, the disease state, individual differences and gender bias. Pain must thus be examined in terms of its severity, temporality and etiology.

Being an unpleasant and emotionally strong colored sensory sensation, pain accompanies any potentially dangerous tissue destruction. It, however, is a necessary integrated part of our life, which protects us from any potentially dangerous thermal, mechanical or chemical injury. By directing the attention towards the injury, further damage of the integrity of the organism is avoided. Pain may be of acute or chronic nature, and it is the major cause why patients visit the doctor, who has the important task to prevent its chronification. This is because over time pain induces a cellular lesion resulting in a disease "sui generis", i.e. a disorder, which in the weeks following cellular destruction, diverts from its creator (Figure I-1). Since the

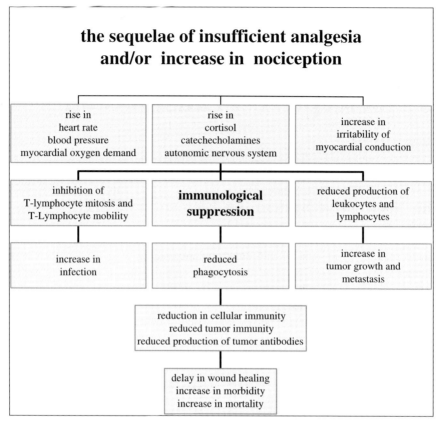

the sequelae of insufficient analgesia
and/or increase in nociception

| rise in heart rate blood pressure myocardial oxygen demand | rise in cortisol catecholamines autonomic nervous system | increase in irritability of myocardial conduction |

| inhibition of T-lymphocyte mitosis and T-Lymphocyte mobility | **immunological suppression** | reduced production of leukocytes and lymphocytes |

| increase in infection | reduced phagocytosis | increase in tumor growth and metastasis |

reduction in cellular immunity
reduced tumor immunity
reduced production of tumor antibodies

delay in wound healing
increase in morbidity
increase in mortality

Figure I-1. Insufficient analgesia and its consequences on the immune system

mechanism of pain sensation is so complex, it becomes an individual experience depending on the emotional condition of the patient, the stage of the disease, the socio-cultural differences, and the respective hormonal cycle. Therefore, immediate and clinically relevant diagnosis is not always possible. While one third of the world population suffers from acute and/or recurrent chronic pain, it affects the respective national health and social system by means of hospital stay, loss of working hours and disability costs. Such consequences can be changed, since only 50% of the patients, who visit the doctor because of unbearable pains, get sufficient treatment. Thus, pain becomes a significant part in the life of an individual; a connotation he first becomes aware of when having pain. Formerly pain was quoted as being "a noble feeling boosting up the morale". Often, however, such claim is forgotten when the philosopher himself has pain. It therefore is mandatory to scrutinize the actual cause of pain in a detective manner in order to treat the patient adequately.

Acute Pain – Sequence of Changes in the Body

Pain as a warning symptom directs the individual's attention to the injury, so that protective measures are taken and everything is done to avoid further damage. However, defensive physical reactions can result in an overcompensation of the individual's capabilities and an additional burden. Thus, pain and fear lead to the release of adrenaline and noradrenaline via an increase of activity of the adrenergic nervous system. Activation of the cortex-hypothalamus-pituitary-axis results in the release of ACTH, inducing a simultaneous rise in the level of gluco- and mineral-corticoids from the adrenal body. Pain and the accompanying stress reaction induce secretion of ADH (antidiuretic hormone) and STH (somatotropic hormone) from the posterior lobe of the pituitary. This is followed by a defense mechanism of the cardiovascular system with:

- hypertonia,
- tachycardia,
- vasoconstriction (peripheral and the splanchnic area),
- increase of heart work,
- rise in cardiac excitability, and
- increase in myocardial oxygen demand (MVO_2).

In addition to catecholamine-related cardiovascular effects, also humeral changes can be observed:

- increase in blood volume
- increase in blood viscosity,
- hyperglycemia (glucocorticoid and adrenaline effect),
- excess formation of lactic acid (hyperlactemia),
- increase of free fatty acids in the plasma (noradrenaline effect),
- reduction in sodium secretion and
- increase of potassium loss (aldosterone effect).

Aside from hormonal changes, as they can be observed in acute pain, particularly in the postoperative period or after acute trauma, such negative effects can result in the malfunctions of organs and organ systems:

- Suppression of immune function, which is due to a long lasting consequence of glucocorticoids with a concomitant rise in the susceptibility for bacterial and viral infections (Figure I-1).
- A raise in the vulnerability of the myocardial conduction system with an ensuing ventricular arrhythmia and/or fibrillation.
- Pulmonary dysfunctions are one of the main postoperative complications, especially after thoracic and intra-abdominal surgery [2, 3]. Due to insufficient ability to cough, atelectasis develops, which, beside an inadequate ventilation-perfusion-ratio with hypoxia, may result in the development of pneumonia,
- Circulatory and metabolic dysfunction lead to an elevation of stroke volume, blood pressure, myocardial metabolism as well as an increase in myocardial oxygen demand,

- Gastrointestinal and urological complications originate in an inhibition of reflex motility, resulting in nausea, emesis and ileus. Pain also induces a reflex-induced hypomotility of the urinal tract, with the sequealae of urinary retention and infection.
- Reflex vasoconstriction in the area of the large joints leads to neglect of use and atrophy with joint stiffening [4].
- Hormonal-related increase in blood viscosity with a decrease in fibrinolysis, especially in the postoperative period in the lower extremities results in the formation of thromboemboli and subsequent pulmonary emboli [4, 5].
- Electrophysiological and morphological changes within the nociceptive system results in the chronification of pain, which may even outlast the actual event [6].

Later, when chronification of pain has developed, it may even become difficult to link it with the actual source [7]. Despite removal of the actual cause, chronification leads to a pain behavior, which requires the entire attention of the patient. Thus, chronified pain has lost its actual function as an alarm signal, because it accompanies the patient over years and even decades [8, 9, 10].

The importance of pain transmission is underlined by the fact that half of all skin nerve fibers with their peripheral nociceptors can be activated by means of thermal (heat or cold), mechanically (push, pressure), and even chemically (acids, lye) stimuli. This for instance is highlighted by the affection of locomotion, where pain has warning function. For instance, after trauma such as bruise, strain, inflammation as well as thermal or electric injury a barrage of so-called pro-nociceptive compounds are being released, which excite the peripheral nociceptors (anatomically free nerve endings). These nociceptors are activated directly or indirectly through different kinins, such as bradykinin, kallidin, T-kinin and/or prostaglandin E. The kinins are body-made compounds the concentration of which is increased through inflammation, tissue damage, or directly through trauma. It is only by inhibition of the enzyme, cyclooxygenase (COX), a necessary step in the formation of prostaglandin from arachidonic acid, peripheral analgesics (NSAIDs) induce their

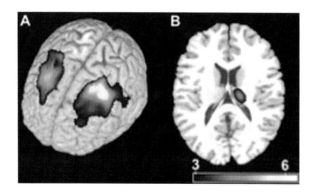

Figure 1-2. Decrease in prefrontal and thalamic gray matter during chronic pain Adapted from [12]

action. In addition, it has been demonstrated, that aside from their peripheral mode of action, peripheral analgesics also induce a centrally related analgesic effect [11].

Following transition from acute to chronic pain, it can be regarded as an ailment of itself and has to be treated accordingly. This has been demonstrated in patients with chronic pain. By using magnetic resonance imaging (MRI) an irreversible loss of brain tissue has been demonstrated. For instance patients with long-lasting neuropathic pain, showed a reduction in neocortical tissue (prefrontal cortex and thalamus) by as much as 11%, which is equivalent to a loss in the grey matter following 10–20 years of normal ageing. In addition, cortical tissue loss was directly related to the duration of pain. These findings are in accordance with other imaging studies that demonstrated a decrease in brain tissue in the specified areas. These studies provide compelling evidence for the early identification and appropriate management of pain (Figure I-2).

Differences in Pain Quality

When diagnosing pain it can be categorized into the following qualities:
1. Physiological pain
2. Acute or chronic pain
3. Inflammatory pain, and
4. Neuropathic pain.

On the other hand pain can be divided into different categories depending on its origin:
1. Transient-stimulus induced pain
2. Pain from tissue damage
3. Pain from injury of afferent neurons
4. Pain from injury of central neurons.

Everything should be done in order to identify the mechanisms of chronification, which may be due to:
1. Nociceptor activation
2. Nociceptor sensitization
3. Central sensitization
4. Disinhibition
5. Ectopic activity
6. Structural reorganization, and/or
7. Phenotype switch

Acute pain sensations are transmitted from the periphery to the brain. At the level of the spinal cord, ascending pain signals are modulated by afferent signals from touch receptors. Nociceptors release glutamate and substance P in layers I, II (substantia gelatinosa) and III that stimulate both NMDA- and AMPA-(glutamate) receptors and NK1-(neurokinin) receptors on spinal output neurons. As a consequence of NMDA receptor activation, two potent mediators of pain, nitric oxide and adenosine, are produced. The glutaminergic neurons (Aß-fibers) carrying somatosensory information from touch receptors synapse in laminae III and IV onto dendrites of spinal output neurons that become the contralateral spinothalamic tract carrying the pain, temperature, and touch signals to the higher levels of the CNS (Figure I-3).

The mechanisms underlying chronic pain (i.e. neuropathic pain) may be either peripheral (e.g. reflex sympathetic dystrophy) or central (e.g. postherpetic neuralgia). For instance, following peripheral injury and inflammation, repetitive firing of C-fibers lead to activation of NMDA glutaminergic receptors, and C-fiber-evoked "wind-up" in which the C-fiber response is highly augmented to subsequent input. NMDA receptor antagonists can block this phenomenon. The C-fiber-evoked "wind-up" results in hypersensitization with expansion of receptive fields of nociceptive input and hence the induction of spontaneous pain and hyperalgesia (excessive sensitivity to noxious stimuli). In addition, allodynia, a condition under which an ordinarily non-painful stimulus evokes pain, results from the activation of Aß-fibers by innocuous tactile stimuli. Peripheral mechanisms also include collateral sprouting from primary nociceptive afferents.

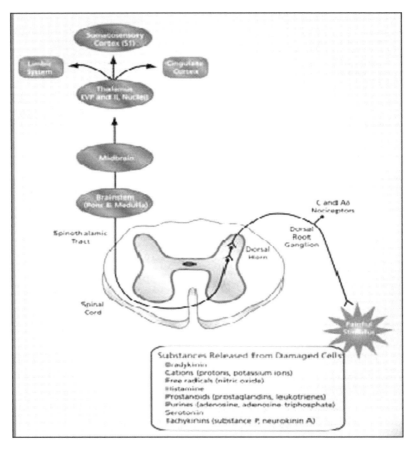

Figure I-3. The ascending pain pathways (Il = intralaminar nucleus of the thalamus; VP = ventroposterior nucleus of the thalamus)

All these mechanisms add up to "wind up", including:

1. Excitotoxicity in layers 1 and II of dorsal horn neurons;
2. reorganization of dorsal horn synaptic connectivity, characterized by sprouting of large myelinated Aß-afferents into lamina II of the dorsal horn;
3. spontaneous discharge in spinal cord neurons, and
4. a lowered threshold in the spinothalamic tract neurons and the next relay station, the thalamus.

Aside from commonly known transmitters in mediation of afferent pain sensation, such as substance P, recent discoveries have identified a number of additional mediators and target sites, all of which presently are under scrutinization for possible therapy:

1. Neurotropins, with its typical ligand, the nerve growth factor and the respectable receptor site.
2. Interleukin 6, interferon-γ receptors, PGI_2 and its receptors, B_2 bradykinin receptors, tachykinin receptors, A_{2A} adenosine receptors as peripheral mediators of nociception and hyperalgesia.
3. Opioids and their receptors: e.g. ß-endorphin, enkephalins, orphanin FQ/nociceptin, dynorphin, μ-, κ- and δ-opioid receptors.
4. Non-opioid neurotransmitter receptors like adrenergic and serotonin receptor ligands.
5. Intracellular molecules participating in signal transduction such as protein kinase A and protein kinase C_g, nitric oxide synthetase (NOS), heterotrimeric G_o proteins.
6. Selective ligands for the CB_1 cannabinoid receptor.
7. Selective ligands for the VR_1 vanilloid receptor.
8. A fatty acid amide hydrolase.
9. Calcium ion channels of the N- and R-type, as well as voltage-gated (or inward rectifying) sodium and potassium channels, all of which play an important part in the mediation of nociceptive afferents. In addition,
10. ligands for the H_1-histamine receptor, a
11. specific galanin-like mediators, and
12. ligands that bind to the $P2X_3$ (nucleotide-gated, inotropic) receptors.

All such ligands presently are under investigation as new targets in pain therapy.

Anatomy of Pain and Analgesia

At the site of injury, tissue damage leads to the release of several chemical factors such as adenosine 5′-triphosphate (ATP), bradykinin, substance P, chemokines, neurotrophic factors, histamine, prostaglandins, leukotrienes, serotonin, epinephrine, acetylcholine, protons and potassium ions. Any of these factors may stimulate the sensory neurons (nociceptors) that carry pain signals to the central nervous system (CNS; Figure I-3). There are two major types of nociceptors, unmyelinated and myelinated. Unmyelinated nociceptors are small-diameter, slow conducting C-fibers, which transmit burning or dull pain (Figure I-4). Myelinated nociceptors

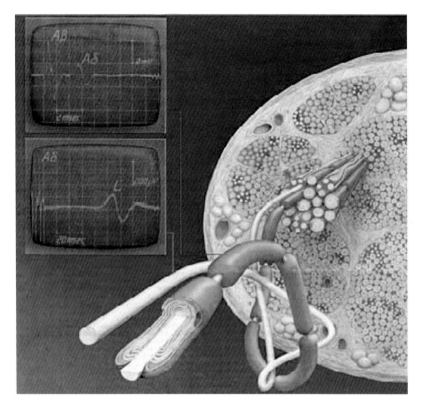

Figure 1-4. The two afferent nociceptive pathways with different conduction velocities. Small diameter cells contain non-myelinated C-, and thinly myelinated A-fibers, functionally and pharmacologically identified as mediating the long-lasting pain sensations. Contrary, the myelinated Aδ-fiber transmits the initial sharp-like pain sensations

are medium to large diameter, fast-conducting Aδ-fibers, which sense prickling pain. Both types of nociceptor carry pain signals from the peripheral site of injury and synapse on interneurons in the dorsal horn of the spinal cord. In addition to the speed of conduction, nociceptors can differ in the neurotransmitters they contain, the receptors and ion channels they express, and their capacity for sensitization during injury or disease. Approximately 70% of all nociceptors are C-fibers, while Aß-fibers comprise the remaining 30%.

SIGNIFICANCE OF C-FIBERS IN PAIN TRANSMISSION

C-fibers that express TrkA (a nerve growth factor receptor) and do not bind isolectin B4 (a lectin from a shrub, Griffonio simplicifolia) project to the outermost layers of the dorsal horn (lamina 1 and outer lamina II). Isolectin B4-positive C-fibers project to the inner lamina II and also express fluoride-resistant acid phosphatase and P2X3 receptors. Nociceptors expressing neurokinin (NK1) receptors constitute projection neurons and are clustered in lamina I of the dorsal horn. Small diameter nociceptors that do not express NK1 receptors seem to target interneurons in lamina II.

SIGNIFICANCE OF Aß-FIBERS IN PAIN MODULATION

Medium and large neurons that innervate low threshold mechanoreceptors mediate the response to tactile and vibrational stimuli via Aδ- and Aß-fibers that synapse in laminae III–V (Figure I-5). Neurons in the dorsal root ganglion are further classified physiologically based on the type of stimuli by which they respond. In the superficial dorsal horn, nociceptive cells are unresponsive to innocuous stimuli (i.e. gentle stimulation) because of their relatively high threshold, and thus respond only to painful stimuli. In the deep dorsal horn, a wide range of neurons responds to both innocuous and noxious stimuli. Some information is also carried in parallel by myelinated Aß-fibers, which are responsible for relaying sensations of touch [10].

Transmission of Pain with Different Qualities

Already at the periphery where stimulation of nociceptors is induced by the trauma, an inhibitory activity will come into play, affecting the advanced transmission along the selective pain tract. At the peripheral site selective pain receptors are only excited once serotonin and prostaglandin are present. The excitatory substance bradykinin promotes prostaglandin synthesis, which explains why a lowered pain threshold is present in inflamed areas. Subsequent pain afference can be differentiated into distinct qualities of pain:

1. A superficial sensation of pain with a piercing-like, intense, short and well localized quality.
2. A secondary type of pain with a delayed temporal quality. It is of longer duration, has a dull quality and can hardly be localized.
3. Pain from the viscera is of dull and of colic-like nature. It is difficult to localize and is accompanied by vegetative sensations.
4. Deep-sited pain from the subcutaneous areas like muscles, joints, and bones. It is dull and radiates into the surroundings.

Such different pain qualities are mediated via two diverse nervous pathways tracks, which project to the spinal cord (Figure I-4):

- The Aδ-fibers with a relatively fast (15–20 m/s) conduction velocity; they mediate superficial, knife-like, and well localized pain sensations.
- The C-fibers, which result in a dull and less well localized pain quality, are characterized by a slow conduction velocity (1 m/s).

Transmission of peripheral, painful primary afferents (Aδ- and C-fibers) from the first order to the second order neuron (spinothalamic and spinoreticularis tract) occur in the posterior column of the spinal cord. In the substantia gelatinosa, fast Aδ-fibers terminate in the lamina II, III and IV (Figure I-5); the slow C-fibers end in the Lamina I and II of the spinal cord [13].

The relevant transmitter, which synapses at the spinal dendrites is a neuropeptide called substance P. Substance P is an undecapeptide consisting of 11 amino acid sequences, which can also migrate retrograde to peripheral terminals, resulting in a local irritation with swelling and reddening of the skin. Transduction from the first order to the second order neuron is an important center, where facilitation, modulation, sensitization, and decision-making of all incoming painful stimuli take place (Figure I-5). There sensory afferents are collected from different segments, being integrated and modulated. Repetitive stimuli result in lowering of action potential thresholds with a prolonged and enhanced after

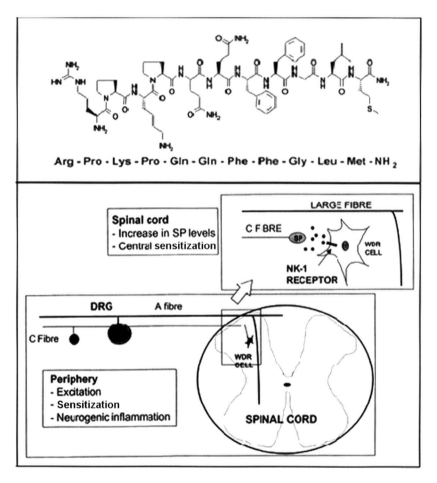

Arg - Pro - Lys - Pro - Gln - Gln - Phe - Phe - Gly - Leu - Met - NH$_2$

Figure I-5. Substance P, an undecapeptide and a member of the tachykinine family, with a molecular weight of 1346, is an important neurotransmitter and neuromodulator in pain processing at the periphery and the spinal cord, which binds to the NK$_1$-receptor. Through stimulation of wide-dynamic range neurons (WDR), additional excitatory cells are recruited resulting in an increased area of pain discharge (spinal sensitization with primary hyperalgesia) and an activation of prior dormant wide-dynamic range (WDR) receptors (Figure I-5). Peripherally this is characterized by a lowering in pain threshold, an increased sensitivity to threshold stimuli with evolving spontaneous pain, resulting in a larger areas of hyperalgesia and allodynia that surround the primary site of injury (secondary hyperalgesia).

Substance P, a Mediator of Pain and a Member of the Tachykinin Family

The spinal cord also is the area where the reticulospinalis tract projects (corticospinalis tract), which descends down from higher cortical areas, using serotonin or noradrenaline (serotinergic tract) as transmitter substances.

At the spinal relay station local endorphinergic interneurons with their transmitters endorphin, and enkephalins, inhibit ascending afferences, resulting in an increase of pain threshold (Figure I-6). It is the area where the enkephalins inhibit the release of substance P as well as other excitatory transmitters such as glutamate or the "calcitonin gene-related peptide" (CGRP), resulting in a reduction of transduction. Also, in response to an inflammatory stimulus, CGRP, an important 37 amino-acid vasodilatatory peptide is released from peripheral nerve terminals, often leading to hyperalgesia. CGRP is synthesized increasingly during inflammation and

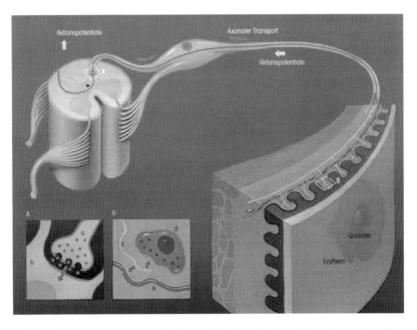

Figure I-6. In addition to the release of substance P in the spinal cord, there is a retrograde axonal transport, which results in an increased permeability of local vessels, and the formation of wheal and erythema in the area surrounding injury

being co-expressed with substance P at the spinal cord level, it's release can be reduced by the administration of opioids at the spinal or epidural space. This is because such agents bind to the same receptors as enkephalines, where the target cells can be found on interspinal enkephalinergic neurons (Figure I-7). Thus, the spinal cord site can be considered as an important site of communication where among others, central analgesics exert their antinociceptive action.

During pain, the ascending spinoreticularis tract projects from both sides of the spinal cord to the reticular formation as well as to the intralaminary nuclei of the right and left thalamus, resulting in an arousal reaction. In addition, there are connections to the anterior cortex, the cinguli gyrus and structures of the limbic system (nucleus amygdalae and hypothalamus). While the latter are related to the emotional (fear) and autonomic reactions (hypertension, tachycardia), the anterior cortex is linked to individual negative sensations of pain; the cingulus is accountable for the release of endogenous opioids resulting in a reduction of pain (Figure I-8). Fibers of the spinothalamic tract also project to the brain stem (medulla and mesencephalon) where it interacts with synapses of the ventero-posterior and intrathalamic nuclei of the thalamus. Thereafter, fibers from the thalamus project to the primary somatosensory area (S1 and S2) of the cortex, where fibers connect to the rear, and the parietal section of the cortex, are ending in the nucleus amygdalae, the perirhinal cortex and the hippocampal area (Figure I-8).

It is important to point out that the primary fibers of the spinothalamic tract are composed mainly of so-called "wide dynamic range" neurons and specific

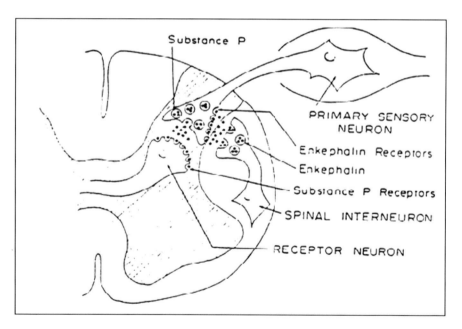

Figure I-7. Antinociceptive effect of inhibitory enkephalinergic interneurons at the spinal cord level

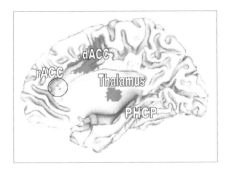

Figure I-8. Neuroimage of relevant subcortical areas of the brain during pain using magnetic resonance imaging (MRI): Rostral and dorsal anterior cingulate cortex (rACC/dACC), thalamus and parahippocampal cortex (PHCP) Adapted from [14]

neuronal pain pathways. Especially during long-term irritation, there is an additional acquisition of afferent pain-related fibers and additional nociceptive afferences.

Several researchers have questioned if the specific nociceptive afferent fibers are accountable for the sensitization of pain. According to the theory by Melzack and coworkers [15], pain is the final result of an imbalance in the neuronal network distributed over the whole body. It therefore can be regarded as the ultimate result of the body's own neuromatrix and, to a lesser degree, it is the result of an injury within the sensory nervous system. This theory was confirmed in so-called phantom pain, which appears in up to 70% of patients following amputations. There cortical reorganizations by means of a mirror image of the missing extremity resulted in a significant reduction of pain. Such data underline the proposition that **clinical pain is the *manifestation of a modified nervous system*.**

In this context it has to be pointed out that insufficient reduction in pain, especially in the post-operative period, results in an increase in postoperative morbidity and mortality [16, 17, 18], followed by chronification of pain. It is imperative in order to sufficiently block the process of chronification and the accompanying nociceptive-adaptive alterations in the nervous system, to block all nociceptive afferences *before* the barrage of afferent stimuli arrive at the spinal cord, the brain stem, and/or subcortical pain-related centers. Once nociceptive discharges are sufficiently reduced, temporary or permanent neuronal transformations at different areas of the CNS can be eliminated.

Supraspinal Processing of Pain

Peripheral nociceptive stimulation has been shown not only to trigger spinal neuronal signaling of the ascending nociceptive system, but also supra–spinal areas are activated. From the layers I and V of the posterior column, second order neurons originate and ascend to supraspinal pain-modulating centers (Figure I-8). Via the lateral projecting neospinothalamic tract large myelinated fibers pass cephalically to the ventro-posterior-lateral-thalamic nuclei (VPL). From there axons synapse

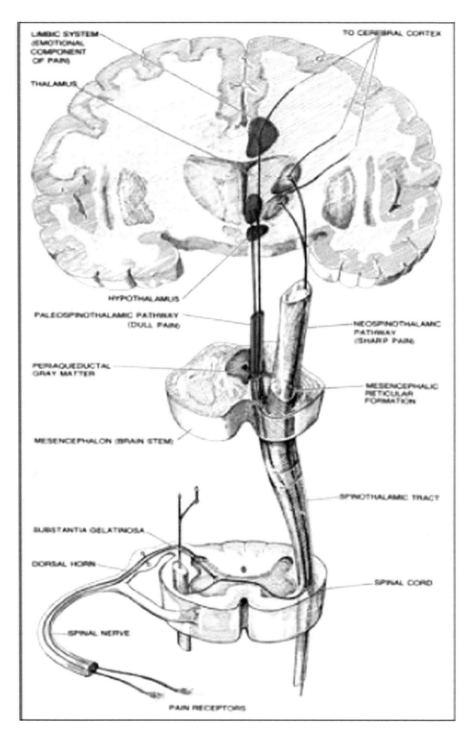

with third relay of fibers projecting to the somatosensory cortex (Figure I-9). The cell-bodies of the medial part of the ascending spinothalamic tract, also called the paleospinothalamic tract, originate in the deep layer of the spinal cord. They have thin fibers, project to the reticular formation, the periaqueductal gray (PAG), the hypothalamus, and the medial as well as the intralaminar thalamic nuclei. These fibers then connect with neurons of the limbic forebrain system, which thereafter project diffusely to other parts of the brain (Figure I-9). Functionally, the phylogenetically older medial system consists of thin fibers. They lack somatotopic organization, and are of slower transit than the lateral system. They determine the level of arousal, mediate the specific unpleasant nature of pain, affect the general behavior in fostering rest, protection, and care of the damaged area. They thereby promote healing, and recuperation. The lateral system composes relatively long and thick fibers that conduct rapidly (Figure I-10). They functionally convey discriminating information, have a discrete somatotopic organization about the onset of injury, its precise location, its intensity, and duration. It quickly can bring about a response that prevents further damage.

There is evidence that the ventrobasal thalamus and the somatosensory cortex, which receive input from the rapidly conducting lateral ascending pathway, have anatomic and physiologic characteristics that permit processing of sensory discriminative information. Moreover, the reticular formation (e.g., hypothalamus, medial thalamus, and limbic system) is involved in motivational and affective features of pain. They are strategically connected to activate and influence the hypothalamic and the limbic forebrain systems, which are responsible for the activation of supraspinal autonomic reflex responses such as ventilation, circulation, neuroendocrine function and the motivational drive, triggering the organism into action (fight or flight reaction) while at the same time acting as a watchdog during sleep.

The myelinated fibers of the neospinothalamic tract, end in the nuclei ventrocaudalis-parvocellularis (Figure I-11). From there fibers project directly to the rear gyrus of the cerebral cortex, the somatosensory cortex, involved in the localization of the origin of pain. The somatosensory cortex shows an exact somatotopic arrangement, a reverse "homunculus" necessary for exact localization of the injury. However, more importantly in pain therapy are the endings of the unmyelinated fibers of the paleospinothalamic tract, which project to intrathalamic nuclei, especially to the nucleus limitans, which lies at the border of the mesencephalon and the tegmentum (Figure I-11).

The nucleus limitans and the intrathalamic nuclei are part of the non-specific projection system of the thalamus, which, via basal ganglia, project diffusely to practically to all cortical areas. The nucleus limitans mediates the alarming, timeless,

Figure I-9. The ascending nociceptive pathways originating in the dorsal horn of the spinal cord, give rise to the spinothalamic tract. The trigeminal nucleus of the brainstem carries afferents from the face and the trigeminal nerve, where fibers cross and ascend to the thalamus along the trigeminal lemniscus

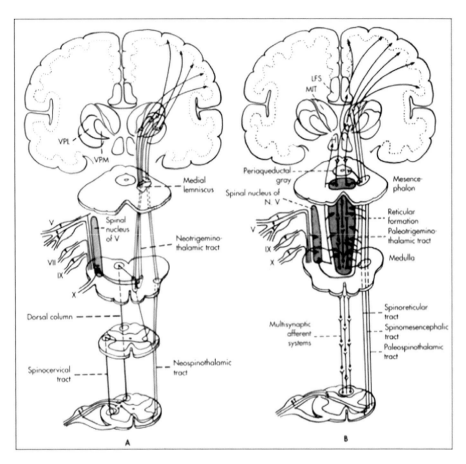

Figure I-10. Origin and course of the lateral (A) and the medial (B) ascending spinothalamic tract with its different interconnections

dull, and less localizable feeling of pain ("it hurts" = identification of pain). From the nucleus limitans and the intrathalamic nuclei, fibers project to the limbic system consisting of the nucleus amygdalae, and the hippocampal area, which give pain an aggravating, negative connotation with a dysphoric component (painful emotion). The pallidum in this respect is not only a center of motor impulses; it can be considered as a psychomotor center for conscious movements transmitting the emotional, affective component of pain [19, 20]. Between both nociceptive afferents, the fast one for localization of pain and the slower system for mediating the feeling of pain, there is an inhibiting interaction. Thus, the faster conduction system is capable to inhibit the slower system within the substantia gelatinosa of the spinal cord and the thalamus, resulting in a modulatory balance among each other [19].

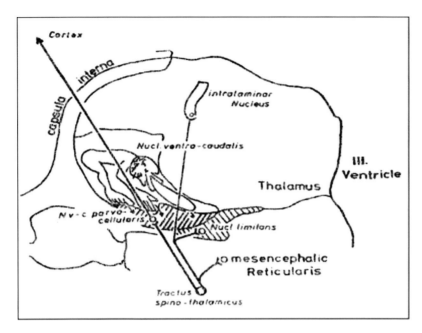

Figure I-11. Topography of the nucleus limitans, an important relay station in the transmission of nociceptive afferents to higher pain modulating and discriminating centers of the CNS. This area, which mediates the unspecific feeling of pain, and contrary to the adjacent nucleus ventro-caudalis, does not show a topography (homunculus). It is closely coupled with emotions and shows a dense accumulation of opioid binding sites (Nucl. vc.pc. = nucleus ventro-caudalis parvo-cellularis). Adapted from [24]

TRANSDUCTION OF NOCICEPTION VIA THE SPINOTHALAMIC TRACTS

The spinothalamic tracts (Figures I-9 and I-10) send fibers through the brainstem (medulla, pons) and midbrain to synapses in the ventroposterior and intralaminar nuclei of the thalamus. Projections from the thalamus finally terminate in the primary somatosensory cortex (S1 and S2 region). From the S1 and S2 regions, the pathway proceeds to the posterior parietal cortex and insular cortex, and finally to the amygdala, the perirhinal cortex and the hippocampus. It is important to note that the types of neurons originating in the dorsal horn that give rise to the spinothalamic tract are predominantly wide dynamic range neurons together with some nociception-specific neurons. These two types of neurons are important for processing different dimensions and stages of pain. Thus, the spinothalamic tract is critical not only for sensory processing of nociceptive information, but for pain affect as well.

The sensation of pain and temperature from the head and face is carried by the trigeminal nerves that synapse in the trigeminal nucleus of the brainstem. The fibers then cross and ascend to the thalamus along the trigeminal lemniscus. Recently, a new visceral pain pathway that projects in the dorsal column of the spinal cord has been identified.

While acute pain has a meaningful purpose in the framework of tissue damage, it functions as a warning signal. At the same time it is an important diagnostic tool for the physician and the pain specialist. Contrary, chronic pain is the corollary of continuous tissue damage such as a tumor or a degenerative destruction in a joint. It does not serve as a warning signal, and often it has totally lost its connection to the origin, developing into a disease of itself.

It is apparent that the mechanisms underlying the perception of pain implicate many brain regions. In the 1960s, Melzack and Wall proposed a gate theory of pain, which postulated that certain neurons in the dorsal horn that project in the spinothalamic tract are stimulated by both large diameter sensory axons and unmyelinated axons carrying the pain signal [21]. The dorsal horn projection neuron is inhibited by an interneuron that is stimulated by the large diameter sensory axons and blocked by unmyelinated pain axons. In this fashion, activity in the axon carrying the pain signal maximally stimulates the projection neurons. However, if the mechanoreceptive sensory axons fire concurrently, they cause activation of the interneuron and suppress the nociceptive signals. Another theory proposed by Melzack suggests that pain is the result of the output of a widely distributed neural network (the body's own neuromatrix), rather than being the direct result of sensory input evoked by injury [15]. The phenomenon of phantom limb pain (pain sensed from a nonexistent limb) experienced by 70% of individuals after amputation or severe nerve damage (e.g., brachial plexus transection) supports this hypothesis [22, 23].

Opioids directly affect the pain modulating and pain discriminating centers within the CNS, especially via the nucleus limitans, an accumulation of small neurons with opioid binding sites, which lie close to the nucleus ventro-caudalis-parvo-cellularis (Nucl. v-c. p-c). The nucleus limitans is responsible for the recognizing an impulse as being painful (Figure I-11). Thus, during pain therapy with an opioid, the afferent impulse may be felt; however, it has lost its aggravating, negative character and is not recognized as being painful.

THE DESCENDING ANTINOCICEPTIVE SYSTEM

Another, clearly defined and important system, that modulates nociceptive input at the spinal cord level, is the descending tract. It originates at three different locations:
1. In the periaqueductal gray of the midbrain structure and the nucleus raphe magnus of the medullary reticular formation [25].
2. At the lateral hypothalamus, where descending fibers originate
3. In the basolateral amygdalae, where an inhibitory tract originates.
All these fibers do not project directly to the dorsal horn. Some fibers project only through connection via the rostral ventromedial medulla (RVM), and the

dorsolateral pontine tegmentum (DLPT). Others project via detour to the nucleus raphe magnus and the locus ceruleus from the periaqueductal gray directly to the posterior column of the spinal cord (Figure I-12).

It also had been demonstrated that the analgesic effect of both μ- and δ-opioid ligands work in union, resulting in an activation of this descending tract. This additive/synergistic action can be observed following systemic or local injection into the central gray or the RVM. This is also the site, where Ach-receptor sites have been identified, explaining the analgesic mode of action of cholinergic agents. The neuronal cells, which project to the posterior column of the spinal cord, are of serotonergic and noradrenergic origin, (Figure I-13). Via desensitization they selectively modulate the activity of the nociceptive posterior column neurons by means of inhibitory, enkephalinergic interneurons and α_2-adrenoreceptors relay neurons [26]. Being part of the descending inhibitory fibers, the reticulospinal tract releases different neurotransmitters such as glutamate, aspartate, serotonin and neurotensin, all of which had been demonstrated in the periaqueductal central gray [27, 28].

Finally, the substantia gelatinosa of the posterior column in the spinal cord also is the "gate-control", as originally described by Melzack and coworkers [15]. Being activated by fast acting Aß-fibers projecting from mechanoreceptors of the skin, it is the relay station where other inhibitory mechanisms propagate inhibitory interneurons in the posterior column. If nociceptive action potentials from slower Aδ- and C-fibers hit upon these cells, their transmission is

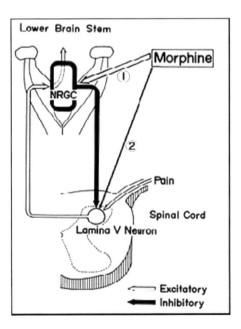

Figure I-12. The descending inhibitory tract being activated by opioids originating in the nucleus reticularis gigantocellularis (NRGC) of the ventromedial medulla (RVM)

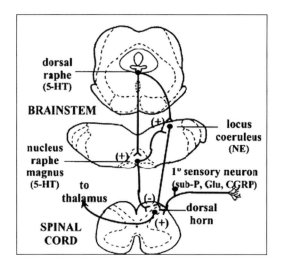

Figure I-13. The descending, inhibitory pathways influencing afferent nociceptive input at the spinal cord and the transmitters affecting transition (sub $-$ P $=$ substance P; Glu $=$ glutamate; CGRP $=$ calcitonin gene related peptide; $5-$ HT $=$ serotonin; NE $=$ norepinephrine)

blocked [29]. This mechanism explains the therapeutic value when pain sensations can be relieved through simultaneous tactile or thermal activation (TENS $=$ transcutaneous electrical nerve stimulation; Figure I-14). At the same time it is also an explanation of electrical spinal cord or dorsal cord stimulation (SCS), thalamus stimulation and of electroacupuncture, all of which inhibit nociceptive afference by means of electric stimulation, also termed counter irritation therapy. Following the "gate-control" theory, ascending nociceptive impulses from Aδ- and C-fibers connect with the descending inhibitory efferent input of Aβ-fibers at the substantia gelatinosa of the spinal cord, which collects all nociceptive input. There, pain impulses are suppressed, diminishing the actual sensation of pain, a therapeutic implication being used regularly in pain treatment by different agents [30].

In summary, within the posterior column of the spinal cord, nociceptive transmission from the first to second order neuron is characterized by three independent operating inhibitory systems:

1. Descending fibers from the locus coruleus, the reticular formation, the reticulospinal tract, the nucleus raphe magnus and the periaqueductal grey. By means of a release of serotonin and norepinephrine at nerve endings of serotonergic and noradrenergic conduction pathways in the substantia gelatinosa, the sensitivity of small relay cells to nociceptive impulses is diminished (Figure I-14).
2. Inhibitory, endorphinergic interneurons in the area of the posterior column block nociceptive transmission (Figure I-14) via the release of endogenous opioids the endorphins, in particular the enkephalins.
3. Pain fibers, which project into the posterior column of the spinal cord, not only excite the second order ascending neurons of the pain tract, they also stimulate

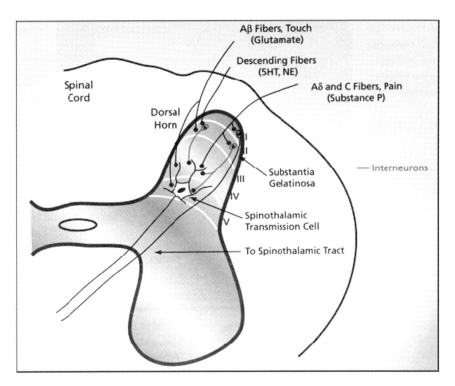

Figure I-14. Modulation of nociceptive transmission in the dorsal horn of the spinal cord, illustrating the interaction of small pain diameter afferents and large diameter mechanoreceptors (touch) afferents, as well as its modulation by descending neurons and enkephalinergic interneurons on afferent pain pathways (5 – STH = serotonin; NE = norepinephrine)

   inhibitory cells. Thus, a self-regulatory mechanism is initiated so that afferent
   stimuli are either facilitated or inactivating on their conduction pathway.
The substantia gelatinosa of the posterior column of the spinal cord, therefore,
can be considered as a main coordinator. It is the place where incoming afferents
are assembled, integrated, and modulated. At the same time it is also the location
where an inhibitory pain mechanism comes into play and where it is decided, if
and at which intensity nociceptive afferents are being transmitted (Figure I-14). In
the context of a meaningful therapy and in order to avoid the transition of acute
to chronic pain and adaptation, the substantia gelatinosa plays a significant role
in any therapeutic approach. Early and sufficient pain inhibition with an opioid is
one of most imperative components of useful antinociceptive strategy, where the
agents not only block the transmission, but also the transfer within the spinal cord.
The spinal cord is the location where an effective and twofold pain management
is instigated; directly through potentiation of the endogenous mechanisms of pain
control through binding at local opioid receptor sites, and indirectly by means of
activation of inhibitory descending pain system.

Because nociceptive afferents regularly are modulated by descending pathways originating in
a. the basolatral amygdalae,
b. the lateral hypothalamus,
c. the periaqueductal gray,
any reduced activity and/or destruction of the descending inhibitory pathways results in an increase in nociception. Especially the midbrain structure, and the periaqueductal gray, inhibit either directly the pain signals at the neurons of the dorsal horn or indirectly via the raphe magnus nucleus of the medullary reticular formation and via the rostral ventromedial medulla (RVM) all of which project to the spinal cord. Both the serotonergic input from raphe nuclei and the noradrenergic input from the locus ceruleus modulate the output of layer II of the spinal cord by synapsing onto the inhibitory enkephalin neurons of the dorsal horn (Figure I-15). Norepinephrine released from descending fibers act through α_2-adrenoceptors, which in return decrease the sensitivity of dorsal horn relay neurons to noxious stimuli This is also the location where α_2-agonists, when given epidurally, potentiate the effects of opioids such as morphine. Furthermore, agonists at the μ-opioid receptors activate neurons in the periaqueductal gray and rostral ventral medulla by reducing GABAminergic inhibition. In addition, there is a release of a brain-derived neurotrophic factor, which appears to be an endogenous modulator of painful responses in the dorsal horn, and may also contribute to sensory hypersensitivity, especially associated with inflammatory pain.

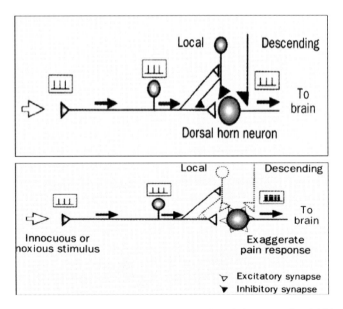

Figure I-15. Schematic representation of insufficient activity of the descending inhibitory pathway compared to control, resulting in an exaggerated response to all incoming nociceptive stimuli at the spinal cord level

Neurophysiology of Pain – Type of Receptor Sites Involved in Therapy

Trauma and damage at the periphery results in inflammation and/or damage of cells, resulting in the release and the formation of so-called nociceptive substances, which activate peripheral nociceptor sites (Figure I-16):
1. Formation of free oxygen radicals (ROS = reactive oxygen species) like peroxides, and nitric oxide (NO),
2. release of prostanoids (prostaglandin D, E, F, I, leukotrienes), thromboxane,
3. formation of purines (adenosine, ATP),
4. release of tachykinins (substance P, neurokinin A, B),
5. increase in the level of kinine (bradykinin, kallidin, T-kinin) as well as
6. increase in local acidity by a rise in H^+- and K^+-protons.

All these tissue-damaging mediators are co-expressed simultaneously. They have been termed "inflammatory soup", which not only maintains the inflammatory process but also results in the initiation of nociception. Within this group prostaglandin E_2 (PGE_2) holds a superior position, because this substance must be present before any activation and sensitization of peripheral nociceptors by other neurotransmitters induces nociceptive sensations. In addition to these algogenic substances, other transmitters like:

- histamine,
- acetylcholine,
- serotonin, and
- bradykinin

also directly affect peripheral afferent nociceptors resulting in the painful sensations. While histamine can only cause pain sensation in relatively high concentrations,

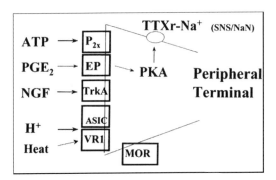

Figure I-16. Schematic representation of main peripheral nociceptors activated by various tissue-damaging stimuli resulting in a nociceptor activation (ATP = adenosinetriphosphate; P = purine/pyrimidine receptor; EP = prostanoid receptor; NGF = nerve growth factor; H+ = acidity; VRI = vanilloid receptor activated by heat, capsaicin; TrkA = tyrosine receptor kinase A; TTXr − Na^+ = tetrodoxin-resistant sodium channel; ASIC = amiloride sensitive proton channel, activated by low pH; MOR = morphine; PKA = protein kinase A)

acetylcholine sensitizes the pain receptors through other mediators already being present in low concentrations.

TRANSDUCTION OF NOCICEPTIVE AFFERENCES VIA ASCENDING PATHWAYS

All peripherally-induced painful stimuli initiate action potentials, which are transmitted to the dorsal horn (lamina l and deep layers V–VI; Figure I-14). From there they ascend to higher cortical areas via two ascending pathways. The spinoreticular tracts ascend on both sides of the spinal cord via the reticular formation and terminate in the intralaminar nuclei of the right and left thalamus. The spinoreticular tracts are responsible for the general arousing effects of pain. They may also influence the perception of pain through their innervation of the anterior cingulate cortex, insular cortex, as well as other structures of the limbic system, such as the amygdala and hypothalamus. The limbic system is implicated in the emotional aspects of pain, with the central nucleus of the amygdala strongly involved in fear and autonomic responses to stress, and the cingulate cortex acting as a center for endogenous opioid activation specific to negative pain affect.

DIFFERENT THERAPEUTIC APPROACHES IN PAIN THERAPY

The most widely used medications for pain management have been opioids with morphine as its prototype (isolated in 1803), and non-steroidal anti-inflammatory drugs, where aspirin (developed in 1899) is a prototype agent (Figure I-17). In addition, a variety of non-specific agents such as anticonvulsants, and antidepressants are also part of the therapeutic armamentarium.

Because neuropathic pain in general is insensitive to morphine and other opioid drugs, it is best managed by antidepressants and anticonvulsants. Non-steroidal anti-inflammatory drugs (NSAIDs) are not only ineffective at ameliorating severe pain, but also produce gastrointestinal side effects and increase bleeding time. Drugs that are at least partially effective in ameliorating pain involve a wide range of compounds affecting different neurotransmitter systems. Receptors modulated by these compounds are often expressed in both the peripheral and central nervous systems. Pain research is currently targeting a complex system of receptors, ion channels and their modulators in an effort to identify newer, safer methods of alleviating pain. Some of the latest research in pain therapy involves the areas of COX inhibitors, bradykinins, opioids and a variety of neuropeptides, such as melanocortins, cholecystokinins, tachykinins, calcitonin gene-related peptide and galanin. Also, the cannabinoid system and vanilloid receptors and their modulators, recently have generated much excitement in the field of pain research. This is followed by modulators of sodium, potassium and calcium channels, P2 receptors, ionotropic glutamate receptors and finally nicotinic acetylcholine receptors, all of

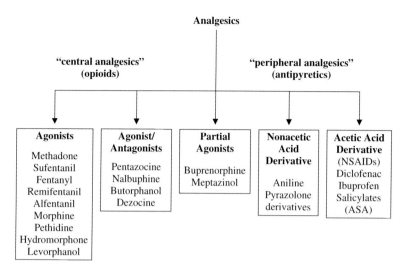

Figure 1-17. Overview of analgesics administered in the treatment of pain

which present other potential therapeutic targets while adjuvant analgesics complete the potential armamentarium in the pharmacology of pain relief.

SIGNIFICANCE OF BRADYKININS IN INFLAMMATORY PAIN

Several kinins, notably bradykinin, kallidin and T-kinin, are involved in inflammation and visceral pain. Bradykinin induces inflammation in part through the receptor-independent release of histamine and serotonin from activated mast cells. B1 and B2 receptors are localized in nociceptive parthways and contribute to inflammation and neuropathic hyperalgesia. B1 receptors are absent in healthy tissue and their expression is evoked by tissue injury or by cytokines, such as tumor necrosis factor α (TNFα), and interleukin 1ß (IL-1ß). The B2 receptor agonist [des-Arg9]-bradykinin produces hyperalgesia that can be blocked by the B1 receptor antagonist [des-Arg′O] HOE-140. B2 receptors are expressed on nociceptors and in central and peripheral sensory ganglia. They appear to be involved in the chronic phases of the inflammation and pain response. Local increase in concentrations at the bradykinin B1- and B2-receptors have demonstrated to be involved in local inflammatory pain and in the development of a late neuropathic painful syndrome with hyperalgesia. While the B1-receptor normally is not present in normal tissue, it is only after tissue damage or an inflammation-related release of cytokines, especially of the tumor necrosis factor (TNFα) and interleukin 1ß (IL-1ß), that this receptor is being expressed. The B2-bradykinin receptor on the other hand has been identified in peripheral as well as central ganglia. This receptor specifically is involved in the chronic inflammatory pain. Following B2 bradykinin receptor activation, the inflammatory response involves the activation of protein kinase C, which in turn increases COX-2 activity and the production and release of PGE_2. Thus, the development of B1, and B2 bradykinin receptor antagonists may yield novel remedies for inflammatory pain. Following B2-receptor activation, intracellular protein kinase C (PKC) initiates an increase of the formation of cyclooxygenase-2 (COX-2) and release of prostaglandin E_2 (PGE_2). PGE_2 especially by itself is ineffective. Only in combination with other mediators does it initiate a painful stimulus. Serotonin also is a transmitter, which holds a central role among all other nociceptive mediators.

COX INHIBITORS IN THE ALLEVIATION OF PAIN

Peripheral nociceptors, sensitive to prostaglandins and other mediators, are not specifically qualified receptors but simple nerve endings. Only by means of pressure on the sensitive nerve fiber ending over a specific threshold, is activation initiated. In chronic tissue injury, or repetitive noxious stimuli however, the nerve endings assume the property of true receptors. Via formation of intracellular cyclic aminomonophosphate (cAMP) they are involved in the area-specified sensitization and hyperalgesia in tissue damage, and during inflammation there is an increased formation of prostanoids. Prostaglandin E_2-synthesis has a significant effect on the initiation of chronic persistent pain. However, prostanoids do not excite the nociceptors directly. Via sensitization, other mediators now manifest an increase in their activity. On the other hand, by means of PGE_2-activation, additional sodium-channels are being generated, resulting in an increase in depolarization and transmission of nociceptive signals. While all local anesthetics such as lidocaine or procaine can block the activated sodium-channels, inhibition of prostaglandin synthesis by means of cyclooxygenase inhibition (COX-1,2-inhibition) represents an imperative analgesic principle that should earn special attention in all peripherally conditioned painful syndromes.

The enzyme cyclooxygenase (COX) is involved in the production of prostanoids, such as prostaglandin PGE_2, which induces inflammation and sensitizes nociceptors, thus contributing to acute pain and hyperalgesia (Figure I-18). Two isoenzymes that have been identified, COX-1 and COX-2, are known to catalyze the rate-limiting step of prostaglandin synthesis and are the main targets of NSAIDs. COX-1 is considered to be constitutive, meaning that the activity of this enzyme is necessary for normal physiologic functions. COX-2 is considered to be inducible and has been shown to be overexpressed during inflammation and neuropathy. NSAIDs, such as aspirin, non-selectively inhibit both COX-1 and COX-2, and the relative selectivity for these isoenzymes varies across the other NSAIDs. Thus, in addition to inducing analgesic and anti-inflammatory effects mediated by inhibition of COX-2, use of drugs, such as aspirin, also leads to gastrointestinal and hematologic side effects, which are mediated predominantly by COX-1. Contrary, agents like refecoxib (Vioxx®, now withdrawn worldwide), celecoxib (Celebrex®) and the prodrug parecoxib (Dynastat®), which is changed intermediary to the active agent valdecoxib, demonstrate high COX-2 selectivity. This is of importance because those agents are largely devoid of the typical NSAID side effects, as COX-1 activity

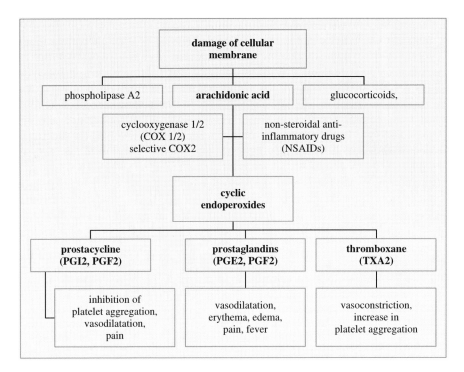

Figure 1-18. The action of non-steroidal anti-inflammatory drugs (NSAIDs) is to inhibit the cascade after peripheral tissue damage. COX enzymes attached to the cell wall, lead to the production of prostaglandins, which result in pain and inflammation. NSAIDs enter the cell where an inhibitory portion detaches and then binds to COX enzymes, blocking the site of receptor binding. The enzyme is then unable to bind to the cell wall resulting in lesser prostaglandin synthesis followed by an inhibition of pain signals

is not inhibited. On the basis of selectivity, the constitutive formation of COX-1 is still possible so that the otherwise common side effects like gastrointestinal ulcerations, hematologic side effects, and renal function impairment, especially in long-term therapy, are minimized. Recently a COX-3 isoenzyme has been identified which appears to be expressed in canine and human cortex and is selectively inhibited by analgesic antipyretic drugs, such as acetaminophen, phenacetin, antipyrine and dipyrone, as well as all other NSAIDs [31], although this notion is still controversial.

THE OPIOID RECEPTOR SYSTEM – MAIN TARGET IN PAIN THERAPY

The endogenous opioid system has a functional role in modulating pain perception and agonists, which bind at G-protein-coupled opioid receptors are potent analgesics. However, opioid receptors are also present in various other locations of the central nervous system where opioid ligands affect other functions of the body. In the hypothalamus they influence temperature regulation and control of hormonal secretion. In the brainstem they are involved in the control of respiration, blood pressure and heart rate. In the forebrain, the endogenous ligands for the opioid receptor are implicated in behavioral reinforcement and they appear to play a role in anxiety and in the expression of emotions. In addition, opioid receptors influence gastrointestinal and autonomic nervous system functions. But most of all, opioid receptors are involved in the transmission of nociception where they represent an imperative part in the strategy of survival.

Opioid peptides are the natural ligands of the opioid receptor, where enkephalin (derived from proenkephalin), dynorphin (derived from prodynorphin) and ß-endorphin (derived from pro-opiomelanocortin) – all appear to modulate pain pathway inputs. They are found in limbic structures, the hippocampus, nucleus of the stria terminalis, the hypothalamus, as well as striatum, substantia nigra, raphe nuclei, pontine-periaqueductal gray (PAG) and the spinal cord. Enkephalins bind predominantly to δ-receptors, the dynorphins have preferential affinity for κ-receptors, but also bind to μ- and δ-receptors. Another endogneous ligand, ß-endorphin activates both μ- and δ-receptors, but has little affinity at κ-binding site. Recently, the highly selective μ-(MOR) receptor agonists endomorphin-1 and endomorphin-2 have been identified in the dorsal horn of the spinal cord. These peptides display potent anti-nociceptive activity in animal models of neuropathic pain. Another endogenous peptide, nociceptin/orphanin FQ (N/OFQ) binds to an orphan opioid-like receptor ORL1. N/OFQ induces allodynia and hyperalgesia, and appears to be involved in PGE2-induced pain responses [50], while the endogenous peptide nocistatin antagonizes N/OFQ pain responses [32].

Recently, novel G protein-coupled receptors that are specific for sensory-neurons have been identified [33] and are activated by a peptide designated bovine adrenal medulla peptide 22 (BAM 22), which is produced by cleavage of proenkephalin A. These novel G protein-coupled receptors are expressed in the dorsal root ganglia and trigeminal ganglia in rats and humans and may play a role in the transmission of pain signals. However, unlike opioid receptors, these receptors are not blocked by the opioid antagonist naloxone.

Inhibitory and Excitatory Effects of Nociception at the Spinal Cord Level

Within the spinal cord, either an enhancement and/or an inhibition of ascending nociceptive afferences come into effect. The spinal cord is also considered as the major site where a number of analgesic agents initiate their mode of action through direct binding at selective inhibitory receptor sites (Figure I-19).

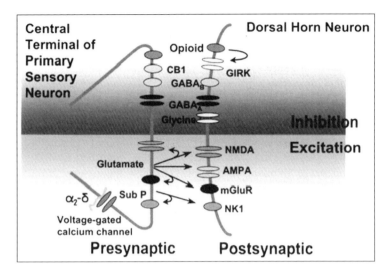

Figure 1-19. Summary of the different receptor sites at the dorsal horn related to inhibition and/or excitation of incoming nociceptive afferent impulses

NEUROHORMONES IN TRANSMISSION OF NOCICEPTION

Melanocortins

Melanocortins are a group of endogenous peptides that are derived from pro-opiomelanocortin. The melanocortins include adrenocortico-tropic hormone (ACTH), and the X- and ß-melanocyte stimulating hormone (MSH). Recent studies indicate that spinal melanocortin receptors (the MC4 subtype) are upregulated in animal models of neuropathic pain. Also, both (X-MSH and ß-MSH have been identified in areas of the spinal cord associated with nociception [34]. The MC4 melanocortin receptor agonists MTII and d-Tyr-MTII increase the sensitivity of rats to painful stimuli following sciatic nerve constriction. In contrast, the pain responses are attenuated following pretreatment with the melanocortin receptor antagonist SHU9119 [34].

Cholecystokinins

Cholecystokinin (CCK) belongs to a gastrin family of peptides. In the central nervous system it is widely distributed and predominantly exists as CCK-8, which binds to CCKs or CCKz receptors. In the periphery, the receptors that normally bind CCK are CCKA or CCK1. Axotomy leads to an upregulation of CCK in rat dorsal root ganglion. Antagonism at the CCK receptor by YM022 has been shown to produce analgesia following constriction injury to rat sciatic nerve. Administration of another CCKz receptor antagonist, L-365,260 has been shown to reverse tactile allodynia and thermal hyperalgesia [35]. Interestingly, CCK is co-expressed with the μ-opioid receptor in laminae 1 and II of dorsal horn and seems to block the antinociceptive effects of endogenous opioids in models of neuropathic pain. Accordingly, CCK receptor antagonists can thus serve as potentiators of opiate-induced analgesia. One specific antagonist of a CCK receptor, CI-988, has been found to enhance the effects of morphine [36].

Calcitonin-Gene-Related Neuropeptide

The calcitonin-gene-related peptide (CGRP) is a 37 amino-acid vasodilatory peptide, of which two isoforms, αCGRP and βCGRP, have been described. CGRP is released from peripheral nerve terminals in response to an inflammatory stimulus, such as local application of capscaicin, often leading to hyperalgesia. Some 80% of substance P trigeminal and other sensory ganglia contain CGRP. However, CGRP is also found alone in C-fiber nociceptors. Both CGRP and substance P are increased during inflammation, but decrease following dorsal root ganglion lesions. CGRP is also co-expressed with galanin. CGRP antagonists, such as CGRP8-37, when injected into the dorsal horn lead to analgesia. Another antagonist of the aCGRP receptor specifically, BIBN4096BS, reduces vasodilatation and thus has potential for treating migraine pain [37].

Galanin

In humans, galanin is a 29 or 30 amino acid residue peptide that is widely distributed in the nervous system and like CCK has been implicated in nociception. Galanin along with CGRP and substance P is expressed in small size sensory neurons in dorsal root ganglion. In acute pain state, galanin displays antinociceptive effects, reduces spinal hyperexcitability and decreases the nociceptive effects of Substance P [63]. In lamina II, galanin is also co-expressed with enkephalin and potentiates the antinociceptive effects of morphine, especially when co-administered with the CCKz receptor antagonist PD 134,308 [38]. A nonspecifie galanin receptor antagonist, M35 enhances C-fiber "wind-up" and spinal sensitization during inflammation. Following axotomy the expression of GalRz receptor mRNA is reduced, while recent evidence suggests that the GalR1 receptor is upregulated in dorsal horn neurons following nerve injury, as well as during inflammation (Figure I-20). Thus,

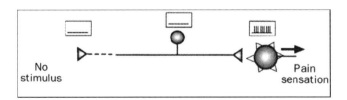

Figure I-20. Excitability in the dorsal horn neurons is determined by balance between excitatory input from periphery and inhibitory inputs (local and descending). Loss of sensory function after nerve injury results in spontaneous firing of dorsal horn neurons in spinal cord

a selective GalR1 receptor agonist may constitute a valuable tool for the treatment of neuropathic and inflammatory pain.

Nitric Monoxide, Mediator for Chronic Pain

Nitric monoxide (NO), a gaseous transmitter within the CNS was only discovered in the past years. It also plays a significant part in the process of nociception [39]. NO is generated as an intracellular transmitter with NMDA-receptor activation within the spinal cord. By activation of nitrite oxide synthetase (NOS), long-term release of NO connects to neuronal structures resulting in an activation of genes, followed by chronic pain, its potentiation with wind-up and hyperalgesia (Figure I-21). The significance of NO in the process of chronification especially is set off in tissue injury with accompanying inflammation [40]. This connotation has been corroborated in animal studies, where an increase in morphine-related analgesia could be achieved by intrathecal use of the NO-synthetase inhibitor L-NAME (L-nitroarginin-methylesther), [41]. At the same time, development of tolerance often observed in the process of pain therapy with morphine, experimentally

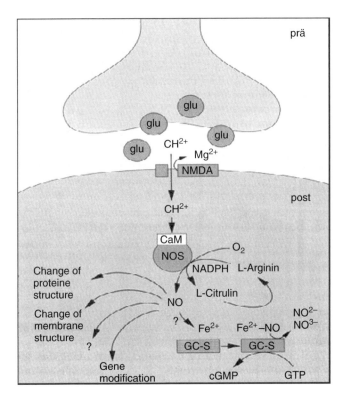

Figure I-21. Increase in synthesis of the gaseous transmitter nitric oxide (NO) in the transition from acute to chronic pain via activation of nitrite monoxide synthetase (NOS)

could be prevented with the NO-synthetase inhibitor [42]. While nitric oxide in acute or neuropathic pain only plays a minor role, it decisively is involved in the process of inflammation with transition to chronic pain. Consequently, agents that regulate the release of nitric oxide in pain therapy in the future may be of importance.

The Cannabinoid System

Cannabinoids derive their name from delta-9-tetrahydrocannabinol (THC), the psychoactive principle in Cannabis sativa (marijuana). Anandamide (arachidonylethanolamine) is the putative endogenous agonist for CB_1 and to a lesser extent the CB_2 cannabinoid receptors. It also acts as an agonist at the VR1 vanilloid receptor [43]. CB receptors are found predominantly in the central nervous system. They are also found on 10–13% of CGRP- and substance P-containing neurons and on interneurons in the dorsal root ganglia [44, 45]. CB_2 receptors are localized primarily on peripheral nerve terminals and on cells of the immune system [46].

Agonists at CB receptors are analgesics and may have therapeutic value in managing allodynia and chronic hyperalgesia such as cancer pain. Antagonists such as SR 141716A block the antinociceptive effects of cannabinoids. However, CB agonists that cross the blood-brain barrier may have the same psychoactive properties as THC. For example, the CB1/CB2 agonist WIN 55,212-2 is self-administered by mice [47]. Interestingly, CB2 agonists, such as HU-308 and AM 121 also possess antinociceptive properties, and AM 121 specifically appears to be devoid of central cannabinoid effects.

ION CHANNEL MODULATORS RESULTING IN FACILITATION/INHIBITION OF NOCICEPTION

The P2X and P2Y Receptor System

Several animal models of inflammation and pain indicate that ATP facilitates the transmission of pain input and modulates pain signals via the activation of ionotropic purine/pyrimidine receptors referred to as P2X receptors. ATP is released extracellularly in the vicinity of nociceptors under a variety of conditions, including tissue injury, visceral distension and sympathetic activation [48]. Heteromeric P2X2/3 and homomeric P2X3 and P2X2 receptors are selectively distributed within pain pathways. P2X3 receptors are almost exclusively expressed on small diameter sensory neurons that conduct nociceptive inputs from the periphery and have also been localized in the dorsal horn and lamina II of the spinal cord, as well as in the trigeminal ganglia. Other ionotropic P2 receptors, P2X2, P2X4 and P2X6 also appear to be involved in central nociceptive pathways[48, 49].

Metabotropic P2Y purinergic receptors may also be implicated in pain transmission. Unlike the ionotropic P2X receptors that seem to be involved in enhancing pain transmission, the P2Y receptor agonists UTP and UDP reduce spinal pain transmission in several rat models [50]. However, a pronociceptive effect of UTP also has been reported. These studies indicate that ionotropic receptor P2X3 antagonists or P2Y agonists may represent new approaches to explore in search of more effective pain treatment.

The Vanilloid Receptor System

The best-known vanilloid is capscaicin, the main pungent ingredient extracted from Capsicum frutescence chili peppers. Capscaicin activates VR1 vanilloid receptors that are present on afferent nerve fibers involved in pain transmission and neurogenic inflammation (Figure I-22). Although an endogenous ligand for the VR1 vanilloid (also known as TRPV1) receptor has not been identified, the endogenous cannabinoid anandamide activates VR1 receptors via a mechanism that is independent of cannabinoid receptor activation [51]. However, evidence suggests that N-arachidonyl dopamine may be the best endogenous VR1 ligand. In addition, VR1 receptors are known to be activated by noxious heat, low pH and calcium depletion. Studies with gene knock out mice indicate that the VR1 receptor is essential for normal thermal nociception and for thermal hyperalgesia induced by inflammation.

VR1 receptors are expressed on C- and Aδ-sensory fibers projecting to the dorsal horn of the spinal cord and on trigeminal afferents projecting to the hypothalamus, limbic system and neocortex. They are also expressed in non-neural tissues such as kidney, lung and spleen. The VR1 receptor is coupled to a non-specific membrane cation channel that is preferentially permeable to calcium and sodium ions. This channel is not affected by conventional channel blockers, but can be blocked by ruthenium red [52]. Activation of VR1-positive fibers by capscaicin, resiniferatoxin (RTX) and their analogs evokes sensations ranging from heat to burning pain. Activation is followed by loss of further sensitivity to capscaicin, insensitivity to noxious heat and chemical stimuli and loss of the ability of the fibers to release neurochemicals, such as substance P and CGRP, and elicit inflammation. This agonist-induced desensitization has been exploited in the use of capscaicin and capscaicin analogs as topical analgesics. VR1 antagonists may also be useful in the treatment of inflammatory hyperalgesia and pain. Capsazepine is the prototype competitive VR1 antagonist. The recently identified antagonists, JYL 1421 and 5-iodo-RTX, are 25–60 times more potent than capsazepine. The role in pain management of compounds such as arvanil, with dual CB1NR 1 agonist properties is currently an area of great research interest [50].

Recently the vanilloid receptor homologs VRL-1 (TRPV2) and VRL-2 (TRPV4) have been identified. Both are non-selective cation channels. VRL-1 channels are localized on Aδ and C-fibers in laminae 1 and II of the dorsal horn. They appear to mediate high threshold heat responses. The affinity of VRL-2 is less defined, but may be involved in responses to pressure or stretching [50]. It is suggested that the VR1-receptor sensitizes heat response by opening the channel where NGF also contributes to the heat pain responses.

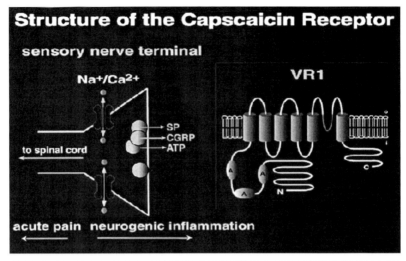

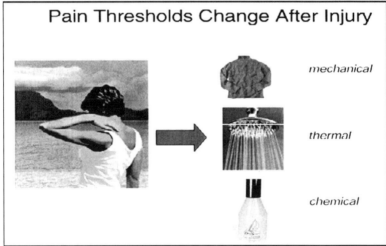

Figure I-22. The capscaicin-vanilloid receptor at the peripheral site, involved in thermosensations (e.g. sun burn) where protons augment the mediated heat responses

Voltage-Gated Sodium Channels as Ion Conduit Modulators

Voltage-gated sodium channels are present in most excitable cell membranes. Their activation supports neuronal depolarization and plays a crucial role in the generation and propagation of the action potential. Voltage-gated sodium channels are composed of a large IX subunit (approximately 260 kDa) and a variable number of small ß subunits (approximately 35 kDa). Brain sodium channels comprise three subunits, designated α, ßl and ß2. Skeletal muscle sodium channels include IX and a ß1-like subunit. While it is known that sodium contributes to nerve impulse

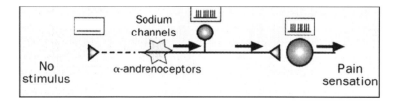

Figure I-23. Spontaneous firing along axon via increase in sodium channels

propagation, it is now accepted that inflammation evokes changes in sodium channel isoform expression in the periphery and the dorsal root ganglia (Figure I-24). This results in the formation of additional sodium channels along the nerve tract resulting in lowered threshold, leftward shift of stimulus-response curve function, increase of impulse propagation, spontaneous (ongoing) discharge, and hyperexcitability (Figures I-23 and I-24). Classically local anesthetics, such as lidocaine and procaine, are sodium channel blockers. Also, certain tricyclic antidepressants (TCA) are excellent sodium channel blockers, which explain their efficacy in chronic inflammatory pain. One of the most potent and selective sodium channel blockers is the toxin tetrodotoxin (TTX) produced by the Japanese puffer fish. TTX sensitive sodium channels are found in the brain and peripheral nerves, in sympathetic ganglia, and in skeletal muscle. In contrast, cardiac muscle and dorsal root ganglion neurons are associated with fibers that express TTX-insensitive sodium channels. These TTX-insensitive channels in the dorsal root ganglion, designated PN3/SNS (Nav 1.8), comprised of IX and ß3 subunits, and NaN/SNS2 (Na$_v$ 1.9), whose ß subunit composition is not known, play important roles in nociception. Selective blockers of these sodium channels may possess analgesic activity. PN3/SNS channels have a higher activation threshold and slower inactivation kinetics than NaN/SNS2 channels. Thus, it is likely that PN3/SNS channels

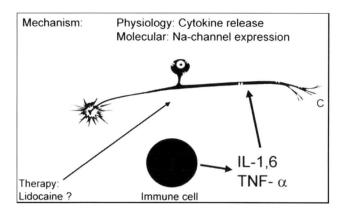

Figure I-24. Formation of inflammatory-related cytokines affecting sodium-channel expression with hyperalgesia

play a role in neuropathy, inflammation and chronic pain states, while NaN/SNS2 channels are involved in acute pain [53].

Most local anesthetics block sodium channels by binding either to the voltage sensor site or to a receptor that blocks the sodium pore, both of which are localized to the IX subunit. However, it appears that sites on the ß subunit may also constitute viable targets for therapeutic intervention in pain.

Non Voltage-Gated Potassium Channels

The pore-forming potassium channels, TREK, TRAAK, TWIK and TASK, differ structurally from ion-gated potassium channels. They are widely distributed in the central nervous system and are targeted by arachidonic acid and other unsaturated fatty acids [89]. Volatile anesthetics (e.g., halothane, ether, chloroform) seem to stimulate these channels, especially TREK, leading to depression of neural activity. Local anesthetics that target sodium channels (e.g. lidocaine, bupivacaine, mepivacaine) also activate the TASK channel.

Activation of high-threshold voltage-dependent L-, P-, Q- and N-type calcium channels on spinal neurons is involved in the mechanisms underlying acute pain, hyperalgesia and allodynia induced by a variety of stimuli [90]. Most research interest has focused on N-type calcium channels. Rats lacking the ß3 subunits of this channel show reduced C-fiber "wind-up" of spinal cord activity in response to sensory nerve stimulation and a reduced response to neuropathic pain. N-Type calcium channels appear to be localized on presynaptic nociceptive terminals where they serve to enhance the release of substance P and glutamic acid [54]. Blockade of N-type channels with ω-conotoxin GVIA reduces spinal cord hyperexcitability due to both innocuous and noxious sensory nerve stimulation. However, the concentrations at which these compounds are effective also induce toxic effects, thereby limiting their clinical utility as analgesics.

Like N-type calcium channels, P/Q-type channels also appear to be localized presynaptically on glutamanergic neurons. P/Q-type blockers inhibit pain induced by the stimulation of glutamanergic fibers, but not that induced by the ionotropic glutamate receptor agonist NMDA [54].

L-type calcium channels appear to be localized post-synaptically where they serve to enhance substance P-evoked neurotransmission [54]. L-type calcium channel antagonists potentiate analgesia produced by κ-opioid agonists and block the induction of opioid tolerance.

Ionotropic Glutamate Receptor Ion Channel Modulators

The development of allodynia and hyperalgesia following nerve injury and inflammation is in part due to increased synaptic excitability manifested by long-term potentiation (LTP) in central pain pathways mediated by NMDA ionotropic glutamate receptors [55]. Thus, LTP may underlie the plastic changes that occur in nociceptive pathways in neuropathy and other chronic pain states [56] and may be modulated by NMDA receptor antagonists.

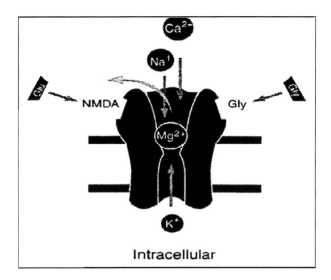

Figure I-25. The kainate receptor complex involved in the mediation of postoperative, incisional pain. Different ligands acting upon this non-NMDA receptor site

The NMDA receptor consists of NR1 subunit combined with one or more NR2 (NR2A, NR2B, NR2C or NR2D) subunits and has two amino acid recognition sites, one for glutamate, and the other for glycine, both of which must be occupied to allow channel opening. Antagonists of the NMDA receptor that have been identified selectively compete for either the glutamate or glycine site (Figure I-25). Subunit-selective (e.g. NR2B) antagonists have also been identified. Several high affinity NMDA antagonists and channel blockers, such as CPp, MK-801 and ketamine, may reduce hyperalgesia in animal models. However, the psychotomimetic effects, memory and motor impairment, induced by these compounds limit their utility. Selective glycine receptor and NR2B antagonists display analgesic properties that are devoid of deleterious side effects [57]. Low affinity NMDA channel blockers, such as memantine, also attenuate neuropathic pain in animal and human models without psychotomimetic side effects [58].

Other glutamate receptors have also been implicated in the transmission of pain inputs (Figure I-25). For example, kainate receptors located on sensory neurons may play a role in sensitizing pain states. The kainate receptor antagonist LY 293558 is antinociceptive in a capscaicin model of hyperalgesia.

EXCITATORY GLUTAMATE RECEPTOR; MEDIATOR OF PRONOCICEPTIVE EFFECTS

With every nociceptive stimulus neurokinins are being released in the posterior column of the spinal cord. Besides the tachykinins substance P, neurokinin A and B, excitatory amino acids like glutamate and glycine also are being released. The latter interact with specific receptor sites, which can be divided into ionotropic and metabotropic glutamate receptors. Following binding of the ligand at the ionotropic receptor, an ion channel is opened (Figure I-26) affecting the G-Protein, which causes secondary intracellular change with the propagation of action potentials.

Because of this G-protein-related mediation of effects, and contrary to the metabotropic receptor, the ionotropic receptor is characterized by a fast response. The metabotropic glutamate receptor is much slower by several orders of magnitudes, resulting not in propagation but in modulation of the receptor response.

Both, the ionotropic as well as the metabotropic glutamate receptor can be subdivided into several subtypes. The ionotropic glutamate receptor exists as a NMDA-(N-methyl-D-aspartate) and of the non-NMDA-type. Depending on the nature of the transmitter involved in the transmission, the receptors can be differentiated into both the kainite- and the AMPA-receptor (α-amino-3-hydroxy-5-methyl-4-isoxazole-propionic acid) respectively (Figures I-27 and I-28).

The NMDA-receptor in regard to the mediation of pain is of importance, because it is a fast-acting ion channel that regulates the outward shift of sodium and calcium ions and the inward shift of potassiumions. Only a minute binding at the NMDA-receptor via the two excitatory amino acids glycine and glutamate results in marked potentiation of excitatory effect, and a propagation of nociceptive action potentials. It is because of this activation, that the NMDA-receptor is considered to be closely related to the so-called "wind-up-phenomenon", where repetitive

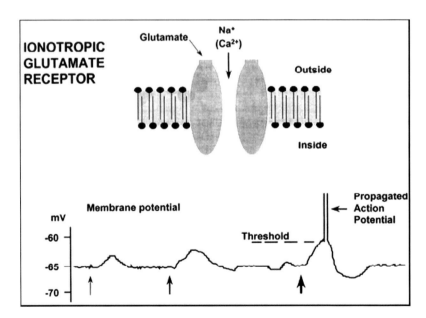

Figure I-26. The excitatory receptor site where glutamate binds resulting in a propagation of action potential in the afferent nociceptive system

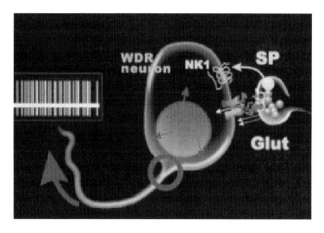

Figure 1-27. Nociceptive afferents to the cells of the spinal cord result in the release of excitatory transmitters substance P (SP), which bind to the NK1 receptor, and glutamate (Glut), which binds to a separate excitatory receptor. Both induce an acquisition of dormant wide-dynamic-range neurons (WDR) resulting in an increase in the propagation of action potentials in the spinal tract

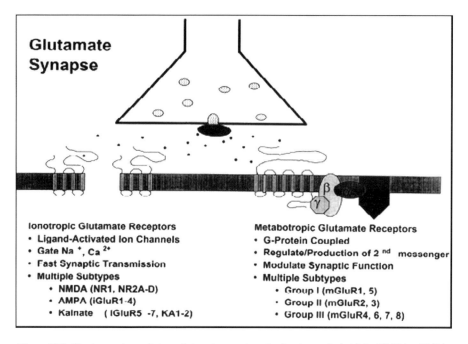

Figure 1-28. The two main excitatory glutamate receptors, the fast iontropic (with its NMDA-, AMPA- and kainite subtypes) and the slower metabotropic binding site, involved in the transmission of painful stimuli with its subsites

non-noxious stimuli result in an augmentation, which finally ends in a nociceptive reaction. Because the NMDA-receptor is a voltage-type ion channel, any increase of inward transmission of calcium ions results in an increase of nociceptive transmission. And because the increase of Mg^+-ions results in a receptor blockade, this "second-messenger" is of paramount importance in the process of pain transmission. This is because the inward Ca^{2+}-current results in activation of enzyme changes within the cells of the posterior spinal column, and an activation of the genetic machinery of the nucleus, which is correlated with chronic pain conditions. The NMDA-receptor also has an additional PCP (phencyclidine)-modulating site, through which the receptor-dependent ion channel can be blocked. Such a mechanism is used clinically when ketamine interacts with the PCP-binding site, while magnesium and doziciplin (MK-801) inhibit transmission via a separate unit (Figure I-29).

Following binding of the excitatory ligand glutamate at the voltage-gated, and fast acting ionotropic AMPA- and neurokinin-receptor, it initiates an increase of sensitivity of the slower metabotropic NMDA-receptor. As a consequence there is an increase of current of Ca^{2+}-ions through the NMDA-channel resulting in an increase of intracellular Ca^{2+}-ions. Since this process is initiated by substance P through binding of neighboring neurokinin receptors, co-activation of glutamate- and tachykinin- (substance-P) receptors instigate neuroplastic changes within the neuronal matrix (Figures I-29 and I-30).

Within the cell, the increase in calcium ions reinforces a postsynaptic *c-AMP-response element-binding protein* (CREB) synthesis of c-fos and c-jun, the target genes that increase the synthesis of amino acids in the formation of receptor sites. As a result, additional receptors are now available for binding, resulting in an increase of nociceptive transmission, which is reflected clinically in "augmentation" phenomenon with hyperalgesia (Figure I-31).

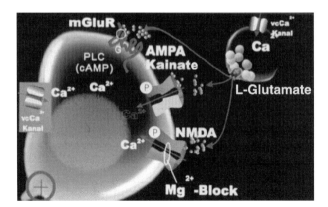

Figure I-29. The different type of pro-nociceptive receptor sites (NMDA-, AMPA-kainate-receptors) involved in chronic pain

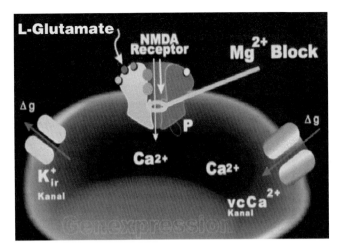

Figure 1-30. Following activation of the excitatory NMDA receptor, an increased inward current of Ca^{2+}-ions via selective ion-channels induces gene expression is intracellularely

The Nicotinic/Acetylcholine (NAchR) Receptors

Nicotinic/acetylcholine receptors are widely distributed throughout pain pathways in the central nervous system. Evidence suggests that the cholinergic cells in the pedunculo-pontine tegmental nucleus that project to the nucleus raphe magnus are a

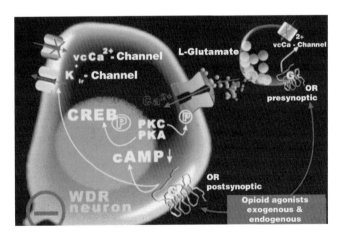

Figure 1-31. In chronic pain, protein kinase C (PKC) and protein kinase A (PKA) results in the activation of intracellular CREB (c-AMP-response element-binding protein), which expresses an increase in synthesis of excitatory receptor sites. A higher number of receptor sites results in higher transmission of action potentials responsible for the initiation of spontaneous, neuropathic pain, which can be blocked by opioids. OR-opioid receptor

source of descending inhibitory input to the dorsal horn. In addition, the descending cholinergic pathway that modulates pain signals seems to contain Ach receptors. Stimulation of these receptors leads to analgesia in models of acute and chronic pain. Nicotine, the prototypic agonist of nicotinic receptors, displays antinociceptive properties at high doses, but this effect is of short duration. The nicotinic receptor agonist epibatidine is 100–200 times more potent than morphine at producing analgesia in preclinical pain models. However, epibatidine also produces ataxia, hypothermia and seizures, which preclude it from potential therapeutic use [59]. Recently, a nicotinic receptor agonist, diazobicyclooctane (DBO-83) has been shown to have analgesic effects [60]. ABT-594, an analog of epibatidine that binds to the Ach subunit of the nicotinic receptor (Figure I-32), also exhibits analgesic properties, but is devoid of the side effects characteristic of epibatidine [61]. However, due to its side-effects in clinical trials new derivatives of the agent are under investigation.

Nerve Growth Factor (NGF) in Mediating Hyperalgesia

The NGF was the first neurotrophic factor to be discovered and purified. During the past 50 years, work on NGF established the concept that the survival of neurons in the developing nervous system is regulated by, and dependent on, neurotrophic factors [62]. Until recently the pervasiveness of this concept has hindered the recognition of the role of NGF as a key pain mediator. However, these roles of NGF are not contradictory. The dependence of some populations of sensory and sympathetic neurons on NGF for survival is restricted to a brief window of development when they are establishing functional contacts with their targets. NGF is the founding member of the neurotrophin family of structurally related secreted proteins that includes brain-derived neurotrophic factor (BDNF), neurotrophin 3 (NT-3) and NT-4. Mature neurotrophins are homodimers that are derived by proteolytic cleavage from precursor proteins encoded by separate genes. They bind to two types of receptor: a common receptor, p75NTR, which binds all neurotrophins with a similar affinity; and members of the trk family of receptor tyrosine kinases, trkA, trkB and trkC, which bind different neurotrophins. TrkA is the receptor tyrosine kinase for NGF. TrkA mediates the survival-promoting and neuron growth-promoting effects of NGF during development and its later pain-provoking actions (Figure I-33). The NGF also regulates the activity of several transcription factors, including c-FOS, c-JUN, ELK-1, forkhead-1, nuclear factor KB (NF-KB) and cAMP-dependent response-element-binding protein (CREB), which leads to alterations in gene expression [63].

Induction of the expression of NGF is an early event in injured and inflamed tissues, and elevated levels of NGF are sustained in chronic inflammation (Figures I-33 and I-34). These changes in the synthesis of NGF appear to be caused, in part, by the action of pro-inflammatory cytokines, many of which induce the synthesis NGF in several cell types in vitro and in vivo [64]. NGF also sensitizes nociceptive neurons directly to several pain-provoking stimuli. This is caused by

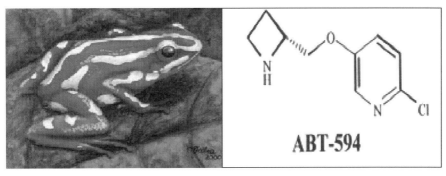

Radioligand binding	epibatidine	ABT-594
Neuronal		
α4ß2	0.042	0.037
α7	3.2	1780
Muscle		
α1ßδγ	2.4	16,600
Functional activity (nM)		
Ganglionic (α3ß4)	7	460
(% efficacy)	153%	124%

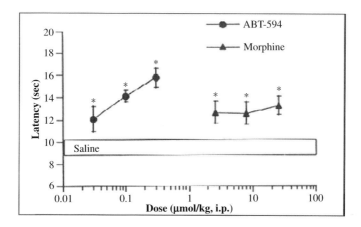

Figure 1-32. Difference in receptor affinity of epibatidine, derived from skin secretions of the south american poison arrow frog (Epipedobates tricolor), and its derivative ABT-594, a highly selective AChRs-ligand, to neuronal, muscle and ganglionic binding sites. ABT-594 shows selectivity to neuronal subsites involved in the modulation of pain, being 20fold more potent than morphine in the thermal hot box model

rapid post-translational changes in the transient receptor potential vanilloid receptor 1 (TRPV1) cation channel and by modulating the expression of genes that influence nociceptor function. NGF also sensitizes nociceptors indirectly by activating mast cells.

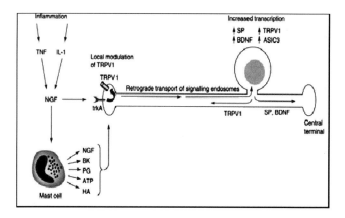

Figure I-33. The main mechanisms by which NGF enhances pain and hypersensitivity following inflammation. The local production of inflammatory cytokines such as interleukin-1 (IL-1) and tumor necrosis factor (TNF) promotes the production of NGF by several cell types. NGF binds to trkA receptors on a major subset of nociceptive terminal. Retrograde trafficking of signaling endosomes to the cell body results in an enhanced expressions of proteins that further increases excitability and facilitates the activation of second-order neurons in the CNS (ASIC = acid sensing ion channel; BDBF = brain- derived neurotrophic factor; BK = bradykinin; HA = histamine; PG = prostaglandin; SP = substance P)

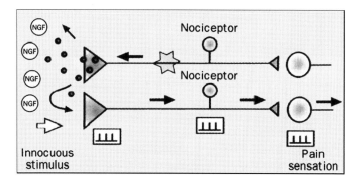

Figure I-34. Partial denervation in injured neurons increases release of neuronal growth factor (NGF) affecting activity in nearby primary Aß-afferents with peripheral sensitization (phenotype switch to C-fibers)

SIGNIFICANCE OF THE IMMUNE SYSTEM AND MICROGLIA IN CHRONIC PAIN

The inhibitory role of glycine and $GABA_B$ (γ-aminobutyric acid type B)-receptor activation in spinal neuronal circuits has long been established. The same applies to the inhibitory effect of morphine-like molecules, which have an analgesic action. However, the recent discovery of the importance of microglia in pain sensation opens new avenues for investigating the effects of endogenous inhibitory mediators and pathways. The concept of anti-inflammation has been suggested to be an important determinant in the therapy of inflammatory pathology: malfunction or absence of one or more endogenous anti-inflammatory pathways and mediators could lead to persistent pain and inflammation, and prolonged disease.

The central role of immune cells in pain associated with peripheral neuropathy has been established. Peripheral nerve injuries can lead to neuropathic pain states caused not only by a pathology in the damaged peripheral nerve and dorsal root ganglia (DRG), but also by a series of changes in the central processing of sensory information, which are best characterized at the spinal level. These changes are indirect, as the CNS itself is not damaged including changes in immune cell function. Two types of immune cell have been studied in this context – haematogenous leukocytes and resident microglia. Although there have been many studies of immune cell extravasations in the periphery, few have focused on the infiltration of immune cells into the spinal cord after peripheral nerve injury. For instance, extravasations of leukocytes (macrophages and/or T cells) occurs in the lumbar spinal cord 3–14 days after peripheral L5 nerve transaction. While the specific role of these infiltrating cells is not clear, they could even have neuroprotective or antihyperalgesic functions.

In addition, microglia express the same surface markers as macrophages/monocytes, which are derived from the periphery. Microglia are activated by events such as CNS injury, microbial invasion and some pain states, which leads to an increase in the production of various inflammatory cytokines, chemokines and other potentially pain-producing substances. Although microglial activation has been found to be beneficial in some circumstances, substantial evidence now indicates that it can contribute to neuropathic pain after peripheral nerve injury (Figure I-35). This is substantiated by several studies showing that specific microglial inhibitors and/or modulators can block and/or reverse neuropathic states. The most commonly used compounds are fluorocitrate and minocycline. Interestingly, pre-emptive and curative fluorocitrate treatment, which selectively blocks astrocyte and microglial metabolism, also inhibits neuropathic pain, whereas minocycline (a specific microglial inhibitor) blocks the development of neuropathic pain states but does not reduce pain that is already established. The latter study indicates that microglia might be more important in the initial phases of neuropathic pain. Recently, Watkins et al. in a model of sciatic inflammatory neuropathy and acute spinal immune activation with intrathecal HIV-1, reported that intrathecal minocycline was much more effective in delaying the induction of allodynia than in reversing it. Various findings indicate that microglial activation is necessary, but not sufficient, for the emergence of neuropathic pain behaviour. Microgial activation might be just the first step in a cascade of immune responses in the CNS. Therefore, microglia might be responsible for the initiation of neuropathic pain states, and astrocytes may be involved in their maintenance. This occurs at the central nervous

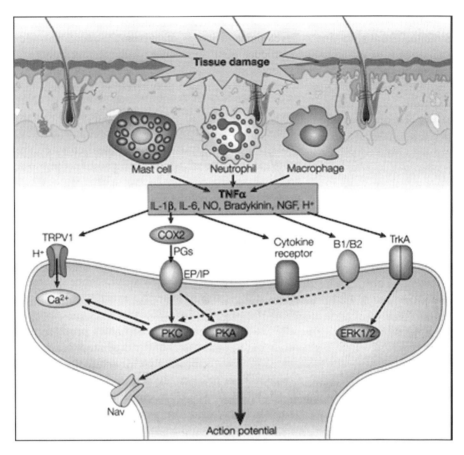

Figure I-35. Activation of mast cells and macrophages by inflammation results in the release of various immune mediators such as tumor necrosis factor-α (TNF-α), interleukin-1ß (IL-1ß), interleukin-6 (IL-6) nitric oxide (NO), bradykinin, nerve growth factor (NGF) and protons, acting directly through receptor binding or indirectly through the release of other modulators such as prostanoids

system, where MAP-kinase activates glial-formation, which in return results in the release of a number of neuroactive substances.

It is not clear which factors activate microglia in the spinal cord in peripheral neuropathic pain states. On the basis of antisense and pharmacological evidence, Tsuda et al. showed that the activation of microglia in neuropathy requires P2X4 receptors, which are upregulated and specifically expressed by microglia in neuropathic pain models. Other evidence indicates that P2X7 receptors are expressed on microglia and that their activation by ATP can lead to the production and release of inflammatory cytokines. Indeed, mice that lack this receptor show an impaired ability to develop neuropathic pain. The released cytokines (TNFa and 1L-6) might themselves be involved in microglial activation.

Despite some inconsistencies and uncertainties, microglial activation very likely is the important factor in the development of neuropathic pain. However, presently it is not clear how microglia produce pain and which mediators are involved. Activation of astrocytes in the relevant spinal cord segments seems to be crucial for the full emergence of neuropathic pain behaviour. In pathophysiological conditions, microglia can release various mediators, such as IL-lß, TNFα, PGE$_2$ and nitric oxide. While some evidence indicates that intrathecal administration of IL-lß or TNFα can lead to symptoms of neuropathic pain in normal rats, the expression of both these cytokines is increased in models of neuropathic pain. Blockade of these cytokine increase reduces pain and hyperalgesia. Despite the lack of strong evidence about their source (i.e. neurons and/or microglia), these cytokines can modulate spinal pain processing in several ways. Activation of their receptors on spinal neurons can lead to rapid changes in neuronal excitability. IL-Iß or TNFα might also act indirectly through the release of nitric oxide and PGE$_2$. However, spinal cord cytokines alone are probably not sufficient to explain neuropathic pain, which work in concert with other pro-nociceptive compounds (i.e. substance P and glutamate). Also, there is conflicting evidence about the roles of COX2 and PGE$_2$ in the spinal cord after nerve injury.

Injuries and diseases that directly affect the CNS can also induce an intense immune reaction. Aside from spinal cord injury (SCI), multiple sclerosis (MS) can be associated with abnormal pain sensitivity. Loss of function is usually the main consequence of SCI. However, pain severely compromises the quality of life in up to 70% of patients with SCI. Mechanisms of SCI-associated pain, although poorly understood, are likely to be manifold. Direct injury of the spinal cord leads to local breakdown of the blood-brain barrier, the release of many intracellular constituents, such as ATP, and the production of reactive oxygen species (ROS). As in other tissues, injury of the spinal cord leads to local inflammatory responses and the activation of immune cells, which are similar to those described above (Figure I-36). Although direct evidence is still lacking, similar factors and mechanisms might contribute to the abnormal pain state that occurs in SCI. In response to injury, neutrophils, monocytes/macrophages and lymphocytes are recruited to the injury site, and microglia are activated at and beyond this site. The invasion of neutrophils and haematogenous macrophages peaks at 12 and 5–7 days after SCI, respectively. There might be two phases of microglial activation. The mechanism of action of the antibody is unclear, but might involve changes in intraspinal serotonergic innervation. Soon after SCI, the TNFα/CD95 (FAS) complex is secreted, and leads to the auto-activation of microglia and macrophages. TNFα might have a double role in pain after SCI: a function in the activation of immune cells and a direct effect on pain-processing neurons. Almost all of the factors that are released by immune cells and have an effect on pain after peripheral nerve injury might also affect pain processing after SCI. So, TNFα might be involved in SCI pain through the mechanism described above. Other pro-inflammatory cytokines (such as IL-lß and IL-6) and prostaglandins that are produced by COX2 and nitric oxide cannot be excluded. IL-lß could activate macrophages and microglia, which could, in turn,

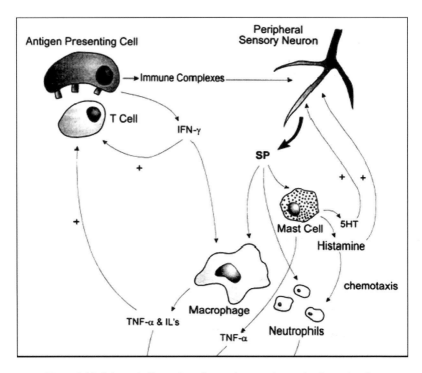

Figure I-36. Schematic illustration of neuro-immune-interaction in nociception

release pronociceptive compounds and/or directly influence pain pathways. Another mechanism might be neuronal apoptosis. IL-1ß can trigger inflammatory apoptotic outcomes through nuclear factor-KB (NF-KB) transcriptional activation, which, in turn, increases the expression of caspase 3. Moreover, it has been shown that after SCI, apoptosis occurs in an important pain pathway, the spinothalamic tract. This is through a prompt decrease in BLC2-like protein 1 levels, which are also under the control of NF-KBI32. So, IL-1ß could affect pain-signaling function through a pro-apoptotic effect on neurons of pain pathways.

Multiple sclerosis (MS) is the most common chronic inflammatory disease of the CNS in humans. It is classically associated with demyelization and more recently with neuronal degeneration. Almost 50% of patients with MS experience significant pain at some point during the course of the disease and it is plausible that immune cell factors also contribute to MS-associated pain. More than 90% of patients with MS have high immunoglobulin G (IgG) concentrations in the brain or cerebrospinal fluid (CSF), which is indicative of the presence of an active inflammatory reaction. Also, histological studies of post-mortem material have shown that inflammatory infiltrates are present at the periphery of MS plaques, with features not dissimilar to those that are characteristic of active infection T and B lymphocytes, mast cells, macrophages, microglia and astrocytes, and all are recruited and/or activated. The role of these types of immune cells in the genesis of pain in MS remains largely unexplored, but the participation of microglia is an attractive possibility. It is not clear which mediators are released and how they affect the pain processing pathways in MS. The activated immune cells can release all the pro-inflammatory cytokines that are involved in neuropathic pain of peripheral origin. It is well documented that the concentrations of cytokines are elevated in clinical cases and in animal models of MS, but which of these cytokines are important in the pain caused by MS is not clear.

In summary, glial activation induces the development and maintenance of nerve injury-induced neuropathic pain by means of different machanisms:

1. Both microglial and astroglial cells are activated by spinal cord or peripheral injury; they express receptors and locally release neuroactive substances, which result in chronic pain.
2. Activation of signaling molecules (MAP-kinases, and chemokine receptors) by spinal microglia or astroglia.
3. Astrocytes within the spinal cord enhance pain afferences of neuropathic origin.
4. Phenotype switch from microglia to astrocytes, resulting in a change of symptoms in neuropathic pain.
5. Astroglia as well as microglia release chemokines (TNFa, IL-2, IL-6, IL-1ß) being activated by Schwann cells, result in an increased response of voltage-gated ion-channels (Na^+, Ca^{2+}, K^+, Cl^-) with either an increase in excitability and/or pronounced hyperalgesia.

Reflectory, Segmental Mediation of Pain Afferents

Once nociceptive activity in the spinal cord is above threshold levels, action potentials from the first order neuron are transmitted to the second order neuron of the spinothalamic tract. From there they are transmitted to higher pain-regulating centers In the substantia gelatinosa of the posterior column of the spinal cord, pain afferent stimuli directly, via interneuronal connections, interact with the lateral column of the spinal cord and transfer to the motor tract of the anterior column. It is here, where in the same segment or via collateral fibers to several neighboring segments, nociceptive impulses are switched to vegetative as well as motor neurons (= conversion afferents; Figure I-37b). This explains the development of muscle spasms of the abdominal wall during pain, the expansion of visceral-sensitive pain (Figure I-37c), accompanying vegetative circulatory effects, activation of sweat glands, and the projection of pain from deep visceral structures to specific areas of the skin ("head zones"; Figure I-37a). The latter are transmitted from the same spinal cord segment as the affected internal organ. Nociceptive visceral activity can be transmitted on to motor neurons with activation of smooth muscle activity and contraction, resulting in a vicious circle. Such a development is elucidated by free nerve endings within the smooth muscle, which are sensitive to contraction, resulting in a reinforcement of the nociceptive barrage and an increase in pain sensation (Figure I-38).

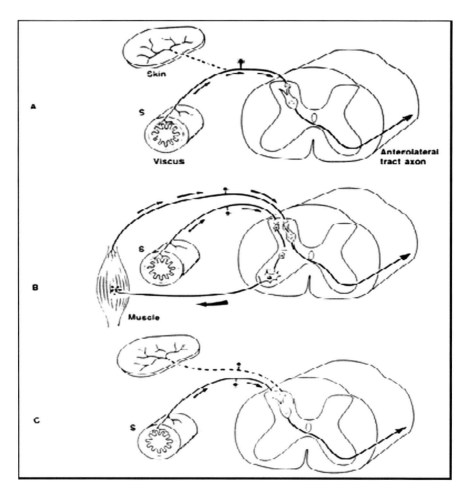

Figure I-37. Principle of referred pain with reflectory innervation of sensory fibers to the skin referred to as head zones (A, C) and positive reinforces muscle activity via motor fibers (B)

Sequence of Resulting in Neuropathic Pain

Therefore prevention of such transition from acute to chronic pain with opioids is the major goal in pain therapy. Also, intracellular gene expression can be prevented most successfully, if opioids are administered before nociceptive stimuli reach the cells [65], and before neuroplastic changes within the cells are being initiated. It is because of such intracellular changes, that acute pain can become chronic if it not sufficiently treated from the start. If however, during the process of initiation of pain a neuropathic component is diagnosed, it is of clinical importance that in addition to an opioid, an unspecific NMDA-antagonist such as ketamine is given in sub-anesthetic doses, to reduce pain. Such considerations are of significance,

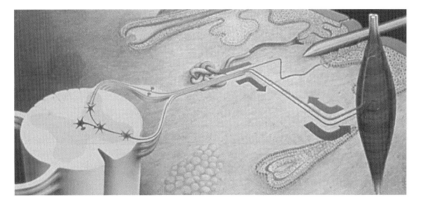

Figure I-38. Transmission of visceral pain to segmental motor neurons, resulting in muscle spasm and the projection of pain to the skin (head zones)

because long-term pain may also result in apoptotic degeneration of interspinal neurons with their attached opioid receptor sites, resulting in a opioid resistance to any exogenous narcotic analgesic (Figure I-42). It is for this reason that up to 35% of all patients with neuropathic pain of peripheral or central origin may be opioid non-responders. The following disorders with associated pain states may show focal/diffuse neuropathic pain (Table I-1).

The phenomena of insufficient pain relief with opioids demands an additional and multimodal therapeutic approach. In such situations additional antiepileptic and/or antidepressive agents should be given. Those agents primarily act at the GABA receptor site with increase in GABA-synthesis, diminution of intracellular Ca^{2+}-ions, and an increase in the release of GABA. In addition to NMDA-antagonists,

Table I-1. Classification of neuropathic pain disorders

- Phantom limb pain,
- Post-herpetic neuralgia,
- Entrapment syndrome,
- Post-traumatic neuralgia,
- Chronic radiculopathy,
- Complex regional pain syndrome (CRPS),
- Central post-stroke pain (CPSP),
- Multiple sclerosis (MS),
- Painful diabetic neuropathy (PDN),
- Ischemic neuropathy,
- Polyarteriitis nodosa,
- Polyneuropathy in long-term alcohol abuse,
- Toxic reaction due to vincristine, taxoids, cisplatin,
- Neuro-borrelliosis
- AIDS neuropathy
- Amyloid, plasmacytoma, morbus Fabry

interventional blocks with local anesthetic (sodium-channel blockers), topical therapy with lidocaine or capscaicin are used as adjuncts in neuropathic pain. Certain cases will respond to neuromodulation with TENS (transcutaneous electrical nerve stimulation) or SCS (spinal cord stimulation), while physical and occupational therapy as well as psychobiological treatment, regularly are implemented in the therapeutic armamentarium of neuropathic pain.

Description of Neuropathic Pain Deafferentiation

Symptoms: Burning, shooting, stabbing, paroxysmal, vice-like, electric-shock-like pain, paresthesias

Causes: Injury to peripheral nerves leading to spontaneous and paroxysmal discharges, loss of central inhibitory modulation, interaction of sympathetic to somatic afferent nociceptors

Treatment: Opioids, antidepressants, anticonvulsants, antiarrhythmics, local anesthetics, topical capscaicin or lidocaine

---

Neuropathic pain is often described as burning, shooting, stabbing, paroxysmal, vice-like, electric-shock-like, or an abnormal sensation such as that of ants crawling on the skin. Neuropathic pain is often associated with sensibility changes such as allodynia and hyperalgesia or paresthesia. Neuropathic pain is caused by aberrant somatosensory processing induced by injury to an element of the nervous system. This may result from compression, destruction, or penetration injury of the nervous tissue or by an intrinsic disease process. Spontaneous paroxysmal discharges, loss of central inhibitory modulation, and sympathetic to somatic afferent nociceptor interaction may all contribute to the genesis of neuropathic pain.

Some common types of neuropathic pain include trigeminal neuralgia, post-herpetic neuralgia, reflex sympathetic dystrophy, lumbosacral plexopathy, phantom limb pain, nerve avulsion after trauma, and diabetic peripheral neuropathy. Damage to thalamic sensory relay neurons (as might occur after a stroke) can also give rise to intense neuropathic pain referred to the body surface.

Unlike nociceptive pain, which tends to decline with the cessation of the noxious stimulus, neuropathic pain persists for prolonged periods. Mechanisms involved in sustaining neuropathic pain are thought to include cellular and molecular changes in the pain pathway. For example, ephaptic stimulation of sensory fibers by adjacent autonomic fibers can lead to a perception of pain in the absence of any noxious stimulus (Table I-2). In addition, changes at the level of the spinal cord and brain, such as hypersensitivity to stimuli and excessive release of neurotransmitters, can lead to molecular changes, changes in gene expression, and changes in the receptive fields of neurons involved in perception of pain.

Neuropathic pain appears to develop by the following mechanisms: activated C fibers release glutamate or substance P, or both, in the dorsal horn of the spinal cord. These neurotransmitters have excitatory effects on second-order neurons, mediated

Table 1-2. Postulated mechanisms involved in sustaining neuropathic pain

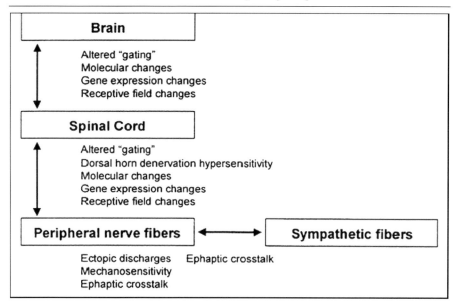

by AMPA and NMDA receptors. Glutamate activates AMPA receptors, resulting in an influx of cations (sodium, potassium, calcium) and depolarization of the postsynaptic neuron. These excitatory effects are rapid and short-lived. Repeated stimulation of primary afferent fibers can also lead to membrane depolarization via tachykinin receptors, which may be additive with stimulation of AMPA receptors. In the second-order neuron, membrane depolarization releases the inhibition (by magnesium) of voltage-gated calcium channels coupled to NMDA receptors and releases the inactivation of NMDA receptors, both of which contribute to a rise in cytosolic calcium. Glutamate activates the metabotropic aminocycIopentane-1, 3-decarboxylate (ACPD) receptors coupled to inositol phosphate, which mobilizes microsomal calcium, and this also contributes to the increase in intracellular calcium. Substance P stimulates IP3 (inositol triphosphate) synthesis and activates voltage-dependent channels.

The increased calcium concentration in the cell activates various enzyme cascades (e.g. phospholipase A2 and nitric oxide synthetase, which synthesize prostaglandin and nitric oxide) and induces transcription of immediate-early genes (C-fos, C-jun), all of which impair synaptic efficiency between primary afferent fibers and second-order neurons. The second-order neurons are gradually depolarized, and their responses increasingly amplified. This is referred to as the "wind-up phenomenon". Glutamate-initiated hyperactivity, or wind-up, leads to a vicious cycIe of pain. It is because of this glutamate-related neuronal hyperactivity, which is also the principal cause of epilepsy, that antiepileptic drugs are useful agents in neuropathic pain.

CAUSES OF POTENTIATION AND TRANSITION
FROM ACUTE TO CHRONIC PAIN

The posterior column of the spinal cord can be regarded as a gate, through which nociceptive afferents must travel, in order to reach higher supraspinal pain-processing centers in the CNS. However, it is also the gate, where modulation of pain impulses takes place, resulting in either in diminution or fortification. Also, it is a commonly accepted belief, that opioid receptors and their endogenous ligands, endorphins or enkephalins, play a critical part in the reduction of incoming pain impulses [66, 67, 68]. In particular pro-nociceptive transmitters are of importance, as they cause a fortification of arriving nociceptive afferences [65]. The principle pronociceptive mediators are related to the group of excitatory amino acids, comprising of glutamate, aspartate and the tachykinin group. The latter consists of substance P, the endogenous ligand for the NK_1-receptor, as well as neurokinin A, B and C, which bind to the NK_2-, NK_3- and NK_4-receptor respectively. Thus, besides initial nociceptive-related electro-physiological and hormonal changes, sensitivity of peripheral and central nociceptors increases [69, 70], resulting in the initiation of a chronic pain process (Table I-3). Because long-term nociception results in a facilitation of afferent pain afferents [71], they eventually induce morphological changes in the sense of a prevailing condition, a change within the matrix of spinal cord [6, 7, 72].

All C-fiber-related nociceptive afferents first bind to the excitatory tachykinin receptors. Via this receptor the intracellular G-protein is activated, which can be considered as the main intracellular, "second messenger". It is the G-protein, which converts into adenylcyclase (AC), and the activation of adenosinetriphosphate (ATP) into cyclic amino monophosphate (c-AMP). This activation results in the formation of several c-AMP-dependant kinases, especially protein kinase A (PKA) and protein kinase C (PKC), resulting in phosphorylation and opening of voltage-dependent Ca^{2+}-ion channels. The increased shift of Ca^{2+}-ions from the extra – to the intracellular space results in an increased excitability of the neuronal cell (Figure I-40). Repetitive long-term activation, however, in particular

Table I-3. Time-dependent levels in the development of chronic pain

First level:	transient stimulus-induced pain
Second level:	tissue damage
Third level:	injury of primary afferent neuron
Fourth level:	injury of central neuron
Fifth level:	activation and sensitization of nociceptors and central pain pathways with
	– disinhibition,
	– ectopic activity
	– structural reorganization
	– phenotype switch (Aß- via NGF − > C-fiber)
	– sympathetic sprouting
	– central sensitization

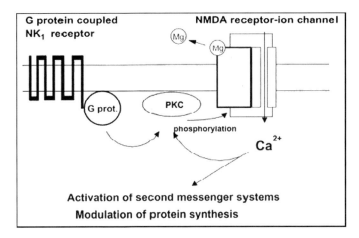

Figure 1-39. Substance P binds to the NK_1-receptor, which via PKC (protein kinase C) activation increases Ca^{2+-}-transfer through the N-methyl-D-asparate (NMDA) receptor channel, ensuing in the transition of acute to chronic pain through increase through activation of second messenger systems [73]

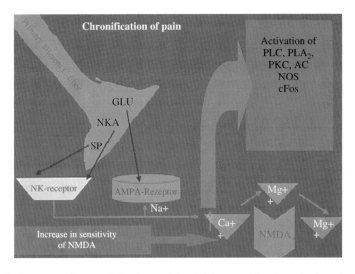

Figure 1-40. Summary of events following peripheral injury resulting in activation of neurokinin- and AMPA-receptors, which after Mg^+-displacement leads to sensitization of the NMDA-receptor. This is followed by an increase of intracellular Ca^{2+}-transfer. The latter activates several intracellular biochemical mechanisms resulting in the initiation of chronic pain (NK-Neurokinin; AMPA = α-amino-3-hydroxy-5-methyl-4-isoxazole propionic acid; PKC = Proteinkinase; PLA_2 = Phospholipase A_2; NMDA = N-methyl-D-aspartate; PLC = Phospholipase C; NOS = Nitric oxide synthetase; c-fos = target gene)

the activation of glutaminergic synapses of the spinal neurons, results in potentiation of the NMDA-(N-methyl-D-aspartate)-receptor (Figure I-39), participating in the transmission of nociceptive afferents [73, 74].

NEUROPHYSIOLOGICAL CHANGES TAKING EFFECT DURING EVOLUTION OF PAIN

The skin is the site where approximately 90% of over 3 million nociceptors are located. The peripheral tissue damage, in order to develop into pain of chronic nature, peripheral nociceptors of the skin are irritated over a long period of time. In order to be transmitted, a certain threshold level has to be surpassed, before so called multimodal "wide-dynamic-range" (WDR)-receptors pick up tactile sensation like pressure, heat, distension, and pain is transmitted to the spinal cord. There, aside from inhibitory transmitters such as endorphins, so-called pro-nociceptive transmitters such as substance P, neurokinin A and B, glycine, and glutamate are being released. As in higher central nervous system structures, synaptic potentials activate glutamate receptor (NMDA-receptor, AMPA-receptor), with the consequence that repetitive irritation results in a learning process at the level of the nerve cell. This is because repetitive impulses result in facilitation with spontaneous electrical discharge of action potentials (wind-up-phenomenon), accounting for the increase in output.

Such long-term increase in activity will cause the cell to react to a given stimulus at a higher rate in the near future. This is because nociceptive transmitters act on postsynaptic neurons, resulting in an increased inflow of Ca^{2+}-ions into the cell with the consequence of initiating a deleterious cascade: following opening of the voltage-gated ion channel the increase in Ca^{2+}-ions induce activation of so-called "second messenger" within of the nerve cell. Calcium ions therefore can be considered as important messengers, which guide a series of cell functions, responsible for central sensitization. Via activation of phosphorylation, transcription factors like CREB (c-AMP responsive element binding protein) are initiated, which govern activation of genes and the phenotype formation of nociceptive posterior column cells. In addition, transcription factors will induce specific amino acids to form "immediate-early-genes", necessary to transmit their genetic information into structural information of genes. As a result c-fos and c-jun are synthesized which induce the synthesis of amino acids necessary for the formation of new receptor sites. The consequence of additional binding sites is linked to the process of central sensitization. Since adding new binding sites for transmitters, which are released as the consequence of a nociceptive input, amplification of excitation is initiated with an increase of impulse transduction (Figure I-41). Thus, the neuronal cell being equipped with additional receptors, is put into a permanent state of "attention" (= phase of sensitization and hyperactivity), where neurotransmitters and neurohormones are released spontaneously. Despite a low but constant impulse from the periphery, previously inactive synapses are now being recruited so that the signal information now is transmitted faster and to a higher extent to other spinal cord neuronal cells.

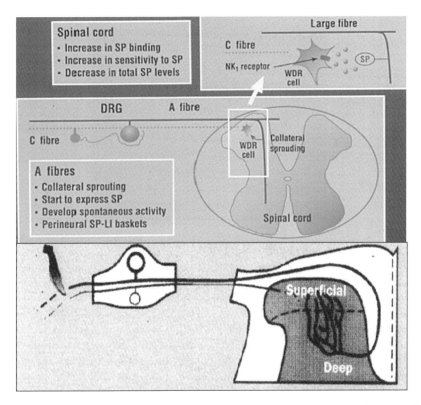

Figure I-41. Following peripheral nerve injury of C-fibers with atrophy there is collateral sprouting into the dorsal root ganglia (DRG), Also, terminal sprouting in the dorsal horn, as well as phenotype switch of Aß-fibers to C-fibers is postulated, all of which results in the transition from acute to chromic pain

In addition nociceptive afferents are functionally interconnected with low-threshold mechano- and thermo-receptors. As a result, there is an expansion of sensitive zones into previous insensitive areas of the skin, and light impulses such as touch, which originate far away from the area of destruction, become painful (development of allodynia). At the final stage, the nervous cell is unable to forget the painful information and a chronic hyperexcitatory state is the consequence. This leads to a long lasting recollection of pain, which is even active when the original trigger stimulus for pain no longer is in existence (Figure I-42). Henceforth, all impulses originally referred to as harmless (e.g. temperature or pressure changes) are now being sensed as painful (=phase of chronic hyperexcitability).

At this moment, opioids such as morphine [30], but also 5-HT$_2$, and 5-HT$_3$-receptor antagonists [75], as well as peptidase inhibitors, that potentiate the action of endorphins by means of an inhibition of enzymatic degradation [76], come into play. These agents are able to prevent the formation of specific amino acids ("immediate-early-genes") and their subfamilies c-jun and c-fos, which usually would result in the formation of additional excitatory receptors. During chronic nociceptive irritation

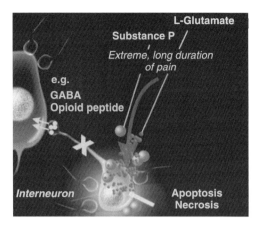

Figure I-42. Long term and excessive release of excitatory transmitters, due to apoptotic degeneration and necrosis of inhibitory interspinal cells, clinically results in opioid non-responders

at the spinal level such increase in the expression of c-fos experimentally could be blocked by morphine, and equianalgesic doses of the κ-ligand U50,488H [77]. Such data can be transmitted into the clinic, suggesting that diverse visceral, nociceptive afferences can be blocked adequately by opioids with different receptor affinity. On the other hand antidepressants and anticonvulsants also mediate an antinociceptive effect in humans. The principal mode of antidepressants is activation of the descending inhibitory tract, while anticonvulsants (e.g. carbamazepine, valproate acid, lamotrigine, gabapentin) have a GABAnergic effect. By reducing excessive Ca^{2+} inflow, programmed cell death (apoptosis) of inhibitory interneurons, which normally release γ-amino butyric acid (GABA) as a transmitter, is prevented. And because the usual loss of GABAnergic inhibition results in intense hyperalgesia and allodynia as well as spontaneous pain arising in the spinal cord level, consequences of an insufficient pain therapy have to be avoided. If such a loss is apparent, it however, can be balanced by compensatory activation of receptors interacting with anticonvulsants and/or benzodiazepines. This is why such "non-analgesic agents" are capable of initiating an analgesic effect. Such compensatory mechanism has been demonstrated in spinal as well as supraspinal areas, where the use of antiepileptic agents resulted in an increase in γ-aminobutyric acid (GABA) [78, 79], deleting the "memory of pain", an effect which clinically goes with a fading of pain sensations.

Such clinical as well as preclinical results indicate that aside from the inhibitory opioids, the GABAnergic system plays an important part in pain therapy at the spinal cord level [80, 81, 82]. This may also explain why baclofen has antinociceptive effects, because it is the prototype $GABA_B$-receptor ligand and muscinol, being the prototype $GABA_A$-receptor subtype ligand. Both GABA-agonists decrease the biochemical cascade within the posterior column of the spinal cord, which follows somatic or visceral nociceptive input, thus avoiding sensitization [83]. Besides direct activation of the $GABA_A$-receptor, also the enzyme glutamatdecarboxylase (GAD),

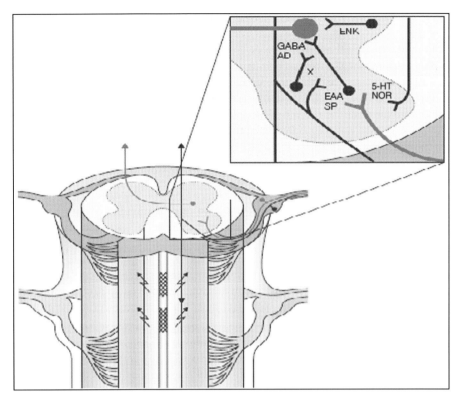

Figure I-43. Schematic representation of some of the putative neurotransmitters involved in spinal cord stimulation with orthodromically electrical impulses resulting in the release of GABA, which in return decreases excitatory amino acids (EAA = glutamate and aspartate). Also, SCS activates enkephalin (ENK) interneurons, and induces the release of norepinephrine (NOR) and serotonin (5-HT) from descending fibers Adapted from [85]

necessary for the synthesis of GABA, is another potential analgesic agent [78]. In addition, this is how the analgesic effect of a benzodiazepine such as midazolam is being mediated, resulting in an antinociception via the $GABA_A$-receptor [84]. Such results are conclusive in that the GABAnergic inhibitory interneurons in the spinal cord play an significant part in the process of antinociception. They also seem to be the result of spinal cord stimulation, where electrical stimuli induce a release of the inhibitory transmitter GABA (Figure I-43).

SUPRASPINAL ENGRAMS RELEVANT IN TRANSITION FROM ACUTE TO CHRONIC PAIN

Nociceptive afferent signals from damaged peripheral tissue are relayed to the posterior column where they transmit to second order neurons of the spinal cord where they are being modulated. Nociceptive simuli originating in the head or the face are conveyed via the trigeminal nerve to the trigeminal nerve nucleus in the brain stem. There, all afferent signals are being modulated after which they cross to the opposite side, further ascending to the thalamus. From there, fibers ascend rostrally to lemniscal and thalamic structures, before they reach the somatosensory cortex (Figure I-44). Each long-term or even a paroxysmal increase of activity of afferents to the posterior column of the spinal cord or to the trigeminal nerve nucleus also induce an activity-dependent adaptation of the rostrally located thalamic and neocortical structures [86]. In the process of development of chronic pain, besides adaptive peripheral changes, also an alteration at the cortical level is instigated resulting in central sensitization (Table I-4).

For instance, hyperexcitability of cortical neurons was documented in patients with chronic pains, where experimentally pain-related stimulation with sensory-evoked potentials resulted in an augmented response in the primary cortical projection area. Such response could be derived within 80–129 ms after the stimuli. Such increase in excitability of specific cortical areas in pain patients was also reflected in the augmentation to acoustic stimuli. Similar to the process of sensitization at the peripheral site, non-nociceptive stimuli are felt as painful. And simple words or even thoughts can cause pain sensations. This is because during the process

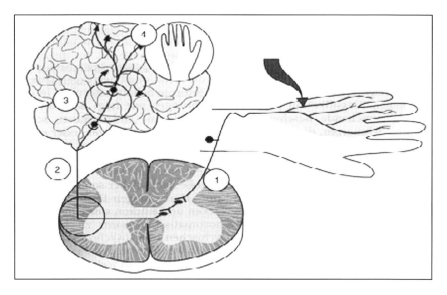

Figure I-44. In chronified pain the touch at the skin induces activation at the corresponding sensory cortical area (cueing of nociception). Because of an elevated basal activity even minor stimuli are able to induce a hyperexcitatory state resulting in allodynia 1 = Aδ- and C-fibers; 2 = spinothalamic tract; 3 = intrathalmic pain-related nuclei; 4 = sensory cortex

Table I-4. The changes within the supraspinal system, resulting in central sensitization

1. Reduction of threshold to incoming excitatory stimuli
2. Expansion of receptive fields within the corresponding sensory cortical area
3. Lowering of threshold of cortical cells for excitability followed by hyperalgesia
4. Synaptic long-term potentiation of cells in the hippocampal area with prolonged memorization

of nociceptive propagation, within cortical structures, a localized recollection of pain impulses is set-off, which can be activated without peripheral stimulation. Excitatory amino acids (e.g. glutamate, tachykinins) seem to play a significant role in such situation, because painful reactions can be induced experimentally following microinjection into different mesencephalic and diencephalic parts involved in pain transmission [87].

Therefore pain without any doubt, is also a subjective experience where the first level of consciousness is due to a connection between the intralaminary nuclei to the pallidum and the second level of consciousness, the cerebral cortex. It is here where the activity of sensory organs will be translated into pain, while at the same time resulting in an individual complexion of painful afferences. In chronified pain conditions, aside from neurochemical changes within the first transmission site in the spinal cord in the spinal cord, as demonstrated by Beechy and McKenzie [88] also a learning effect at the ventral area of the hippocampus. This is because the hippocampus is an area where traces of memory are being consolidated permanently into so-called engrams. They result in an attitude of expectations in the chronic pain patient. On the other hand during nociceptive processing, the pallidum is responsible for the affective component of pain. It is therefore not too surprising, that aside from the striatum and the nucleus coeruleus, the pallidum is rich in opioid receptor sites and a place where endogenous opioids bind [89, 90]. Opioids given for the suppression of pain exert their primary site of action in the pallidum by blocking the negative and agonizing character of pain. Such agents are also of value when the neuronal stored information on a previous pain experience is to be deleted. On the other hand, it also becomes clear why unsolved conflicts, aggressions, fear, resignation and passiveness, contempt, and psychological imbalance reinforce pain sensations. On the other hand psychic balance, satisfaction, joy, enforcement strategies, all result in a reduction of pain intensity. Consequently, pain experience is not comparable with one another. It is an extremely individual feeling, subjectively colored, emotionally tuned and assessed differently by each person. According to the individual experience and its sequences pain is difficult to measure and can hardly be classified as such. Lastly, such considerations underline the theory of Melzack [21], in that pain is an individual sensory feeling, which incorporates the neuronal networks of the entire body, being affected by cultural, genetic, socio-economic as well as individual experiences in the past.

Preventing Transition from Acute to Chronic Pain – Use of Analgesics with Different Pharmacology

An intense nociceptive impulse transmitted to the dorsal horn of the spinal cord, always results in the release of excitatory neurotransmitters and peptides. Aside from activating interneuronal cells, they also stimulate the cells of the spinothalamic tract resulting in a prolonged sensitization and augmentation of all incoming further nociceptive impulses. Such an effect can outlast the original impulse [7], a phenomenon called central hypersensitization or "wind-up" [91, 92]. Clinically this is related to hyperalgesia in the damaged area accompanied by dysesthesia in the surrounded skin with prolonged pain [6, 69].

RATIONALE FOR THE USE OF OPIOIDS

Based on such knowledge, the need for a sufficient pain therapy is inevitable. However, such changes in nociceptive transmission ask for "pre-emptive", or rather "preventive"-analgesia. Opioids are agents, which after binding to and a conformational change of their respective receptor site result in secondary inhibition of adenylcyclase (AC) are able to prevent calcium inflow through voltage-dependent ion channels (Figure I-45).

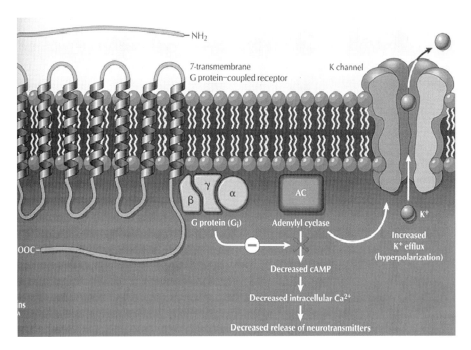

Figure I-45. The interaction of the opioid receptor with the potassium ion-channel, which after activation results in an increased outward shift of potassium resulting in a hyperpolarized state

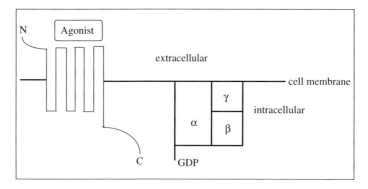

Figure 1-46. Schematic representation of the dormant opioid receptor, a 7 helix transmembrane, G-protein-coupled receptor. Following binding, the intracellular mediator G-protein with its α-, β- and γ-subunit is activated resulting in the decreased formation of cyclic AMP
GDP-Guanidine dip

A secondary and important messenger of opioid action is G-protein, which after activation results in formation of guanidindiphosphate (GDP) to guanidintriphosphate (GTP; Figures I-46 and I-47).

This transformational process, as a consequence, results in the dissociation of G-protein from the receptor and a reduction of affinity of the ligand. If this process lasts for a long period of time, it results in the development of tachyphylaxis. By dissociation of the α-GDP subunit from the remaining β/γ-complex of G-protein,

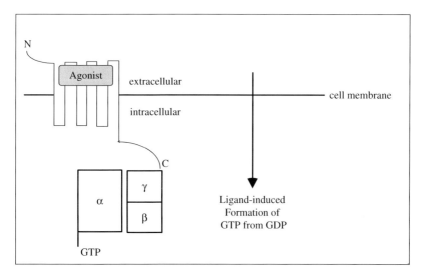

Figure 1-47. Following binding of an opioid ligand to the receptor site, guanidine-diphosphate (GDP) is activated resulting in the formation of guanidine-triphosphate (GTP)

by means of enzyme phosphorylation of AC and a reduction in cAMP, it interacts with the effector site, a calcium/potassium-channel (Figure I-48). This results in permeability changes of the voltage-gated ion channel, with an inward shift of potassium, and an outward shift of calcium ions, resulting in hyperpolarization.

Such changes result in a reduced response to all incoming nociceptive afferents as the neuronal cell no longer can be depolarized. GTP releasing its phosphate constituent, results in the dissociation of the α-unit from G-protein, and ends opioid action. After merger of the α- with the remaining β/γ-complex, the cell again returns into its dormant state. Such opioid-related analgesic effect first is initiated at the spinal cord level, where analgesics bind to opioid receptors. Via intraneuronal links a reduction in response of cellular reactions to all incoming nociceptive afferences is initiated. The spinal cord nerve cell no longer responds to subsequent afferent impulses from the periphery, no excitatory transmitters are being released at the synaptic cleft, interrupting nociceptive transmission.

The neuromolecular changes induced by opioids support the need for sufficient blockade of pain *before* nociceptive afferents arrive at the scene. Clinically, in the framework of anesthesia for example, such knowledge demands sufficient analgesia before a surgical intervention, as well as a prolonged postoperative and/or posttraumatic pain relief with an opioid. These facts also demand a sufficient high dosage of a narcotic analgesic in order to bind all opioid existing receptors. Then the nociceptive impulse is effectively blocked by an opioid before arrival of nociceptive afferents. Instead of trying to cancel out an already started process of chronification

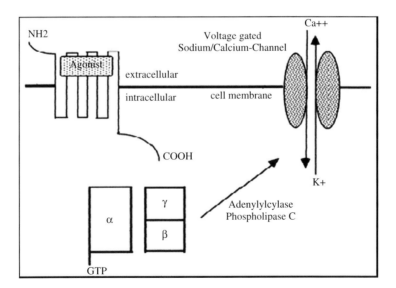

Figure I-48. The secondary intracellular messenger G-protein being activated after binding of a narcotic analgesic, resulting in a secondary transmembrane flux of electrolytes of voltage gated ion channels with hyperpolarization

and neuroplastic changes with higher doses than necessary, lesser doses are needed when opioid therapy is initiated before exposure to pain [23].

REASONS FOR INSUFFICIENT OPIOID USE – THE 11 MYTHS IN OPIOID THERAPY

Because pain in many therapeutically interventions cannot be prevented, it is the utmost priority of the medical personnel to deal with pain in its diverse manifestations and consider all possible therapeutic concepts. Analgesics are available for the treatment of pain, especially centrally active analgesics – the opioids – represent a group, which not only are most effective, but also take a "essential" position in the therapeutic regimen.

Such consideration appears to be more and more necessary, since governmental regulations have not eased the legal prescription of opioids. Enforcement agencies and regulatory legislature in the past years have impeded their early use [93]. And although prescription of opioids such as morphine in the western world is characterized by a steady increase (Figure I-49), there is still prejudice when it comes to the use of opioids for treatment of chronic pain. The following arguments often are stated as an explanation to refrain from regular opioid use or writing out prescriptions:
- Consolidation of prejudices in regard to opioid use,
- Stigmatization of patient, when taking an opioid

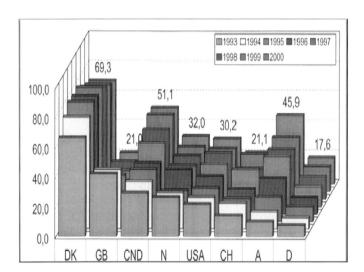

Figure I-49. Morphine consumption in kg/Mio. Inhabitants in western countries from the year 1993–2002 (DK = Denmark, GB = Great Britain, CND = Canada, N = Norwegian, CH-Switzerland, A = Austria, D = Germany)
Source: International Narcotics Control Board

- connection of opioid use as being "hooked" or "addicted",
- concern of patient that if they take too much of the opioid they will stop functioning properly,
- the amount of paper work, necessary to comply with regulatory requirements.

All these reasons prevent sufficient pain therapy instead of promoting it. On the other hand, there still exists "opiophobia" with an extensive and persisting ignorance – even in specialists – of how to sufficiently take advantage of the group of opioids in therapeutic strategy. Often, the possible development of dependency is quoted as an explanation, for not providing a sufficient supply of analgesics, and that the expected benefit is opposed by the risk of addiction development [94]. The danger of dependency development can be bypassed by using simple guidelines in opioid therapy. Thus,

- use by the clock, at fixed time intervals before the pain breaks through,
- use of a delayed release formulation, resulting in constant plasma concentrations, and
- Adequate information of the patient, that no addiction, and no sedation or other side-effects are caused when opioids are used in long-term treatment.
- The patient needs to be informed that his/her therapy can be adjusted to the individual pain level, using either moderate to potent opioids.

Such elucidation still is mandatory, because numerous prejudice and myths still predominate. For instance, a representative survey demonstrated that there still is strong opposition to the use of potent analgesics, resulting in an in-appropriate treatment, with 13% of the people interviewed still believing, that chronic persistent pain is normal in the age population, and has to be tolerated. While 3% even think chronic pain as being psychologically related, 30% consider chronic pain as a separate entity disease that needs to be treated. The majority of those (60%) however, expressed the opinion, that the underlying disease has to be treated in chronic pain, while almost one third wrongly believed, that opioid agents deaden all senses and induce a state of addiction. However, 59% of citizens are confident that opioids should be given to patients with severe pain, while 34% would give such medication only to cancer patients in their final stage.

Because 70% of patients with a tumor in the advanced stage complain of pain as the major symptom, by giving an analgesic in sufficient amounts with a sufficient potency, it would result in a 90% relief of pain. In England, where opioids can be prescribed on a normal prescription formula, 90% of the tumor patients are pain-free. Contrary, according to Zimmermann [95] in Germany the ghost "of addiction development and shortening of life through the use of opioids (opiophobia)" still lingers in the heads of doctors, and health-care providers. Also, regulatory issues from local or federal state medical boards with fear of sanctions, loss of license, loss of prescribing rights and the remote possibility of imprisonment and fines consistently are identified as primary reasons for physicians and other health care professionals not to treat or undertreat pain with opioid analgesics. It is for all these reasons, that 100,000 of cancer patients in Germany are not being provided with sufficient pain medication, and roughly less than 10% receive sufficient amounts of opioids to control their pain.

Different myths circulate about the use of opioids, which have to be clarified by the health care professional:

Myth 1: Opioids depress respiration and therefore are too dangerous to be considered as safe.

Fact is, that opioid-related respiratory depression indeed represents a potentially serious side-effect. It, however, does not appear in patients if opioid dose is prescribed according to pain intensity, and that dose is titrated to efficacy. In addition, controlled-release formulations when taken by mouth, result in less peak plasma levels than after intravenous injection.

Myth 2: Opioids lead to addiction with compulsive use (physical dependence) representing a major problem in their therapeutic administration in patients.

Fact is, this a very rare event and overestimated. When retarded release formulations of the opioid are being used, true addiction does not develop and there is an overall incidence of only 1/1000.

Myth 3: Regular opioid use results in the fast development of tolerance, with a never-ending increase in dosages.

Fact is, that tolerance development is very slow; it is seldom observed and often is due to a progression of the underlying disease.

Myth 4: Opioids induce an uncontrollable constipation.

Fact is, that constipation is a universal problem, and is present during regular ingestion with any type of an opioid. It, however, can be controlled by laxatives and should not be the reason to withhold opioid therapy from patients.

Myth 5: The majority of patients with opioid therapy prophylactically require an antiemetic.

Fact is, that nausea and emesis usually represent only short-lived side-effects, which subsides within the first days of a therapy.

Myth 6: Marked sedation and confusion are side-effects, repetitively appearing during the use of opioids.

Fact is that the correct use of opioids in moderate or severe pain necessarily does not result in sedation, confusion and a loss of function. They are rare events, which subsides within the first week following initial treatment, as there is the development of tolerance. In addition, cognitive states improve once pain medication is appropriately titrated.

Myth 7: Short-acting opioids with a duration of action between 3 and 6 h represents the ideal analgesic, necessary to master medium to severe pain.

Fact is, that short-acting opioids lead to a faster development of tolerance. Because the patient repetitively has to take the opioid, he may forget the time of intake, resulting in breakthrough pain. Use of a controlled release formulation of 12–24 h such side-effect can be bypassed.

Myth 8: Controlled-release formulations of an opioid agent are only appropriate for use in tumor patients.

Fact is, that the controlled release formulation of an opioid is appropriate for all types of medium to severe pain. Even patients with severe pain due to osteoarthritis, rheumatoid arthritis or with neuropathic pain, can profit from such formulation.

Myth 9: Dose adaptation and precise titration to effect is impossible with a controlled-release formulation of opioids.

Fact is that if one starts with the lowest possible dose in opioid-naive patients, fast adaptation within 1–2 days to the effective dose is possible. Using fixed time intervals during the titration process, doses are being increased by 25–50% to the previous amount. So-called breakthrough pains can be met with a fast-release galenic formulation.

Myth 10: Severe pain in a cancer can be relieved successfully only with the parenteral administration of the opioid.

Fact is, that independent of the underlying disease, the oral formulations of an opioid, according to a statement of the WHO, is the preferred mode of application. If patients are unable to swallow, rather than a motor-pump driven syringe, either the rectal or the transdermal mode of application are recommended.

Myth 11: The opioid dose correlates closely with its plasma level.

Fact is, that an exact correlation between oral dose and plasma concentration does not exist. Only a concentration area between the admitted dose and plasma concentration can be derived.

Achieving an in-depth understanding of the pathophysiology underlying acute and chronic pain syndromes, how and in which way pain originates and how pain can be treated effectively, the sooner a therapeutic starting point of effective therapy may be found. In addition, guidelines and recommendations for acute and chronic opioid use as well as consensus statements are now available, which underlie the accepted and legitimate medical principles to legally practice prescription of opioids. Pain management is now more feasible with scientific breakthroughs in molecular biology, insight into pain at the molecular level, as well as the advances in drug therapy with its drug delivery systems. Together in accord with multidimensional therapeutic options and a multidisciplinary approach, there is a remarkable advancement in the therapeutic strategies to fight pain.

Alternative Therapeutic Targets in Pain Therapy

In addition to the pharmacological agents and their receptors discussed in the previous sections, several other targets for analgesic development have been explored.

Protein Kinase C (PKC) appears to contribute to the long-term changes that underlie injury-associated allodynia and hyperalgesia. Specifically, repeated or prolonged noxious stimulation leads to activation of the PKCy isoform in the dorsal root ganglia [17]. Inhibitors of PKCy may thus possess therapeutic potential in alleviating hyperalgesia and neuropathic pain.

Another therapeutic target is *adenosine kinase*. Via activation of adenosine receptors nociceptive, sensory input is modulated. Adenosine kinase phosphorylates adenosine and maintains low intracellular levels of this neurotransmitter. Adenosine kinase inhibitors (e.g. GP515, GP3269, A-134974 and ABT-702) increase the endogenous levels of adenosine and have been shown to elicit analgesic and anti-inflammatory effects in several animal models. These effects appear to be due to enhanced adenosine receptor activation since they are blocked by adenosine receptor antagonists.

PROTON CHANNELS AS THERAPEUTIC TARGETS IN PAIN THERAPY

Three subtypes of amiloride sensitive proton channels, referred to as ASIC 1, ASIC2 and ASIC3, have been implicated in pain transmission [96]. Specifically, ASIC1 and a splice variant of ASIC2, ASIC1b, are activated by low pH and are expressed in both sensory neurons and the central nervous system. The activation of these channels may be involved in pain transmission, since acid itself produces pain and low pH conditions are associated with chronic joint inflammation, skin ulceration and some tumors. The VR1 vanilloid receptor antagonist, capsazepine, may reduce proton-induced activation of sensory neurons while NPFF appears to increase the sensitivity of ASICs to protons.

ADJUVANT ANALGESICS IN PAIN THERAPY

Adjuvant analgesics are compounds that are not classified as analgesics, but are used clinically for the relief of pain. This class of analgesics contains a wide range of compounds that belong to a variety of chemical families. They are classified according to their use and their mechanisms of action are often not well defined. For example, antidepressants are used to control neuropathic pain, α_2-adrenoceptor agonists (e.g. clonidine, dexmedetomidine) potentiate the anti-inflammatory and analgesic effects of COX inhibitors, while corticosteroids block inflammation and may directly modulate the nociceptive action of substance P. Compounds that have been especially beneficial in the treatment of neuropathic and phantom limb pain include local anesthetics (e.g., mexiletine, flecainide), anticonvulsants (gabapentin, carbamazepine, phenytoin, valproate, clonazepam, lamotrigine), GABA agonists, neuroleptics and calcitonin. Other analgesics such as muscle relaxants and benzo-diazepines are used to relieve musculoskeletal pain.

Difference in Receptor Activation/Inhibition as Drug Targets

Many analgesics affect different sites along neuronal pathways of nociception. Within the CNS neurotransmitters modulate action including synthesis, storage, and release of receptor activation and inhibition. In addition, modulation of intrasynaptic neurotransmitter metabolism or reuptake, and a direct second-messenger pathway can be observed (Figure I-50).

MECHANISM OF ACTION OF TRICYCLIC ANTIDEPRESSANTS

The termination of action of biogenic amines norepinephrine (NE) and serotonin (5-HT) is determined by reuptake into the presynaptic terminal. Drugs that block reuptake, such as tricyclic antidepressants, increase the efficacy of those transmitters by allowing them to remain in the synaptic cleft and activate the receptors longer (Figure I-51).

It should be noted that although the exact mechanism of action of TCAs as analgesics is not known, there appears to be a close relationship between the inhibitory reuptake effects on biogenic amines and analgesic potency. While selective inhibitors of serotonin reuptake are less effective in treating pain, the ability to inhibit norepineprine reuptake is associated more strongly with analgesia. The dose of TCAs is lower than those dosages used to treat depression, suggesting that the analgesic properties are independent of their antidepressant properties.

Aside from TCAs specific antidepressant activity, neuronal hyperexcitability associated with pain is reduced through the mechanism of a decrease in sodium channel activity and $GABA_A$-receptor channel activation. The net effect of these actions by anticonvulsants is to reduce the excitatory synaptic transmission or to enhance the inhibitory synaptic transmission. For instance GABA, which is an inhibitory ligand binds to the $GABA_A$-receptor, thus opening the $GABA_A$-channel, which hyperpolarizes the cell and inhibits further impulse generation. The $GABA_A$-channel has at least five different binding sites (Figure I-52).

In addition, there are three different kinds of sites at which anticonvulsants exert their action:
1. Voltage-gated ion channel of the sodium/calcium type
2. Ligand-gated ion channel receptors
3. Combination of voltage-gated and ligand-gated ion channel/receptors
The ligand-gated ion channel binds excitatory neurotransmitters such as glycine and glutamate on the extracellular portion of the receptor. Via secondary intracellular phosphorylation process of protein kinases, a nearby ion channel opens for Na^+- and K^+-ions, causing an end-plate potential with either depolarization or hyperpolarization of the postsynaptic neuron, depending on whether the ligand which binds to them is of excitatory or inhibitory nature (Figure I-53).

There are four main types of voltage-dependent calcium channels, each composed of several subunits: L-Type, T-Type, N-Type and P-Type. Each type of calcium channel is activated and inactivated at different voltage ranges and at different rates. Representative examples are ethosuximide and valproic acid which inhibit ion flow through the calcium T-channel (Figure I-54). The newer voltage dependent calcium

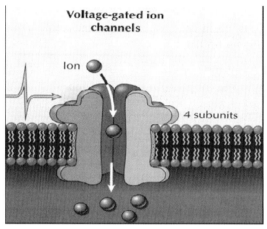

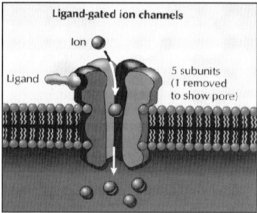

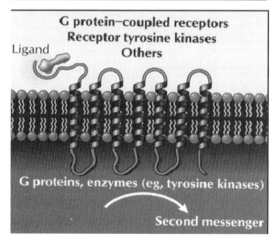

Figure I-50. Summary of schematic representation of the targets receptor sites and their mode of action of different analgesics

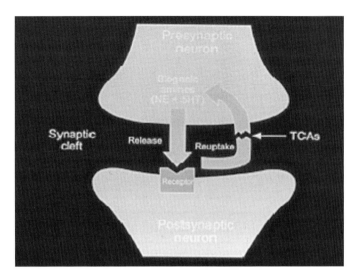

Figure I-51. Tricyclic antidepressants (TCAs) acting at the descending noradrenergic- and serotonergic inhibitory pain pathways, thus relieving pain

channel blocker pregablin acts via the alpha$_2$-subunit resulting in a modulation of the hyperexcited neuron (Figure I-54).

Another type of a voltage-gated channel is selective for the sodium ion. The sodium channels open in response to membrane depolarization, allowing an inward shift of sodium ions into the neuron, thus increasing neuronal depolarization and the spread of action potentials. After the channel closes, it remains inactive for a certain

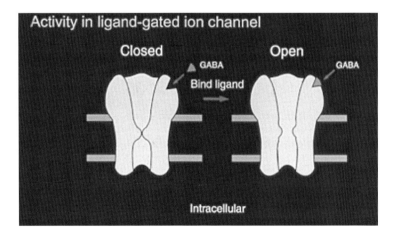

Figure I-52. Basic mechanism of action of anticonvulsants in pain therapy at the GABA$_A$-channel resulting in a hyperpolarization and an inhibition of further impulse generation

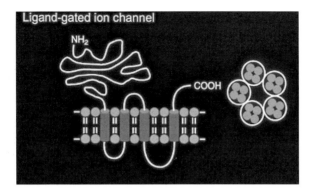

Figure 1-53. Activity of anticonvulsants on ligand-gated ion channels, whereby an agent binds to the extracellular portion of the receptor, and via proteinkinases or phosphatases induced activation of ion channels results in an inward shift of sodium or potassium, resulting in depolarization or hyperpolarization of the postsynaptic neuron

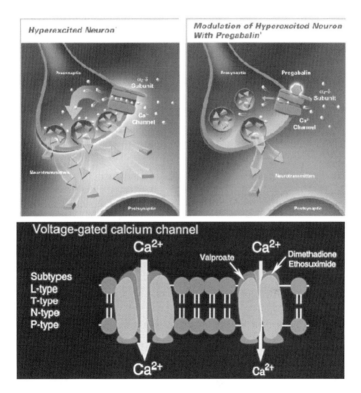

Figure 1-54. Mode of action of analgesics on voltage-gated calcium channels resulting in a closure with a reduced inward shift

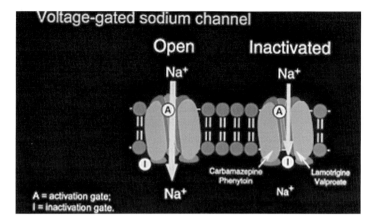

Figure I-55. The voltage-gated sodium ion channel as a target for antiepileptic agents in the treatment of pain via inactivation of the sodium channel

period (it is refractory), during which membrane depolarization cannot reopen it. During neuronal hyperactivity, such as in seizures and in neuropathic pain, the neuron undergoes depolarization and fires action potentials at higher frequencies. Inhibition of firing with drugs is due to the ability of the sodium channel to recover from inactivation, the refractory period is prolonged and the frequency of action potentials reduced. Carbamazepine, lamotrigine, phenytoin and valproic acid all work at this mechanism (Figure I-55).

The NMDA subtype of the glutamate receptor is an ion channel, which operates both by a ligand-gated and voltage gated mechanisms. In order to operate, the NMDA-receptor channel has to bind glutamate in the presence of glycine. In addition, non-NMDA-induced depolarization is needed to remove the magnesium. This is done through activation of the NK1- (substance P) receptor, after which sodium and calcium pass through the open channel. NMDA-receptor antagonists, which are able to inhibit this transfer act as anticonvulsants (e.g. carbamazepine, felbamate), at the same time are potent analgesics (Figure I-56).

In addition to the NMDA subtype of the glutamate receptor, there is the AMPA and the kainite (KA) receptor subtype. Both induce sensitivity and lower the threshold for activation of the excitatory NMDA-receptor. Decreasing the threshold for sensitivity via blockade of the non-NMDA-receptors will result in a reduced excitation with a reduced activation of nociceptive afferents (Figure I-57).

Pharmacologically Resistant – Psychologically Conditioned Pain

"Functional" and feigned pain patients who seem to magnify their physical complaints may be described as exhibiting hysteria, conversion disorder,

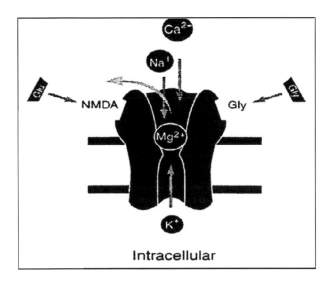

Figure 1-56. Combination of voltage- and ligand-gated ion channel at the NMDA receptor

hypochondriasis, somatization disorder, depression, and malingering or compensatory behavior. These terms are used in a general fashion, without the specificity that a psychiatrist or psychologist would apply. The general practitioner may call the back pain and its manifestations functional overlay or of psychogenic origin, that is, conditions for which no organic origin can be found. Current evidence suggests that the majority of these patients really do perceive disabling pain. Thus,

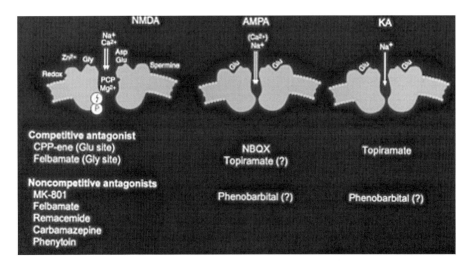

Figure 1-57. Putative effect of anticonvulsants as analgesics on ionotropic glutamate receptors

assuring a patient that the pain is all in the mind offers no benefit. Such labeling creates a negative response in the patient and impairs the working relationship between physician and patient. There is often a strong correlation between inappropriate responses on physical examination and inappropriate response to treatment. These physical responses are (Figure I-58):

1. Tenderness that is nonanatomic and responsive to the lightest touch.
2. Simulation, indicated by inappropriate pain response to light axial loading of the spine by pressure on the head, or pain in the back when the pelvis rather than the spine is rotated.
3. Distraction, in which there is normal straight leg raising in a sitting but not a supine position.
4. Regional abnormalities, such as widespread weakness and sensory disturbance throughout the entire limb or side of the body; and
5. Overreaction to examination, including cogwheel-type resistance to strength testing of an extremity.

All of these responses can be correlated to abnormalities defined on self-report tests such as pain drawings, psychologic tests, depression scales, and pain analogue scales. Once pathologic changes have been ruled out, the best treatment for the mildly anxious patient is reassurance and a time-limited regimen of mild sedatives. In more severe cases, psychiatric referral may be necessary.

The biggest problem in treating pain patients, when therapeutic interventions are without any effect, is that of a functionally related somatization of pain. In the International Classification, a "somatozised pain syndrome" is as follows: "A prevalent symptomatic ongoing, and agonizing pain, that cannot be explained by organic pathology". Pain then appears in connection with psychological and/or psychiatric problems and emotional conflicts, which are of sufficient intensity to become the dominant cause of pain. A large number of patients with apparently

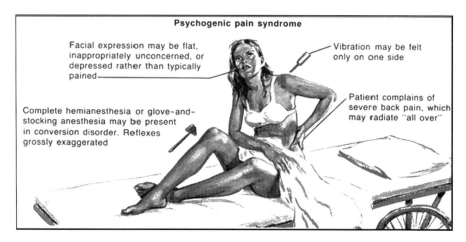

Figure I-58. Patient with psychogenic pain syndrome characterized by typical symptoms

somatoforme pain, is not only seen in the head, the heart, the gastro-intestinal and the genital area, but more frequently in patients with neck and back pain. Patients regularly displace such psychosomatic interconnection, which is very difficult to treat. The patient refuses to acknowledge such cause and demands newer and more extensive medical examinations. Although any premature psychosomatic diagnosis is dangerous, because it impairs the diagnostic assessment and results in a displeased and angry patient, a functionally related ailment has to be suspected when prolonged therapy shows resistance. In the search of an organic cause, ultimately the patient in pain wanders from one doctor to the next ("doctor shopping").

With newer and more costly outpatient, and/or clinical examinations, the patient turns into a "specialist killer" at shorter intervals. This is because with every new step in the ladder of the medical hierarchy, any therapeutic intervention in this psychosomatic disorder is doomed to fail. On the basis of number of various pseudo findings, therapy is only symptom oriented; it could even result in surgical interventions, which the patient is willing to endure without resistance. And although stress reactions resolve within two or three days of a traumatic event, they may be associated with later symptomatology and chronic pain. For instance almost one sixth of all patients involved in a traffic accident develop phobia of traveling in cars trains or even trams subsequent to the accident. The stress of the traumatic event is likely to contribute to later avoidant behavior on standing-learning theory grounds.

A symptom, suggesting a functionally-related pain syndrome, is that of lavished depression, where the depressive symptoms are in the background, while somatic symptoms become evident. Another case of a functionally, psychosomatic-related pain problem is that of a conversion. Here, subconscious conflicts emerge to the surface, disguised as somatic pain (conversion) and where the painful sensations act as an equivalent or a replacement for past stressful events. Such a disorder is difficult to treat because pain has a symbolic character, mirroring subconscious desires, aggressions, and affections, which should to be kept away from the conscious mind. Pain in such sense may also be some kind of self-punishment of uncondoned, not socially accepted desires. This is also reflected in the word "pain" and a linguistic association with the latin word "poena" (penalty), where pain is the attempt of the patient to prevent a nervous breakdown (ailment in the sense of self-healing).

Finally, psychosomatic pain may play an important role in that the patient consciously or unconsciously gains some kind of profit by maintaining the malfunctions. It is there the psychologist comes into play and where the body language points to a problem with his/her significant others, which are not outspoken and otherwise are not confronted. According to some psychoanalysts (Dr. I. Freye/Zürich), such symptoms wrongly often are linked to the everyday "battle of the sexes" as they follow the mainstream of current psychological thinking. Here, the actual problem is misjudged, and where early physical and/or sexual harassment in childhood, chronic pain experiences of family members, psychosocial load such as a divorce, or early personal pain experiences act as predisposing factors in the development of chronic pain. And when somatoform pain is transferred into a partnership symptomatic therapy ultimately does not result in a relief of pain. Contrary, the conflict is further somatized, e.g. it is diffused and further transferred onto the bodies level. As a result, family members spare the sick partner, and any demands upon him/her are avoided. Ultimately however, the patient gains some advantage from the ailment, pain is being misused as an instrument of power resulting in further manifestation if it is not being analyzed. In such patients, principally no physical cause of pain is found, and although they complain of persistent pain, it is described very emotionally, such as if being reported by someone else. In addition, pain typically starts with the stressful situation.

THE MALINGERING PATIENT WITH COMPENSATORY PAIN BEHAVIOR

The malingering patient is motivated by a conscious secondary gain that may be tangible or intangible. It is important to remember that a malingerer may be uninterested in financial rewards and may instead be seeking other forms of reinforcement from employers, coworkers, or family. In contrast, the compensatory patient is interested only in monetary gain. The patient may have been injured at work or may be involved in litigation related to an automobile accident. The possibility of large financial settlements motivates many victims, some with quite minor injuries, to file lawsuits claiming extensive and even ridiculous disabilities. These patients usually give a vague story and try to confuse the examiner by avoiding specific details of their problem or their pain distribution. A bizarre gait, inconsistent with physical findings, is typical (Figure I-59). After bending forward, the patient returns to the erect position in a cogwheel fashion, groaning and complaining of increased pain. These complaints usually indicate that the patient is exaggerating or feigning complaints to impress the examiner. A well-trained examiner should find it relatively easy to identify malingerers and patients with compensatory low back pain. However, it is not advisable to inform the patient of this diagnosis. This can lead to legal action against the physician for defamation of character. The best course is simply to state, "no organic basis can be found for the patient's symptoms."

Therefore when pain is being felt, it can be differentiated between its localization, the feeling of being hurt and the experience of displeasure. And because pain has a strong emotional component, painful sensations are always an individual experience that should be treated individually. The following features significantly affect pain sensations:

1. The current environmental situation when pain is being experienced,
2. the individual genetic make-up
3. the underlying education,
4. the sociocultural environment,
5. the religious environment,
6. the ethnic origin,
7. the level of civilization.

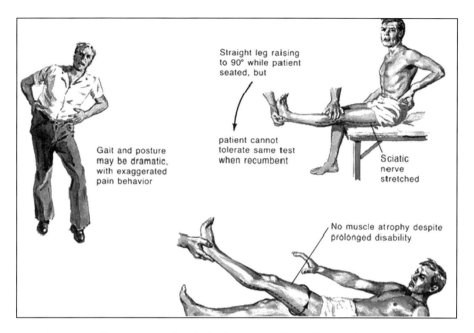

Figure 1-59. Compensatory pain behavior in patients with psychic conditioned nociception

The pain threshold on the other hand can be raised or lowered by the following attributes:

8. fear and/or grief,
9. depression,
10. isolation,
11. insomnia,
12. brooding, and
13. worries.

On the other hand, the following elements increase pain threshold, resulting in a lesser feeling of pain:

1. affection,
2. hope,
3. sleep,
4. distraction,
5. relaxation,
6. career, especially when
7. anxiolytics,
8. antidepressants, and/or
9. opioids

are being used.

Because pain can always be influenced by a number of different features, it can be considered as an extremely subjective experience. Pain gets its individual color in the limbic system, an old phylogenetical system, characterized by a dense accumulation of opioid receptor sites [89]. It is a system, with which the cortex intensively communicates. At the same time, it is a system where all incoming afferent impulses are being assessed and evaluated, receiving an individual attribute.

References

1. Loeser, I.D., et al., *Bonica's Management of Pain*, 2001, Philadelphia: Lippincott.
2. Craig, D.B., *Postoperative recovery of pulmonary function*. Anesth Analg, 1981, 60: pp. 46–52.
3. Spence, A.A., *Postoperative pulmonary complications in general anesthesia*, T.C. Gray, J.F. Nunn, and J.E. Utting, Editors, 1980, Butterworth: London. pp. 591–608.
4. Bonica, J.J., *Current status of postoperative pain therapy*, in *Current Topics in Pain Research and Therapy*, T. Yokota and R. Dubner, Editors, 1983, Exerpta Medica: Tokyo. pp. 169–189.
5. Modig, J., *Thromembolism and blood loss: continuous epidural vs. general anesthesia with vcontrolled ventilation*. Reg Anesth, 1982, 7: pp. S84–S88.
6. Katz, J., B.P. Kavanagh, and A.N. Sandler, *Preemptive analgesia: clinical evidence of neuroplasticity contributing to postoperative pain*. Anesthesiology, 1992, 77: pp. 439–446.
7. Wall, P.D., *The prevention of postoperative pain*. Pain, 1988, 33: pp. 289–290.
8. Cohen, F.L., *Postsurgical pain relief: patients status and nurses' medication*. Pain, 1980, 9: pp. 265–274.
9. Angell, M., *The quality of mercy*. New Engl J Med, 1982, 306: pp. 98–99.
10. Marks, R.M. and E.J. Sachar, *Undertreatment of medical inpatients with narcotic analgesics*. Ann Int Med, 1973, 78: pp. 173–181.
11. Jurna, I. and K. Brune, *Central effect of the non-steroid anti-inflammatory agents, indometacin, ibuprofen, and diclofenac, determined in C fibre-evoked activity in single neurons of the rat thalamus*. Pain, 1990, 41: pp. 71–80.
12. Apkarian, A.V., et al., *Chronic back pain is associated with decreased prefrontal and thalamic gray matter density*. J Neurosci, 2004, 24: pp. 10410–10415.
13. Rexed, B., *Some aspects of the cytoarchitectonics and synaptology of the spinal cord*. Brain Res, 1964, 11: pp. 58–92.
14. Wager, T.D., *The neural bases of placebo effects in anticipation and pain*. Semin Pain Med, 2005, 3: pp. 22–30.
15. Melzack, R. and P.C. Wall, *Pain mechanisms: a new theory*. Science, 1965, 150: p. 971.
16. Kehlet, H., *Surgical stress: the role of pain and analgesia*. Br J Anaesth, 1989, 63: pp. 189–195.
17. Kehlet, H., *The stress response to surgery: release mechanisms and the modifying effect of pain relief*. Acta Chir Scand, 1989, 550 (suppl): pp. 22–28.
18. Scott, N.B. and H. Kehlet, *Regional anaesthesia and surgical mobidity*. Br J Surg, 1988, 75: pp. 299–304.
19. Hassler, R., *Wechselwirkungen zwischen dem System der schnellen Schmerzempfindung und dem des langsamen, nachhaltigen Schmerzgefühl*. Arch Klin Chir, 1976, 342: p. 47.
20. Pert, P.B. and S.H. Snyder, *Opiate receptor: demonstration in nervous tissue*. Science, 1973, 179: pp. 1011–1014.

21. McMahon, S. and M. Koltzenburg, *Wall and Melzack's Textbook of Pain*. 5th edition. 2005, Churchill: London Livingstone, 1280.

22. Ramachandran, V.S. and D. Rogers-Ramachandran, *Synaesthesia in phantom limbs induced with mirrors*. Proc R Soc Lond B Biol Sci, 1996, 263: pp. 377–386.

23. Flor, H., *Phantom limb pain: characteristics, causes and treatment*. Lancet, 2002, 1: pp. 182–188.

24. Hassler, R., *Über die antagonistischen Systeme der Schmerzempfindung und des Schmerzgefühls im peripheren und zentralen Nervensystem, In: Pentazocin im Spiegel de et Entwöhnung*, S. Kubicki and G.A. Neuhaus, Editors, 1976, Springer: Berlin, Heidelberg, New York. pp. 1–17.

25. Basbaum, A.I. and H.L. Fields, *Endogenous pain control systems: brainstem spinal pathways and endorphin circuitry*. Annu Rev Neurosci, 1984, 7: pp. 309–338.

26. Fields, K.L. and S.D. Anderson, *Evidence that raphe-spinal neurons mediate opiate and midbrain stimulation produced analgesia*. Pain, 1978, 5: pp. 333–349.

27. Wiklund, L., et al., *Autoradiographic and electrophysiological evidence for exicitatory amino acid transmission in the periaqueductal gray projection to nucleus raphe magnus in the rat*. Neurosci Lett, 1988, 93: pp. 158–163.

28. Urban, M.O. and D.J. Smith, *Role of neurotensin in the nucleus raphe magnus in opioid-induced antinociception from the periaqueductal gray*. J Pharmacol Expt Therap, 1993, 265: pp. 580–586.

29. Melzack, R., *Pain measurement and assessment*. 1983, Raven: New York.

30. Tölle, T.R., et al., *Effects of Ketalorphan and morphine before and after noxious stimulation on immediate-early gene expression in rat spinal cord neurons*. Pain, 1994, 56: pp. 103–112.

31. Chandrasekharan, N.V., et al., *COX-3, a cyclooxygenase-1 variant inhibited by acetaminophen and other analgesic/antipyretic drugs: cloning, structure, and expression*. Proc Natl Acad Sci (USA), 2002, 99: pp. 13371–13373.

32. Rady, J.J., W.B. Campbell, and J.M. Fujimoto, *Antianalgesic action of nociceptin originating in the brain is mediated by spinal prostaglandin E2 in mice*. J Pharmacol Exp Ther, 2001, 296: pp. 7–14.

33. Lembo, P.M., *Proenkephalin A gene products activate a new family of sensory neuron–specific GPCRs*. Nat Neurosci, 2002, 5: pp. 201–209.

34. Vrinten, D.H., et al., *Chronic blockade of melanocortin receptors alleviates allodynia in rats with neuropathic pain*. Anesth Analg, 2001, 93: pp. 1572–1577.

35. Kovelowski, C.J., et al., *Supraspinal cholecystokinin may drive tonic descending facilitation mechanisms to maintain neuropathic pain in the rat*. Pain, 2000, 87: pp. 265–273.

36. Vanderath, T.W., *Chronic pain and the role of cholecystokinin*. J Neurpath Pain Symtom Palliat, 2004, 1: pp. 89–95.

37. Verheggen, R., K. Bumann, and A.J. Kaumann, *BIBN4096BS is a potent competitive antagonist of the relaxant effects of alpha-CGRP on human temporal artery: comparison with CGRP(8–37)*. Br J Pharmacol, 2002, 136: pp. 120–126.

38. Xu, Z.-Q., et al., *Evidence for galanin receptors in primary sensory neurones and effect of axotomy and inflammation*. Neuroreport, 1996, 8: pp. 237–242.

39. Meller, S.T., et al., *Nitric oxide mediates the thermal hyperalgesia produced in a model of neuropathic pain in the rat*. Neuroscience, 1992, 50: pp. 7–10.

40. Meller, S.T. and G.F. Gebhardt, *Nitric oxide (NO) and antinociceptive processing in the spinal cord*. Pain, 1993, 52: pp. 127–136.

41. Przewlocki, R., H. Machelska, and B. Przewlocka, *Inhibition of nitric oxide synthase enhances morphine antinociception in the rat spinal cord*. Life Sci, 1993, 53: pp. 1–5.
42. Kolesnikov, Y.A., et al., *Blockade of tolerance to morphine but not to k opioids by a nitric oxide synthese inhibitor*. Proc Natl Acad Sci USA, 1993, 90: pp. 5162–5166.
43. Liu, H.X. and T. Hokfelt, *The participation of galanin in pain processing at the spinal level*. Trends Pharmacol Sci, 2002, 23: pp. 468–478.
44. Drew, L.J., et al., *Activation of spinal cannabinoid 1 receptors inhibits C-fibre driven hyperexcitable neuronal responses and increases [35S]GTPγS binding in the dorsal horn of the spinal cord of noninflamed and inflamed rats*. Eur J Neurosci, 2000, 12: p. 2079–2086.
45. Sagar, D.R., et al., *Inhibitory effects of CB1 and CB2 receptor agonists on responses of DRG neurons and dorsal horn neurons in neuropathic rats*. Eur J Neurosci, 2005, 22: pp. 371–379.
46. Griffin, G., et al., *Evidence for the presence of CB2-like cannabinoid receptors on peripheral nerve terminals*. Eur J Pharmacol, 1997, 339: pp. 53–61.
47. Herzberg, U., et al., *The analgesic effects of R(+)-Win 55,212-2 mesylate, a high cannabinoid agonist, in a rat model of neuropathic pain*. Neurosci Lett, 1997, 221: pp. 157–160.
48. Chizh, B.A. and P. Illes, *P2X receptors and nociception*. Pharmacol Rev, 2001, 53: pp. 553–568.
49. Burnstock, G. and M. Williams, *P2 Purinergic receptors: modulation of cell function and therapeutic potential*. J Pharmacol Expt Ther, 2000, 295: pp. 862–869.
50. Di Marzo, V., J.R. Tippins, and H.R. Morris, *Neuropeptides and inflammatory mediators: bidirectional regulatory mechanisms*: Trends Pharmacol Sci, 1989, 10: pp. 91–92.
51. Mezey, E., et al., *Distribution of mRNA for vanilloid receptor subtype 1 (VR1), and VR1-like immunoreactivity, in the central nervous system of the rat and human*. Proc Natl Acad Sci (USA), 2000, 97: pp. 3655–3660.
52. Hough, L.B., et al., *Inhibition of improgan antinociception by the cannabinoid (CB)(1) antagonist N-(piperidin-1-yl)-5-(4-chlorophenyl)-1-(2, 4-dichlorophenyl)-4-methyl-1H-pyrazole-3-carboxamide (SR141716A): lack of obligatory role for endocannabinoids acting at CB(1) receptors*. J Pharmacol Exp Ther, 2002, 303: pp. 314–322.
53. Dib-Hajj, S.D., et al., *NaN, a novel voltage-gated Na channel, is expressed preferentially in peripheral sensory neurons and down-regulated after axotomy*. Proc Natl Acad Sci (USA), 1998, 95: pp. 8963–8968.
54. Kato, A., T. Ohkubo, and K. Kitamura, *Algogen-speific pain processing in mouse spinal cord: differential constitution of voltage-dependent Ca2+ channels in synaptic transmission*. Br J Pharmacol, 2002, 135: pp. 1336–1342.
55. Eglen, R.M., J.C. Hunter, and A. Dray, *Ions in the fire: recent ion-channel research and approaches to pain therapy*. TIPS, 1999, 20: pp. 337–342.
56. Liu, H., P.W. Mantyhy, and A.I. Basbaum, *NMDA-receptor regulation of substance P release from primary afferent nociceptors*. Nature, 1997, 386: pp. 721–724.
57. Parsons, C.G., *NMDA receptors as targets for drug action in neuropathic pain*. Eur J Pharmacol, 2001, 429: pp. 71–78.
58. Williams, K., *Mechanisms influencing stimulatory effects of spermine at recombinant N-methyl-D-aspartate receptors*. Mol Pharmacol, 1994, 46: pp. 161–168.
59. Dukat, M., et al., *Epibatidine: a very high affinity nicotinic receptor ligand*. Med Chem Res, 1994, 4: pp. 131–139.

60. Bannon, A.W., et al., *Broad-spectrum, non-opioid analgesic activity by selective modulation of neuronal nicotinic acetylcholine receptors.* Science, 1998, 279: pp. 77–81.

61. Lynch, J.J., et al., *ABT-594 (a nicotinic acetylcholine agonist): anti-allodynia in a rat chemotherapy-induced pain model.* Eur J Pharmacol, 2005, 509: pp. 43–48.

62. Vrinten, D.H., et al., *Neuropathic pain: a possible role for the melanocortin system?* Eur J Pharmacol, 2001, 429: pp. 61–69.

63. Riccio, A., et al., *An NGF-TrkA-Mediated retrograde signal to transcription factor CREB in sympathetic neurons.* Science, 1997, 277: pp. 1097–1100.

64. Caterina, M.J., et al., *Impaired nociception and pain sensation in mice lacking the capscaicin receptor.* Science, 2000, 288: pp. 306–311.

65. Chattipakorn, S.C., et al., *The effect of fentanyl on c-fos expression on the trigeminal brainstem complex produced by pulpal heat stimulation in the ferret.* Pain, 1999, 82: pp. 207–215.

66. Yaksh, T.L., *Spinal opiate analgesics: Characteristics and principles of action.* Anesthesiology, 1981, 11: pp. 293–346.

67. Goodman, R.R., et al., *Differentiation of delta and mu opiate receptor localization by light microscopic autoradiography.* Proc Natl Acad Sci (USA), 1980, 77: pp. 6239–6243.

68. Yaksh, T.L., *In vivo studies on the spinal opiate receptor systems mediating antinociception. I. mu and delta receptor profiles in the primate.* J Pharmacol Exp Ther, 1983, 226: pp. 303–316.

69. Woolf, C.J., *Evidence for a central component of post-injury hypersensitivity.* Nature, 1983, 306: pp. 686–688.

70. Coderre, T.J. and R. Melzack, *Cutaneous hyperalgesia: contribution of the peripheral and central nervous system to the increase in pain sensitivity after injury.* Brain Res, 1987 (404): pp. 95–106.

71. Cook, A.J., et al., *Dynamic receptive field plasticity in the rat spinal cord dorsal horn following C-primary afferent input.* Nature, 1987, 325: pp. 151–153.

72. Lombard, M.C. and J.M. Besson, *Attempts to gauge the relative importance of pre-and postoperative effects of morphine on the transmission of noxious messages in the dorsal horn of the rat spinal cord.* Pain, 1989, 37: pp. 335–345.

73. Yaksh, T., *Spinal systems and pain processing: development of novel analgesic drugs with mechanistically defined models.* TIPS, 1999, 20: pp. 329–337.

74. Davies, S.N. and D. Lodge, *Evidence for involvement of N-methylaspertate receptors in "wind-up" of class 2 neurone in the dorsal horn of the rat.* Brain Res, 1987, 424: pp. 402–406.

75. Ebersberger, A., et al., *Morphine, 5-HT2 and 5-HT3 receptor antagonists reduce c-fos expression in the trigeminal nuclear complex following noxious chemical stmulation of the rat nasal mucosa.* Brain Res, 1995, 676: pp. 336–342.

76. Kayser, V., et al., *Potent antinociceptive effects of kelatorphan, a highly efficient inhibitor of multiple enkaphalin-degrading enzymes, systemically administered in normal and arthritic rats.* Brain Res, 1989, 497: pp. 94–101.

77. Hammond, D.L., et al., *Morphine or U-50,488H suppresses fos proteine-like immunoreactivity in the spinal cord and the nucleus tractus solitarii evoked by noxious visceral stimulus in the rat.* J Comp Neurol, 1992, 315: pp. 244–253.

78. Higuchi, T., et al., *Effects of carbamazepine and valproic acid on brain immunoreactvce somatostatin and gamma-aminobutyric acid in amygdaloid-kindled rats.* Eur J Pharmacol, 1986, 125: pp. 169–175.

79. Tölle, T.R., et al., *Anticonvulsants suppress c-fos protein expression in spinal cord neurons following noxious thermal stimulation.* Expt Neurol, 1996, 132: pp. 271–278.

80. Sawynok, J. and F.S. La Bella, *On the involvement of GABA in the analgesia produced by baclofen, muscimol and morphine.* Neuropharmacology, 1982, 21: pp. 397–404.

81. Castro-Lopes, J.M., et al., *Expression of GRAD mRNA in spinal cord neurons of normal and monoarthritic rats.* Mol Brain Res, 1994, 26: pp. 169–176.

82. Hammond, D.L. and E.J. Drowner, *Effects of intrathecally administered THIP, baclofen and muscimol on nociceptive threshold.* Eur J Pharmacol, 1984, 103: pp. 121–125.

83. Hao, J.X., et al., *Baclofen reverses the hypersensitivity of dorsal horn dynamic range neurons to mechanical stimulation after transient spinal cord ischemia: implication for a tonic GABAergic inhibitory control of myelinated fiber input.* J Neurophysiol, 1992, 68: pp. 392–396.

84. Aigouy, I., et al., *Intrathecal midazolam versus intrathecal morphine in orofacial nociception – an experimental study in rats.* Neurosci Lett, 1992, 139: pp. 97–99.

85. Linderoth, B. and R.D. Foreman, *Physiology of spinal cord stimulation: review and update.* Neuromodulation, 1999, 2: pp. 150–164.

86. Guilbaud, G., et al., *Primary somatosensory cortex in rats with pain-related behaviors due to peripheral mononeuropathy after moderate ligation of one sciatic nerve: neuronal responsivity to somatic stimulation.* Exp Brain Res, 1992, 92: pp. 227–245.

87. Jensen, T.S. and T.L. Yaksh, *Brainstem excitatory amino acid receptors in nociception: mircroinjection mapping and pharmacological chraracterization of glutamate-sensitive sites in brainstem associated with algogenic behavior.* Neuroscience, 1992, 442: pp. 513–526.

88. Mc Kenzie, J.S. and N.R. Beechy, *The effects of morphine and pethidine on somatic evoked responses in the midbrain of the cat, and their relevance to analgesia.* Electroenceph Clin Neurophysiol, 1962, 14: pp. 501–519.

89. Hong, J.S., et al., *Determination of methionine enkephalin in discrete regions of rat brain.* Brain Res, 1977, 134: pp. 383.

90. Simantov, R., A.M. Snowman, and S.H. Snyder, *A morphine-like factor "enkephalin" in rat brain: subcellular localization.* Brain Res, 1976, 107: pp. 650–655.

91. Wall, P.D. and C.J. Woolf, *The brief and prolonged facilatory effect of unmyelinated afferent input on the rat spinal cord are independently influenced by peripheral nerve section.* Neuroscience, 1986, 17: pp. 1199–11205.

92. Woolf, C.J. and R.J. Mannion, *Neuropathic pain: aetiology, symptoms, mechanisms, and management.* Lancet, 1999, 353: pp. 1959–1964.

93. Portenoy, R.K. and K.M. Foley, *Chronic use of opioid analgesics in non-malignant pain: report of 38 cases.* Pain, 1986, 25: pp. 171–186.

94. Passik, S.D., R.K. Portenoy, and S.L. Ricketts, *Substance abuse issues in cancer patients.* Oncology, 1998, 12: pp. 517–521.

95. Zimmermann, M. and H.O. Handwerker, *Schmerz, Konzepte und ärztliches Handeln*, 1984, Berlin, Heidelberg, New York, Springer: Tokyo.

96. Eglen, R.M., J.C. Hunter, and A. Dray, *Ions in the fire: recent ion-channel research and approaches to pain therapy.* Trends Pharmacol Sci, 1999, 20: pp. 337–347.

Part II

Mechanism of Action of Opioids and Clinical Effects

Treatment with narcotic analgesic is the core of cancer pain management. In addition, opioids are the core in anesthesia as painful afferents are induced by the surgical procedure. Although concurrent use of other approaches and interventions may be appropriate in many pain patients, and necessary in some, analgesic drugs are needed in almost every case. Drugs whose primary clinical action is the relief of pain are conventionally classified on the basis of their activity at opioid receptors as either opioid or non-opioid analgesics.

A third class, the adjuvant analgesics, is drugs with other primary indications that can be effective analgesics in specific circumstances. The major *Opiate* is a specific term that is used to describe drugs (natural and semi-synthetic) derived from the juice of the opium poppy (Figures II-1 and II-2). For example, morphine is an opiate but methadone (a completely synthetic drug) is not.

Opioid is a general term that includes naturally occurring, semi-synthetic, and synthetic drugs, which produce their effects by combining with opioid receptors and are competitively antagonized by naloxone. In this context the term opioid refers to opioid agonists, opioid antagonists, opioid peptides, and opioid receptors.

Narcotic is commonly used to describe morphine-like drugs and other drugs of abuse. The term is derived from the Greek *narke*, meaning numbness or torpor. Since this is an imprecise and pejorative term that is not useful in a pharmacological context, its use with reference to opioids is discouraged.

The source of opium is the opium poppy, *Papaver somniferum*, one of the few species of *Papaver* that produces opium (Figure II-1). Through centuries of cultivation and breeding the poppy for its opium, a species of the plant evolved that is now known as *somniferum*. The genus, *Papaver*, is the Greek word for poppy. The species, *somniferum*, is Latin for sleep inducing.

The psychological effects of opium may have been known to the ancient Sumerians (circa 4000 B.C.) whose symbol for the poppy was hul (joy) and gil (plant). The plant was known in Europe at least 4000 years ago, as evidenced by fossil remains of poppy seed cake and poppy pods found in the Swiss lake dwellings of the Neolithic Age. Opium was probably consumed by the ancient Egyptians and was known to the Greeks as well. References to the poppy are found in Homer's works The Iliad and The Odyssey. Hippocrates (460–357 B.C.), the Father of Medicine, recommended drinking the juice of the white poppy mixed with the seed of nettle.

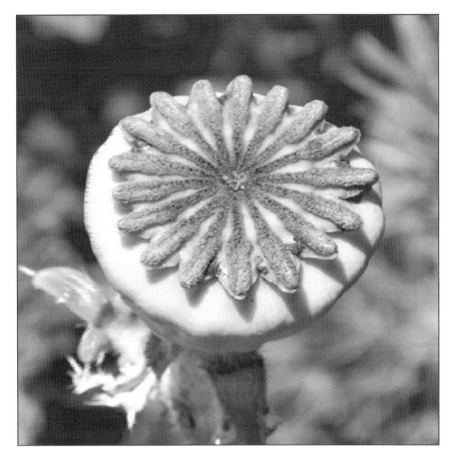

Figure II-1. Fresh capsule of opium poppy plant (*Papaver somniferum*)

The opium poppy probably reached China about the seventh century A.D. through the efforts of Arab traders who advocated its use for medicinal purposes. In Chinese literature, however, there are earlier references to its use. The noted Chinese surgeon Hua To of the Three Kingdoms (220–264 A.D.) used opium preparations and Cannabis indica for his patients to swallow before undergoing major surgery.

The opium poppy, *Papaver somniferum*, is an annual plant, i.e., the plant matures one time, and does not regenerate itself. New seed must be planted each season. From a small seed, it grows, flowers, and bears fruit (a pod) only once. The entire growth cycle for most varieties of this plant takes about 120 days. The tiny seeds (like the seeds on a poppy seed roll) germinate quickly in warm air and sufficient soil moisture. In less than 6 weeks, the young plant emerges from the

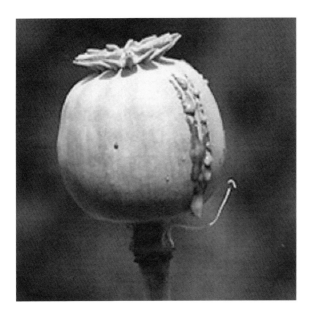

Figure II-2. Cut capsule showing latex exuding from cut

soil, grows a set of four leaves, and resembles a small cabbage in appearance. The lobed, dentate (jagged-edged) leaves are bluish-green with a dull gray or blue tint.

The major legal opium production areas in the world today are in government-regulated opium farms in India, Turkey, and Tasmania (Australia). The major illegal growing areas are in Southwest Asia (Afghanistan, Pakistan, and Iran) and in the highlands of Mainland Southeast Asia (Burma, Laos, Vietnam, and Thailand) – popularly known as the Golden Triangle (Figure II-3). Opium poppy is also grown in Colombia, Mexico, and Lebanon.

Opium poppies containing small amounts of opium alkaloids were, at one time, widely grown as an ornamental plant and for seeds in the United States. The Opium Poppy Control Act of 1942 declared the possession of this plant illegal. From the cut capsule latex is exuded, which is collected and further processed in order to gain the different ingredients (Figure II-2).

Within the secreted latex collectors will find the major constituents of opium poppy, which are as follows:

1. Morphine (10%–17%), the most important alkaloid, which was discovered by the pharmacist Sertürner in a small town of Einbeck, located in Lower Saxonia in Germany in 1803. He decided to name the extract from the opium poppy morphine (Figure A) because it elicited a sedative-hypnotic and sleep inducing effect, related to the Greek god of sleep Morpheus.

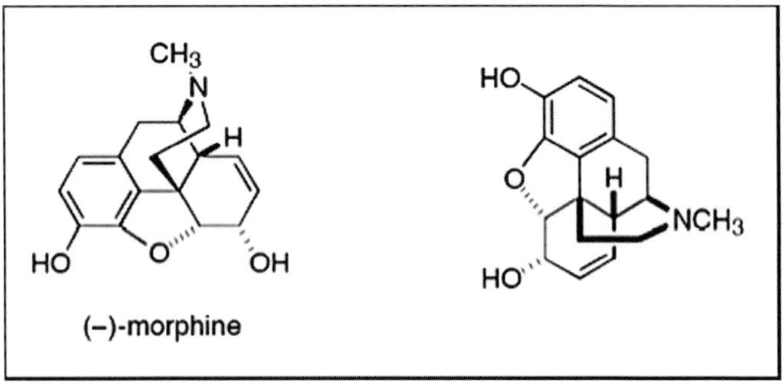

Figure A

2. Codeine (0.7%–4%), chemically a methylmorphinan (Figure B), which today is derived by methylation from the prodrug morphine.

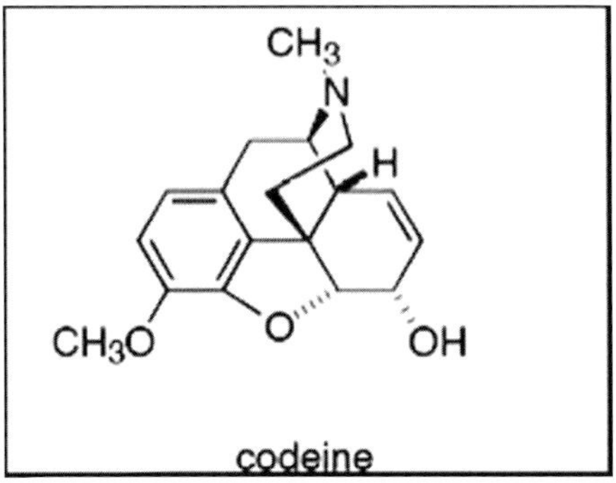

Figure B

3. Thebaine (0.5%–2%) a precursor of many of semi-synthetic opioid agonists (i.e. etorphine, oxymorphone) and antagonists (naloxone, naltrexone, diprenorphine, cyprenorphine), mixed agonist/antagonists (nalbuphine) as well as the partial agonist buprenorphine (Figure C).

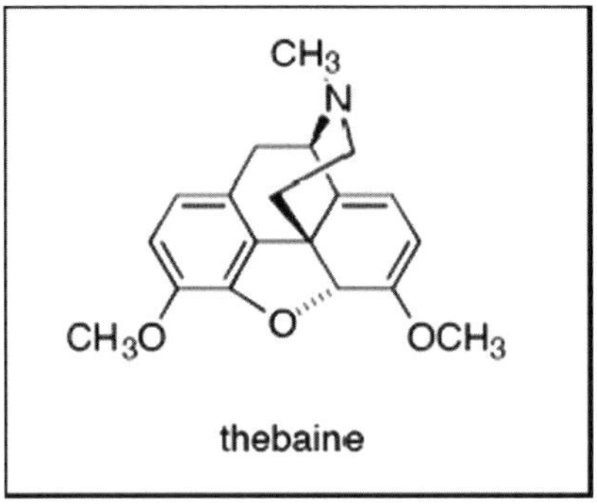

Figure C

4. Benzylisoquinolines are a group of agents, which do not interact with the opioid receptor. The most important one is papaverine (0.5%–1%) a phosphodiestrase inhibitor, which relaxes the smooth muscle, and noscapine (2%–9%), which is used as a cough suppressant (Figure D).

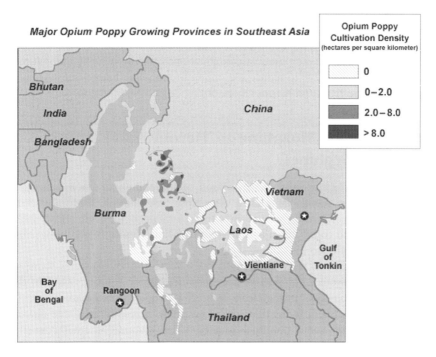

Figure D

Figure II-3. The Golden Triangle where the opium poppy is being harvested

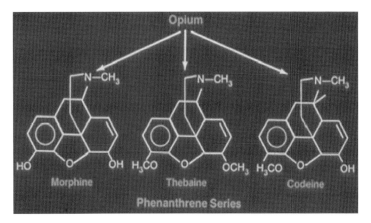

Figure II-4. The major constituents of the poppy plant (*Papaver somniferum*) which are used for the formation of heroin and so called semisynthetic opioid ligands, derivatives of thebaine (e.g. buprenorphine)

Raw or cooked opium contains more than 35 different alkaloids, including morphine, codeine, and thebaine (Figure II-4). In Mainland Southeast Asia, the morphine alkaloid alone accounts for approximately 10% of the total weight of opium. Heroin manufacturers must first extract the morphine from the opium, before converting the morphine to heroin. The extraction is a simple process, requiring only a few chemicals and a supply of water. Morphine sometimes is extracted from opium in small clandestine laboratories, which are typically set up near the opium poppy fields. Since the morphine base is about one-tenth the weight and volume of raw opium, it is desirable to reduce the opium to morphine before transporting the product from the field to a heroin laboratory.

Conversion of Morphine to Heroin (Diacetylmorphine)

The following is a step-by-step description of morphine extraction in a typical Mainland Southeast Asian laboratory. An empty 55-gallon oil drum is placed on bricks about a foot above the ground and a fire is built under the drum. Thirty gallons of water are added to the drum and brought to a boil. Ten to fifteen kilograms of raw opium are added to the boiling water.

With stirring, the raw opium eventually dissolves in the boiling water, while soil, leaves, twigs, and other non-soluble materials float in the solution. Most of these materials are scooped out of the clear, dark brown liquid opium solution.

Slaked lime (calcium hydroxide) or, more often, a readily available chemical fertilizer with a high content of lime, is added to the solution. Lime will convert the water-insoluble morphine alkaloid into water-soluble calcium morphenate. (Other opium alkaloids do not react with lime to form water-soluble calcium salts, as does morphine.) Codeine is an opium alkaloid that is slightly water-soluble and some codeine will be carried over with the calcium morphenate in the liquid. Otherwise, for the most part, the other alkaloids will become a part of the sludge.

As the solution cools, the morphine solution is scooped from the drum and poured through a filter. Cloth rice sacks are often used as filters and can then be squeezed in a press to remove most of the solution from the wet sacks. Liquid saponated cresol (Lysol) is commonly added to the solution to facilitate filtering. The morphine-rich solution is then poured into large cooking pots and reheated but, this time, not boiled. Ammonium chloride (a powder) is added to the heated calcium morphenate solution to adjust the alkalinity to a pH of 8 to 9, and the solution is then allowed to cool. Within 1 or 2 h, morphine base precipitates (crashes) out of the solution and settles to the bottom of the cooking pot.

The solution is then poured off through cloth filters. Any solid morphine base chunks in the solution will remain on the cloth. The morphine base is removed from both the cooking pot and from the filter cloths, wrapped and squeezed in cloth, and then dried in the sun. When dry, the crude morphine base is a coffee-colored coarse powder. This form of morphine is commonly known by the Chinese term pi-tzu in Mainland Southeast Asia.

If morphine base is to be stored or transported to another location, it may be pressed into blocks. Crude morphine base is generally 50%–70% morphine, and is an intermediate product in the heroin process. Addicts do generally not use this morphine base.

This crude morphine base may be further purified (and changed to morphine hydrochloride) by dissolution in hot water and hydrochloric acid, then adding activated charcoal, reheating, and filtering. The solution is filtered several times before being allowed to cool. As the solution cools, morphine hydrochloride precipitates out of the solution and settles to the bottom. The precipitate is trapped (or captured) by filtration.

If the morphine hydrochloride is to be stored or transported to another location, it may be pressed into bricks. Morphine hydrochloride (often tainted with codeine hydrochloride) is usually pressed into brick-sized blocks in a press and wrapped in paper or cloth. The most common block size is 2 in. by 4 in. by 5 in., and weighs about 3 lb (1.3 kg). It takes a full day to extract morphine from opium. As described in the preceding paragraphs, the chemicals used to isolate morphine from opium (known as extraction) include calcium hydroxide (slaked lime) and ammonium chloride. The precursor chemical normally used in the conversion of morphine to heroin (known as acetylation) is acetic anhydride. Chemical reagents used in the conversion process include sodium carbonate and activated charcoal. Chemical solvents needed are chloroform, ethyl alcohol (ethanol), and ethyl ether. Other chemicals may be substituted for these preferred chemicals, but most or all of these preferred chemicals are readily available from smugglers and suppliers.

Laboratory equipment includes large Chinese cooking woks, measuring cups, funnels, filter paper, litmus paper, and enamel (or stainless steel) pots. Only the most sophisticated heroin laboratories use glass flasks, propane gas ovens, vacuum pumps, autoclaves, electric blenders, venting hoods, centrifuges, reflux condensers, electric drying ovens, and elaborate exhaust systems. It is common to find portable, gasoline-powered generators at clandestine heroin conversion laboratories. Generators are used to power various electrical devices.

Heroin synthesis from morphine (either morphine base or morphine hydrochloride) is a two-step process that requires between 4 and 6 h to complete (Figure II-5). Heroin base is the intermediate product. Typically, morphine hydrochloride bricks are pulverized and the dried powder is then placed in an enamel pot. Acetic anhydride is added, which then reacts with the morphine to form heroin acetate. (This acetylation process will work either with morphine hydrochloride or morphine base.) The pot lid is tied or clamped on, using a damp towel for a gasket. The pot is carefully heated for about 2 h, below boiling, at a constant temperature of 85°C (185°F). It is never allowed to boil or to become so hot as to vent fumes into the room. Tilting and rotation agitate the mixture until all of the morphine has dissolved. When cooking is completed, the pot is cooled and opened. During this step, morphine and the anhydride become chemically bonded, creating

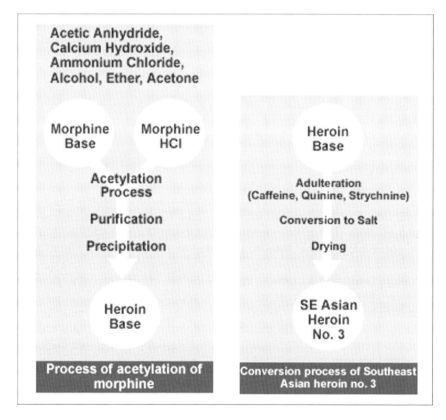

Figure II-5. Summary of the process of acetylation and purification of morphine to heroin

an impure form of diacetylmorphine (heroin). Water is added to the thick, soupy mixture and the mixture is stirred as the heroin dissolves in the solution. Sodium carbonate (a crystalline powder) is dissolved in hot water and then added slowly to the heroin solution until effervescence stops. This precipitates heroin base, which is then filtered and dried by heating in a steam bath. For each kilogram of morphine, 685 g–937 g of crude heroin base is formed, depending on the quality of morphine.

The tan-colored heroin base (about 70% pure heroin) may be dried, packed, and transported to a heroin-refining laboratory, or it may be purified further before conversion to heroin hydrochloride (a water-soluble salt form of heroin) at the same site.

Mainland Southeast Asian heroin base is an intermediate product that can be further converted to either smoking heroin (heroin no. 3) or injectable heroin (heroin no. 4). To make heroin no. 3, the crude base is mixed with hydrochloric acid, resulting in heroin hydrochloride (HCl). Adulterants, including caffeine, are added after this conversion. For each kilogram of crude heroin base, about 1 kg of caffeine is used. Various flavorings such as quinine hydrochloride or strychnine hydrochloride are sometimes added to heroin no. 3. Next, the wet paste mix is stirred to dryness over a steam bath.

The resulting dry heroin no. 3 will be in the form of coarse lumps. The lumps are crushed and passed through a mesh sieve, and the grains (pieces) are then packaged for sale. The entire process takes about 8 h and requires only minimal skill. While extra attention to stirring is required to assure dryness, one person can prepare 1 kg of heroin no. 3 during this time.

The reaction of morphine with acetic anhydride produces heroin acetate. To the heroin acetate mixture in the pot, water is added and mixed by stirring. A small amount of chloroform is added. The mixture is stirred and then allowed to stand for 20 min. Doing so dissolves highly colored impurities and a red, greasy liquid is formed at the bottom of the container. The water layer is carefully poured off and saved in a clean pot, leaving the red grease in the pot. In a clean pot, activated charcoal is stirred into the aqueous solution and is filtered to remove solid impurities. The decolorizing effects of the charcoal, combined with the chloroform treatment, will leave a light yellow solution. The use of charcoal is repeated one or more times, until the solution is colorless.

Sodium carbonate (a crystalline powder) is dissolved in hot water and then added slowly to the heroin solution until effervescence stops. This precipitates the heroin base, which is then filtered and dried by heating on a steam bath. The heroin base is heated until dried. The powder should be very white at this stage. If not white, the base is redissolved in diluted acid, treated repeatedly with activated charcoal, re-precipitated, and dried. The ultimate purity and color of the resulting heroin HCl will depend largely on the quality of the heroin base. The heroin base is then dissolved in ethyl ether. Conversion to the hydrochloride salt is achieved by adding hydrochloric acid in ethanol to the heroin mixture. The heroin then precipitates.

The process of extracting morphine from opium involves dissolving opium in boiling water, adding lime (calcium oxide), or slaked lime (calcium hydroxide), or limestone (calcium carbonate) to precipitate non-morphine alkaloids, and then pouring off the morphine in solution. Ammonium chloride is then added to the solution to precipitate morphine from the solution. The chemicals used to process opium to morphine have a number of legitimate purposes and are widely available on the open market. An empty oil drum, some cooking pots, and filter cloths or filter paper are needed.

In the United States, opium preparations became widely available in the nineteenth century and morphine was used extensively as a painkiller for wounded soldiers during the Civil War. The inevitable result was opium addiction, contemporarily called the army disease or soldier's disease. These opium and morphine abuse problems prompted a scientific search for potent, but nonaddictive, painkillers. In the 1870s, chemists developed an opium-based and supposedly nonaddictive substitute for morphine. The Bayer Pharmaceutical Company of Germany was the first to produce the new drug in large quantities under the brand name Heroin. This product was obtained by acetylation of morphine. Soon thereafter studies showed heroin to have narcotic and addictive properties far exceeding those of morphine. Although heroin has been used in the United Kingdom in the treatment of the terminally ill, its medical value is a subject of intense controversy.

Major Classes of Opioid Analgesics in Clinical Practice

Among the commonly known classes of opioids/opiates being used in practice are morphine, codeine, heroin, and the antagonist naloxone (Figure II-6). Morphine by itself is still made from opium and although there is a major first-pass effect (i.e. degradation by liver enzymes), oral administration is still possible, but requires substantial dosage increase. Codeine, which is also taken orally, has a strong ability to inhibit coughing, but it induces less analgesia. Among the phenylpiperidines a number of synthetic compounds have entered the market. The most known is meperidine/pethidine (Demerol®), which is very similar to morphine, but is more efficacious when given orally for the control of pain. Another derivative is loperamide (Imodium®), an agent being used as a common antidiarrheal, which does not enter the brain, as it is incapable of crossing the blood-brain barrier. Hence it is not abused and therefore is sold as a DOC (drug over the counter). Contrary, fentanyl (Sublimaze®) is an opioid, which is at least 200 times as potent as morphine. This agent is used with nitrous oxide or droperidol (a neuroleptic) in intravenous anesthesia (neuroleptanesthesia), but it is also a used in a transdermal patch for the control of chronic pain. Another known opioid is methadone, which has a good oral efficacy, a much longer half-life than morphine (8–12 h), and in regard to its effect much like morphine. It is used for treatment of heroin addiction and for the control of chronic pain. A methadone congener, which is being used solely in the methadone substitution programs is LAAM (α-levoacetylmethadol), only needs to be taken once every 72 h. The opioid propoxyphene (Darvon®) has

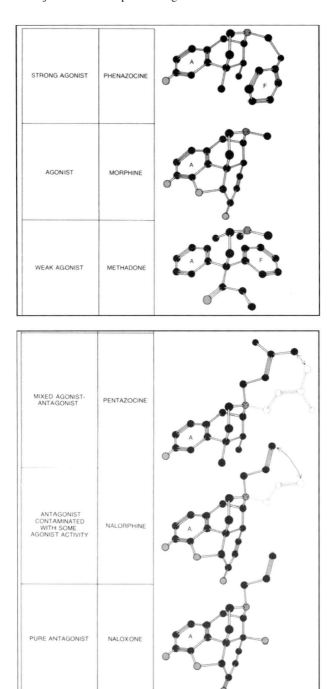

Figure II-6. Molecular structure of different opioid ligands with agonistic or antagonistic properties

the lowest analgesic potency (0.02 times morphine). It is almost always given together with aspirin for the control of mild to moderate pain. It is very popular clinically due to misplaced concerns about the abuse potential of codeine.

MODE OF ACTION OF OPIATES/OPIOIDS

It is interesting to note that all commonly used opioids have a similar structure in regard to their terminal morphine ring and the distance between the ring and the N-substitution. Such common traits suggests that opioids must have a common structure in order to interact with a specific receptor site (Figure II-7).

Thus, central analgesics mediate their action by means of an interaction with specific opioid receptor sites located within specific areas of the central nervous system, which are engaged in the transmission of nociceptive afferences and the identification of pain. There, opioids act as agonists at highly definite receptor sites,

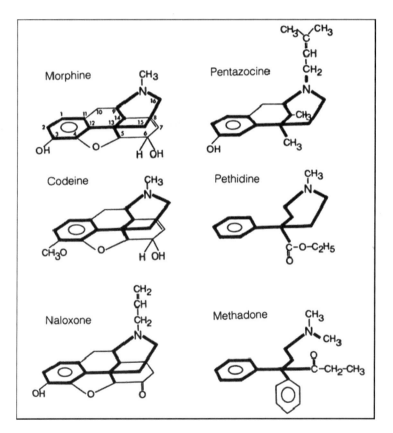

Figure II-7. A similar molecular structure of most opioids implies a structural prerequisite in order to interact with the opioid receptor site

Table II-1. The different population of opioid receptors, their main effects and the ligands that demonstrate a preference of binding

	Opioid receptor	Clinical effects	Preference of binding
μ (mu)	Interaction with this type of receptor results primarily in central depression	Analgesia Resp. depression Bradycardia Hypothermia Miosis Constipation Euphoria	Morphine Fentanyl Alfentanil Sufentanil Remifentanil Lofentanil Endorphin
κ (kappa)	Interaction with this type of receptor results primarily in sedation	Sedation Analgesia Low abuse potential Marginal resp. depression	Nalbuphine Butorphanol Pentazocine Ethylketocyclazocine (EKC) Bremazocine Dynorphin
δ (delta)	Interaction with this type of receptor results primarily in analgesia	Regulation of analgesia Feeling Behavior & Endocrine function	Leu-Enkephalin Met-Enkephalin

and there is general agreement on the existence of at least three types of opioid receptor sites (Table II-1).

1. The morphine mu receptor (μ) at which the prototype morphine binds,
2. The kappa receptor (κ) at which the prototype agonist is ketocyclazocine, and
3. The delta receptor (δ) at which the prototype endogenous opioid ligand enkephalin binds.

OVERVIEW OF THE DIFFERENT OPIOID RECEPTORS AND THEIR SUBTYPES

Opioid receptors are distributed widely in brain and found in spinal cord and peripheral sensory and autonomic nerves. There are the three well-characterized members of the opioid receptor family, designated by the Greek symbols δ, κ and μ. The more recently discovered ORL1 receptor is placed with this family due to its high degree of structural homology. These receptors were renamed OP1, OP2, OP3 and OP4, respectively, by an International Union of Pharmacology (IUPHAR) nomenclature committee in 1996 [1]. This nomenclature has proved unpopular. The nomenclature (X-Opioid Peptide receptor) has been proposed giving μ, mu or MOP; δ, delta or DOP; κ, kappa or KOP and ORL1 or NOP receptors. In order to keep matters straightforward the original nomenclature is used in the following chapters.

The products of endogenous opioid peptide genes activate opioid receptors physiologically: proenkephalin (giving methionine- and leucine-enkephalin; Met-enk and Leu-enk, respectively; Figure II-8), prodynorphin (dynorphins A and B and α-neo-endorphin) pro-opiomelanocortin (β-endorphin) and pronociceptin (nociceptin, also known as Orphanin FQ). Met-enk and Leu-enk have highest affinity

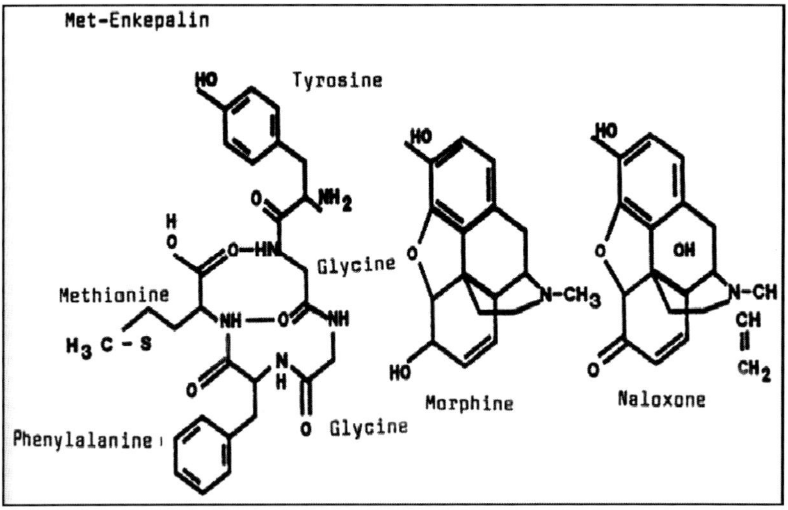

Figure II-8. The tyrosine residue of the endogenous opioid met-enkephalin demonstrates similarity with the molecular structure of morphine and the antagonist naloxone, which is indicative for similar receptor binding sites

for δ-receptors, less affinity for μ, and very low affinity for κ-receptors; the dynorphins have preferential affinity for κ-receptors, but bind to the μ and δ types with high affinity; β-endorphin binds with high affinity to μ and δ receptors, but has little affinity for κ receptors. All the peptides are full agonists at their cognate receptors. Endomorphin-1 and -2, derived from an unknown precursor, are endogenous peptides with high selectivity for μ-receptors. These peptides are unusual in that they are partial agonists. None of the proenkephalin, prodynorphin or pro-opiomelanocortin peptide products or the endomorphins displays affinity for the ORL1 receptor.

Similarly, the ORL1 receptor agonist nociceptin has no appreciable affinity for μ, δ or κ receptors.

The four receptor types have been cloned and shown to be 7-transmembrane receptors activating G proteins of the pertussis-toxin insensitive Gαi/o family, but including Gαz. Evidence for subtypes of μ, δ and κ opioid receptors exists, but the molecular basis for the observed functional and pharmacological differences is unclear. Putative δ1 and δ2 receptors are differentiated by several agonist and antagonist ligands. However, there is only one δ receptor gene, the protein product of which has properties of the putative δ2 receptor. The distinction between the proposed μ2 and μ2 receptors is based largely on the apparent preferential blockade of the μ1 type by the antagonist, naloxonazine [2]. There is only one cloned μ receptor gene, corresponding to the putative μ1 receptor, but several forms of the μ-receptor mRNA arising from alternative splicing have been reported. The receptors these encode differ at the end of the C-terminal tail and show subtle differences in the binding profile of opioid ligands; a role for the variants is not known.

The cloned κ-receptor, with high affinity for U69593 is the κ1 subtype. The proposed κ2 and κ3 subtypes are poorly defined in both molecular and pharmacological terms (Table II-2). A recent explanation for subtypes has evolved with

Table II-2. Summary of the main opioid receptors and the receptor subtypes, their endogenous ligands, their selective exogenous ligands and their functional role

Opioid receptor types and subtypes

Receptor type (Natural ligand)	Selective agonist	Agonist properties	Selective antagonists
μ (enkephalins) (β-endorphin)	morphine sufentanil DAGO (Tyr-ala-Gly-MePhe-NH(CH$_2$)$_2$-OH) also DAMGO) PLO17 (Tyr-Pro-MePhe-d-Pro-NH$_2$) BIT (affinity label)	Analgesia Euphoria Increased gastrointestinal transit time Tolerance and physical dependence Immune supression Respiratory depression (volume) Emetic effects	Naloxone Naltrexone CPT (d-phe-Cys-Trp-lys-Thr-NH$_2$) Cyprodime β-FNA (affinity label)
μ$_1$ (high affinity)	N-(2-pyrazinyl)-N-(1-phenethyl-4-piperidinyl)-2-furamide		Naloxonazine
μ$_2$ (low affinity)	?		N-(2-pyrazinyl)-N-(1-phenethyl-4-piperidinyl)-2-furamides
κ (dynorphins) (β-endorphins)	EKC Bremazocine Mr 2034 Dyn (1–17) Trifluadom	Analgesia Sedation Miosis Diuresis Dysphoria	TENA nor-BNI
κ$_1$ (high affinity)	U-50,488 Spiradoline (U-62,066) U-69,593 PD 117302 UPHIT (affinity label)		
κ$_2$ κ$_3$	Dyn (1–17) ?		
δ (enkephalins) (β-endorphin)	DADLE (d-Ala^2-d-Leu^5-enkephalin) DSLET (Tyr-d-Ser-Gly-Phe-Leu-Thr) DPDPE (d-Pen^2-d-Pen^5-enkephalin) FIT (affinity label) SUPERFIT (affinity label)	Analgesia Immune stimulation Respiratory depression	ICI 174864 Naltrindole

Abbreviations
nor-BNI: nor-Binaltorphimine
BNTX: E-7-Benzylidenenaltrexone

BW373U86:	(±)-(1[S*]2α,5β)-4-(2,5-Dimethyl-4-(2-propenyl)-1-piperazinyl]
	[3-hydroxyphenyl]methyl)-N,N-diethylbenzamide
β-CNA:	β-chlornaltrexamine
CRAP:	D-Phe-Cys-Tyr-D-Trp-Arg-Thr-Pen-Thr-NH2
CTOP:	D-Phe-Cys-Tyr-D-Trp-Orn-Thr-Phe-Thr-NH2
DALCE:	[D-Ala2,Leu5,Cys6]-Enkephalin
DAMGO:	[D-Ala2,N-Me-Phe4,Gly-ol5]-Enkephalin
DPDPE:	[D-Pen2,5]-Enkephalin
DSLET:	[D-Ser2,Leu5,Thr6]-Enkephalin
EKC:	Ethylketocyclazocine
β-FNA:	β-Funaltrexamine
GNTI:	5'-Guanidinylnaltrindole
ICI 174864:	N.N-diallyl-Tyr-Aib-Aib-Phe-Leu
J-113397:	1-[(3R,4R)-1-cycloocylomethyl-3-hydroxymethyl-4-piperdinyl]-3-ethyl-1,
	3-dihydro-2H-benzimidazol-2-one
MCAM:	Methocinnomox
5'-NTII:	Naltrindole 5'-isothiocyanate
Ro 64-6198:	(1S,3aS)-8-(2,3,3a,4,5,6-hexahydro-1H-phenalen-1-yl)-1-phenyl-1,2,
	8-triaza-spiro[4.5]decan-4 one.
SNC80:	(+)-4-[(αR)-α-((2S5R)-4-allyl-2,5-dimethyl-1-piperazinyl]-3-methoxybenzyl]-N,
	N-diethylbenzamide
(-)-TAN-67:	(-)-2-Methyl-4aα-(3-hydroxyphenyl)-1,2,3,4,4a,5,12,12aα-octahydroquinolino
	[2,3,3-q]isoquinoline
TIPP(Ψ):	H-Tyr-TicΨ-[CH2NH]Phe-Phe-OH.
U-69593:	(+)-(5α,7α,8β)-N-Methyl-N-[7-(1-pyrrolidinyl)-1-oxaspiro[4,5]dec-8-yl)
	benzeneacetamide
U-50488:	3,4-Dichloro-N-methyl-N-[2-(1-pyrrolidinyl)cyclohexyl]benzeneacetamide

the identification of opioid receptor heterodimers or hetero-oligomers that appear to have properties different from the monomeric receptors. An interesting addition to ligands that bind to the κ1 receptor is the hallucinogen salvinorin-A. This is a highly efficacious and potent κ agonist, but is most unusual in that it has no nitrogen atom. Endogenous opioid systems have a functional role in modulating pain perception; opioid agonists are therefore potent analgesics. Opioid receptors are also present in hypothalamus (Figure II-9), where they influence temperature regulation and control of hormonal secretion. In the forebrain, endogenous opioids are involved in behavioral reinforcement and appear to play a role in anxiety and in the expression of emotions. In addition, opioids influence gastrointestinal and autonomic nervous system function.

Originally, a fifth binding site, the sigma receptor, was included in this group. However, actions mediated through *this* receptor are not reversed by naloxone so it is not a true opioid receptor. The μ-receptors have been further sub-classified into two distinct subtypes (1 and 2), as have the κ-receptors. Kappa receptors have been divided into 1, 2, and 3 sub-types. Recently, several of these receptors have been cloned successfully. In animal models, some laboratories have cloned up to 10 μ-receptor subtypes [4]. However, the functional significance of these "spliced variants" remains unclear at present. Originally suggested by Martin and coworkers [5], all three opioid receptor types mediate different opiate effects as they

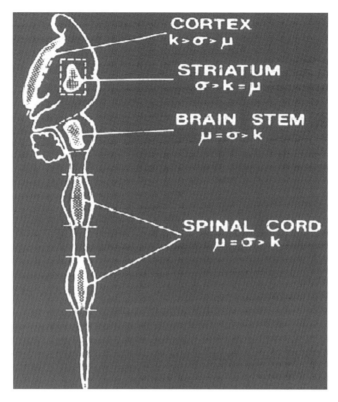

Figure II-9. Difference in topographic density of the three opioid receptor sites within the central nervous system. Adapted from [3]

normally serve endogenous opiates (the endorphins, dynorphins, and enkephalins; Table II-1):

1. Activation of the mu receptors (μ) results in analgesia, euphoria, respiratory depression, nausea, GI slowdown, and miosis. Receptors of this type are mostly located in periaquaductal gray (PAG), spinal trigeminal nucleus, caudate and geniculate nuclei, thalamus, and spinal cord.
2. Binding at the kappa receptors (κ) induces modest analgesia, dysphoria, feelings of depersonalization and disorientation, miosis, and mild respiratory depression. These receptors are mainly found in basal ganglia, nucleus accumbens, ventral tegmentum, cortex, hypothalamus, periaqueductal grey, the spinal cord, and in the periphery.
3. Occupation of the delta receptors (δ) results in anxiolysis and central pain relief, although its overall significance is not all that well understood. They are mainly found in the nucleus accumbens and the limbic system (Table II-2).

Molecular biology techniques have enabled the primary amino acid sequence of the human μ-, κ-, and δ-opioid receptors to be determined. The pharmacological and functional properties of the cloned receptors, the development of "knockout" animals, which are deficient in a receptor or part of a receptor, and the manipulation and substitution of various amino acids in critical domains of the various opioid receptors have provided new insights in opioid action. In this regard, the three opioid receptor genes, encoding mu (MOR), delta (DOR), and kappa (KOR) have been cloned. The binding affinities of a range of opioids to the μ-, κ-, and δ-opioid receptors and also to the cloned *orphinan* receptor have been examined in animals. The animal data indicate that while the commonly prescribed opioids (agonists and antagonists) bind preferentially to the μ-receptor, they also interact with all three receptor types. Morphine and normorphine (a minor metabolite of morphine) show the greatest relative preference for the μ-receptor. Methadone (which also has some NMDA-receptor blocking activity) shows significant binding to μ-receptors, while buprenorphine, and to a lesser extent naloxone, avidly binds to all three receptor types. There is evidence (albeit inconsistent) that the D-enantiomer of methadone blocks the NMDA receptor [6]. The binding affinity of buprenorphine to the μ receptor is much greater than that of naloxone, which explains why the latter only partially reverses buprenorphine overdose.

Animal data also indicate that codeine and diamorphine have very poor binding to opioid receptors, which reinforces the possibility that both are prodrugs where the pharmacologically active species are morphine [7] and 6-monoacetyl morphine, respectively [8]. Oxycodone may also act through an active metabolite, though there are some data, which suggest that this is not the case [9]. Pethidine is considered to be a potent μ-receptor agonist, but it does bind weakly to all three opioid receptors (Table II-1). Ketobemidone has a lower affinity for the μ-receptor than does morphine, but it shows greater discrimination for this receptor compared to κ-receptors. The binding of both of these opioids to the δ-receptor is similar [10].

This difference in opioid action is also mirrored in the difference in affinity of various narcotic ligands interacting with the three relevant opioid receptor sites (Table II-3). It should be noted that some of those ligands, either pure antagonists, mixed agonist/antagonists or partial agonists, are characterized by displacement potency at a specific receptor site.

From the above binding and displacement values it can be seen, that opioid practically bind to all three receptor sites, however with different affinity. The preference in binding to one receptor site manifests itself in the visible clinical effect, which may either be of agonistic or of antagonistic nature.

The binding of morphine, methadone, buprenorphine, and naloxone to the cloned human μ-receptor shows excellent congruence with the animal data [16]. Fentanyl shows a similar binding affinity, while codeine demonstrates greater binding affinity to the cloned human receptor (Table II-3; Figure II-10). Thus, for these commonly administered opioids, there is no great variability in their affinity for the human μ-receptor. The clinical relevance of these data is that different opioids act in different ways. From anecdotal clinical experience there is considerable interindividual

Table II-3. Binding affinity (nmol/l) of various opioids to the three main opioid receptor sites measured in guinea pig brain homogenates. The lower the value the better the fit of the ligand to the respective receptor site and the better their efficacy. Ligands with "*" demonstrate antagonistic potency at the specific receptor site

Opioid ligands	Delta (δ)	Kappa (κ)	Mu (μ)
Morphine	90	317	1.8
Normorphine	310	149	4.0
Levorphanol	5.6	9.6	0.6
Codeine	>1000	no data	2700
Methadone	15.1	1628	4.2
Fentanyl	151	470	7.0
Alfentanil	21.200	>10.000	30
Sufentanil	23	124	1.6
Lofentanil	0.24	0.6	0.023
Carfentanil	3.3	43	0.024
Pethidine	4345	5140	385
Pentazocine	106	22.2	7.0*
Butorphanol	13	7.4	1.7*
Nalbuphine	163	66	6.3*
(±)Pentazocine	467	8.7	39*
Buprenorphine	1.3*	2.0*	0.6
Naloxone	27*	17.2*	1.8*
Naltrexone	9.4*	6.5*	0.46*
Cyprodime	356*	176*	0.4*
(−)Bremazocine	0.78	0.075	0.62*
(±)Tifluadom	290	4.1	22*
(±)U50,488H	9200	0.69	435*
(−)Ethylketazocine	5.2	2.2	2.3
Leu-Enkephalin	1.8	>10.000	150

Adapted from [11, 12, 13, 14, 15]

variability in response to each opioid and this reinforces the need to assess an individual's response to opioid analgesia carefully. It also is premature to extrapolate from laboratory data, which in many instances have not yet been replicated, to the clinic. However, data increasingly inform the clinical use of these drugs and will be particularly relevant to new approaches to their use such as "opioid switching".

Figure II-10 shows the putative analgesic effect mediated by the main μ-opioid receptor depicting that higher affinity also correlates closely with analgesic potency. But aside from μ-receptor interaction, analgesia can also be mediated through a κ-receptor and a δ-receptor site. The classification of different opioid receptor types is based on the original description by Martin and coworkers from 1976 [5]. The effects presumed to be mediated at μ-receptors have been defined as a result of both human and animal studies, while the effects mediated at κ-receptors derive predominantly from animal models. Receptors mediate analgesia that persists in animals made tolerant to μ-agonists. The κ-agonists produce less respiratory depression and miosis than μ-agonists. It is assumed that κ opioid receptors mediate

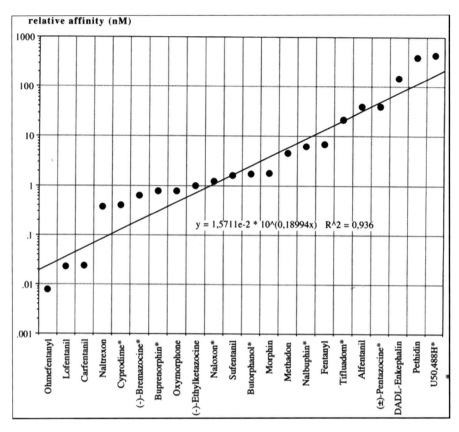

Figure II-10. Difference in affinity of various opioids at the μ-receptor site. Ligands with an asterix reflect antagonistic activity at this site

the sedative and mental clouding effects of opioids, in addition to their other pharmacological actions.

Opioid receptors are found in several areas of the brain, particularly in the periaqueductal grey matter, and throughout the spinal cord (Figure II-9). Supraspinal systems have been described for μ-, κ-, and δ-receptors, whereas μ- and κ-receptors modulate pain at the spinal level [3, 17, 18].

The different distribution of the various opioid subsites suggests different mechanisms of action in the mediation of analgesia. Thus, μ-selective opioids like morphine, fentanyl and sufentanil, due to the high density of binding sites, mediate their main action within the brain stem and the midbrain. Due to their close vicinity to respiratory and cardiovascular regulating centers in the brain stem, selective μ-opioids accordingly induce a marked depression of respiration and blood pressure. On the other hand, due to the main distribution of the κ-receptors within the cortex (lamina V, VI) [19] it is conceivable that these ligands induce a lesser respiratory and cardiovascular depressive effect. As a consequence and contrary to μ-ligands, κ-ligands induce a marked sedative appearance. In addition, there is a lesser addiction liability with κ-ligands, which is easily derived from the fact that the relevant areas in the limbic system show a low concentration of κ-binding sites. Also, the lesser analgesic potency of κ-ligands is enlightened by the fact that most of the κ-selective receptors can be found in the deep lamina VI of the cortex. Since their dendrites retrograde descend to the thalamus, all ascending nociceptive input is modified, resulting in a depression of nociceptive afferences and a reduction in arousal. Certain dendrites of petrosal cells of the cortex also descend down to the brain stem, whereby the activating, ascending reticular system (ARS) is affected resulting in a reduction of vigilance [20].

In summary, due to the dissimilarity of distribution of the three opioid receptor subtypes with the spinal cord and the supraspinal areas of the CNS, a functional differentiation can be expected. This effect is reflected in difference of binding affinities with the brain where 22% of all receptor sites are referred to the μ-, 36% to the κ- and 42% to the δ-opioid receptor [20, 21]. The present understanding of the effect profiles of opioid receptors, however, remains incomplete, as new advances make it clear that their disposition and structure are extremely complex.

Opioids inhibit pain signals by different mode of actions:

- Inhibition of Ca^{++}-influx into the buttons of the presynaptic cell (e.g. the one releasing Substance P; Figure II-11). This is because Ca^{++}-influx is necessary for neurotransmitter release, whereby opioids reduce or prevent Substance P from being released.
- Acting as an inhibitory neurotransmitter, since the opioid hyperpolarizes the postsynaptic cell by enhancing K^+-flow out of the neuron, which makes it more difficult for all incoming nociceptive afferences to stimulate the next neuron, and thus more difficult to send painful information.
- Moderation of central perception of painful information in the limbic system so as to make it less aversive when it is perceived.

Several facts have led to the assumption that opioids interact with specific binding sites in the CNS. A slight molecular substitution at the side chain of the morphine molecule structure results in considerable changes of potency (Table II-5).

Whereas pethidine (meperidine, USP), a piperidine derivative, may be considered a weak analgesic, fentanyl, a piperidine derivative, is about 100–300 times more potent than morphine. The opioid antagonists levallorphan and naloxone are noted for a low and a analgesic effect, respectively. Furthermore, only the levorotator (levo-) isomers of opioids, which appear in their natural form (i.e. compounds which, when in solution, rotate plane-polarised light to the left) are pharmacologically active (e.g. levorphanol). Their dextrorotatory (dextro-) isomers, which can be synthesized in the laboratory (e.g. dextrophane), shows a negligible pharmacological effect. Both substances are structurally the mirror image of each other (Figure II-12).

In this context it is important to note that only the levo-stereoisomer of the racemic mixture is the pharmacologically active ingredient. This observation supports the

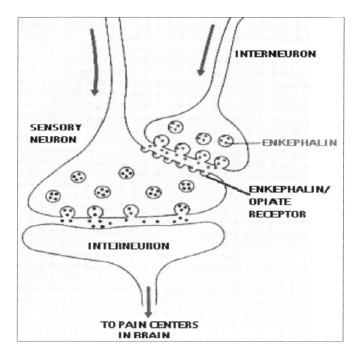

Figure II-11. Mechanism of action of opioids at the central nervous system. By binding at the same receptor site as the endogenous opioids (i.e. enkephalins, endorphins), the release of excitatory neuro-transmitters such as acetylcholine and glutamate is decreased thereby reducing the receiving cells excitatory input. The degree of opiate receptor binding is proportionally to the net release of excitatory transmitters and the reduction of depolarization produced by the arriving nociceptive nerve impulse. This enkephalin inhibitory system normally modulates the activity of the ascending pain pathways within the spinal cord and the brain. Opioid agents act by binding to unoccupied enkephalin receptors, thereby potentiating the analgesic effects of the system

notion that stereroselectivity of an opioid analgesic is a prerequisite in order to bind to the opiate receptor site, thus inducing analgesia.

AGONISTS, ANTAGONISTS, THEIR POTENCY AND MODE OF ACTION

Based on their interactions with the various receptor subtypes, opioid compounds can be divided into agonist, agonist/antagonist, and antagonist classes (Table II-4).

By definition an *agonist* is a drug that has affinity for and binds to cell receptors to induce changes in the cell that stimulate physiological activity. The agonist opioid drugs have no clinically relevant ceiling effect to analgesia. As the dose is raised, analgesic effects increase in a log linear function, until either analgesia is achieved or dose-limiting adverse effects supervene. Efficacy is defined by the

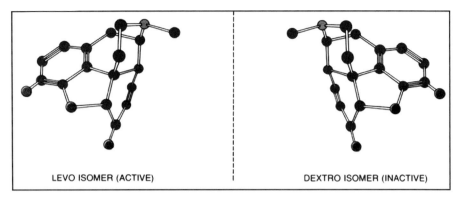

LEVO ISOMER (ACTIVE)   DEXTRO ISOMER (INACTIVE)

Figure II-12. Generally opioids exist in optical isomers, which are a mirror image in the molecular form. Only the levorotatory (levo)-isomer, which in solution rotates plane-polarized light to the left, produces the characteristic analgesic effect of an agent. The dextrorotatory isomer is totally inactive. This sterospecificity of opiate action supports the concept of selective receptor binding to a site, which is able to distinguish in "handedness or goodness of fit" of an opioid molecule

maximal response induced by administration of the active agent. In practice, this is determined by the degree of analgesia produced following dose escalation through a range limited by the development of adverse effects. Potency, in contrast, reflects the dose–response relationship.

Potency is influenced by pharmacokinetic factors (i.e. how much of the drug enters the body systemic circulation and then reaches the receptors) and by affinity to drug receptors. The concepts of efficacy and potency are illustrated in the following

Table II-4. Classification of opioid analgesics into agonists, agonist/antagonists, partial agonists and antagonist classes

Agonists	Antagonists	Agonist/antagonists	Partial agonists
Morphine	Naloxone	Nalorphine	Meptazinol
Codeine	Naltrexone	Pentazocine	Buprenorphine
Oxycodone	Nalmefene	Nalbuphine	
Pethidine	Diprenorphine	Butorphanol	
Diamorphine (heroin)		Dezocine	
Hydromorphone			
Levorphanol			
Methadone			
Fentanyl			
Sufentanil			
Remifentanil			
Tramadol			
Dextropropoxyphene			
Phenazocine			
Dipipanone			

figure, which shows the dose–response curves for two drugs with a full agonistic and a partial agonistic action. If the logarithm of dose is plotted against response an agonist will produce an S-shaped or sigmoid curve. The efficacy of the two drugs, defined by maximum response is the same. The full agonist produces the same response as a partial agonist but at a lower dose, and therefore is described as more potent (Figure II-13).

An *antagonist* by definition is an agent that has no intrinsic pharmacological action but can interfere with the action of an agonist. Competitive antagonists bind to the same receptor and compete for receptor sites, whereas non-competitive antagonists block the effects of the agonist in some other way.

Contrary the mixed *agonist/antagonists* analgesics can, in turn, be subdivided into the mixed agonist/antagonists and the partial agonists, a distinction also based on specific patterns of drug–receptor interaction. Both the partial agonist and the agonist/antagonist drugs have a ceiling effect for analgesia, and although they produce analgesia in the opioid-naive patient, in theory they can precipitate withdrawal in patients who are physically dependent on morphine-like drugs. For these reasons, they have been considered generally to have a limited role in the management of patients with cancer pain.

The *mixed agonist/antagonist* drugs produce agonist effects at one receptor and antagonist effect at another. Pentazocine is the prototype agonist/antagonist: it has agonist effects at the κ-receptors and weak to medium antagonistic action at the

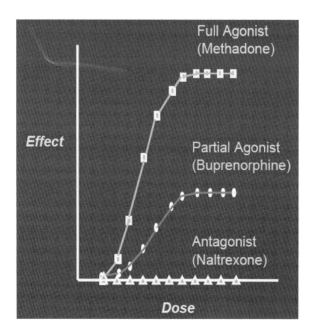

Figure II-13. Typical dose-response curves of a full agonist, a partial agonist and an antagonist on opioid-related effects

μ-receptor Thus in addition to analgesia, pentazocine may produce σ-mediated psychotomimetic effects not seen with full or partial agonists. When a mixed agonist/antagonist is administered together with an agonist, the antagonist effect at the μ-receptor can generate an acute withdrawal syndrome.

A *partial agonist* has low intrinsic activity (efficacy) so that its dose–response curve exhibits a ceiling effect at less than the maximum effect produced by a full agonist (Figure II-11). Buprenorphine is the main example of a partial agonist opioid. Increasing the dose of such a drug above its ceiling does not result in any further increase in response. This phenomenon is illustrated in the figure in which buprenorphine is the partial agonist. The full agonist is more potent than the partial agonist (in the lower part of the curve it will produce the same response at a lower dose), but is less effective than both coadministered ligands because of its ceiling effect.

When a partial agonist is administered together with an agonist, displacement of the agonist can cause a net reduction in pharmacological action, which may be sufficient to generate an acute withdrawal syndrome. While this is a theoretical possibility with morphine and buprenorphine, no such interaction has been reported clinically. Similarly, it has been suggested that the effects of morphine may be blocked in a patient switched from buprenorphine, because of the prolonged action of buprenorphine and the assumption that it will "antagonize" the effect of morphine. This has been one of the reasons, why buprenorphine has not been in cancer pain management. However, the recent development of a transdermal formulation of buprenorphine may encourage its use in chronic cancer pain (and chronic non-cancer pain). An analgesic ceiling with buprenorphine is only reached at doses of 8–16 mg or more in 24 h [22, 23]. When used in usual recommended doses (e.g., two patches of 70 μg/h of transdermal buprenorphine, equivalent to 3–4 mg per 24 h) buprenorphine can be considered a full μ-agonist since at these doses its effect will lie on the linear part of the dose–response curve [24].

RELATIVE POTENCY AND EQUIANALGESIC DOSES

Relative potency is the ratio of the doses of two analgesics required to produce the same analgesic effect. By convention the relative potency of each of the commonly used opioids is based upon a comparison with 10 mg of parenteral morphine. Data from single- and repeated-dose studies in patients with acute or chronic pain have been used to develop an equianalgesic dose table (Table II-5) that provides guidelines for dose selection when the drug or route of administration is changed. The information contained in the equianalgesic dose table does not represent standard doses, nor is it intended as an absolute guideline for dose selection. Many variables may influence the appropriate dose for an individual patient, including intensity of pain, prior opioid exposure in terms of drug, duration, and dose (and the degree of cross-tolerance that this confers), age, route of administration, level of consciousness, metabolic abnormalities (see below), and genetic polymorphism in the expression of relevant enzymes or receptors.

Table II-5. The analgesic potency of different opioids in comparison to morphine (= 1) on a mg-level

Analgesia	Opioid	Analgesic potency
	Sufentanil	1000
	Fentanyl	100–200
Very strong	Remifentanil	100–200
	Alfentanil	40–50
	Phenoperidine	10–50
	Oxymorphone	12–15
	Butorphanol	8–11
	Hydromorphone	7–10
	Diamorphine	1–5
	Dextromoramide	2–4
	Racemorphane	2.5
Medium	Levomethadone	2
	Methadone	1.5
	Isomethadone	1–1.3
	Piminodine	1
	Piperidine	1
	Morphine	1
	Nalbuphine	0.5–0.8
	Hydrocodeine	0.35
	Pentazocine	0.3
Weak	Meptazinol	0.15–0.2
	Codeine	0.2
	Pethidine	0.1
Very weak	Levallorphane	0.07–0.1
	Tramadol	0.05–0.07

SPECIFIC BINDING SITES FOR OPIOIDS IN THE CNS

In addition, a substitution at the side chain, for example the substitution of a methyl-group by an allyl-group or the substitution by a cyclopropyl-group results in the new opioid antagonist naloxone, diprenorphine and naltrexone respectably, or mixed agonists/antagonists (nalorphine, levallorphane), which have the capability of antagonizing the effect of the parent compound (Figure II-14).

Similarly, when the N-methyl group of the highly potent opioid oxymorphone or the pure agonist etorphine (1000 times of morphine) is replaced by a cyclo-propylmethyl group, the highly potent antagonists naltrexone and diprenorphine are derived. These compounds are 2.5 times as potent as naloxone and while the former is used as an oral preparation in the rehabilitation of the earlier opiate addict, the latter is used in veterinary medicine for the reversal of immobilization of wild animals. In addition, diprenorphine is also the original substance of buprenor-phine where additional three methyl groups are incorporated in the molecule (Figure II-15).

Such minor changes in the molecular structure and their resultant major pharma-cological effect suggest, that similar to hormones and catecholamines, opioids

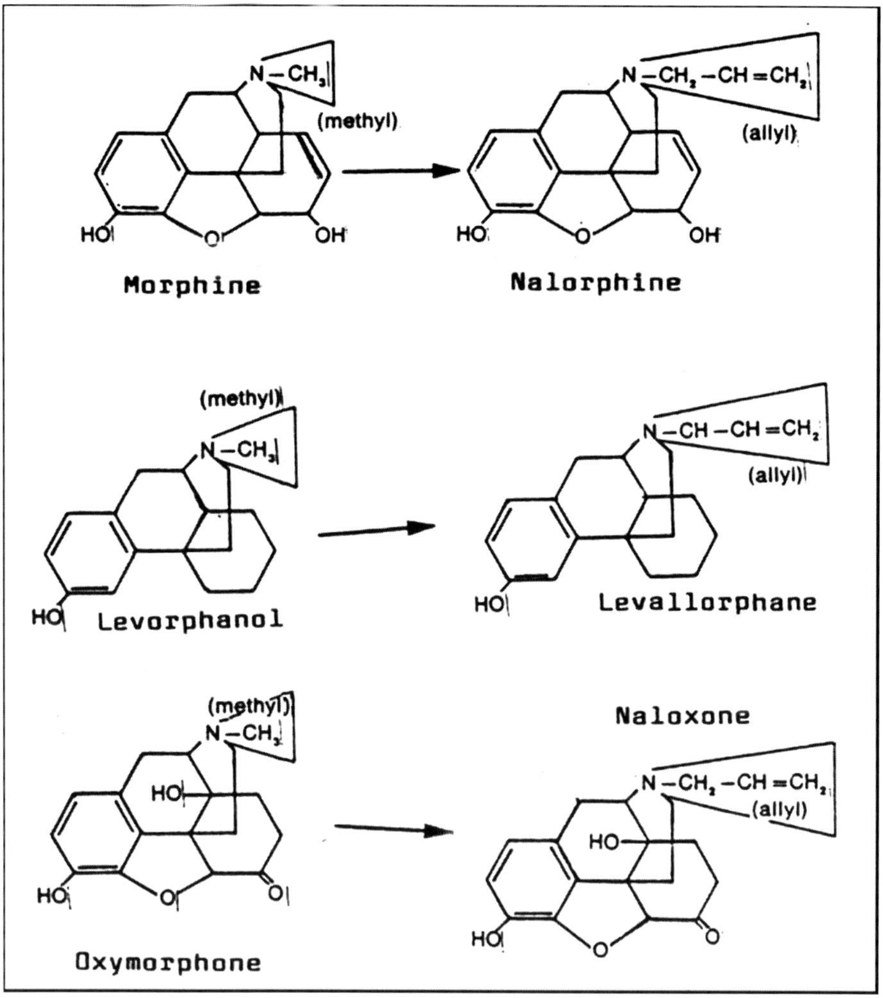

Figure II-14. Molecular structure of the mother compounds morphine, levorphanol and oxymorphone (15 times morphine), all pure agonists, where substitution of the N-methyl group by an allyl-group results in mixed agonists antagonists (nalorphine, levallorphane) or the pure antagonist naloxone

bind with specific receptor sites which results in the characteristic effects such as analgesia. Various research groups corroborated this hypothesis almost simultaneously. Pert and Snyder [17], Terenius [25] and Kosterlitz [26] were the first research group to identify selective binding sites in the CNS using radioactive labeled opioids. These so-called opiate binding sites were found mainly in neuronal structures and nervous pathways involved in the transmission of nociceptive signals such as the first relay station of pain transmission, the substantia gelatinosa of the spinal column. In the posterior horn the impulse is passed over to the second

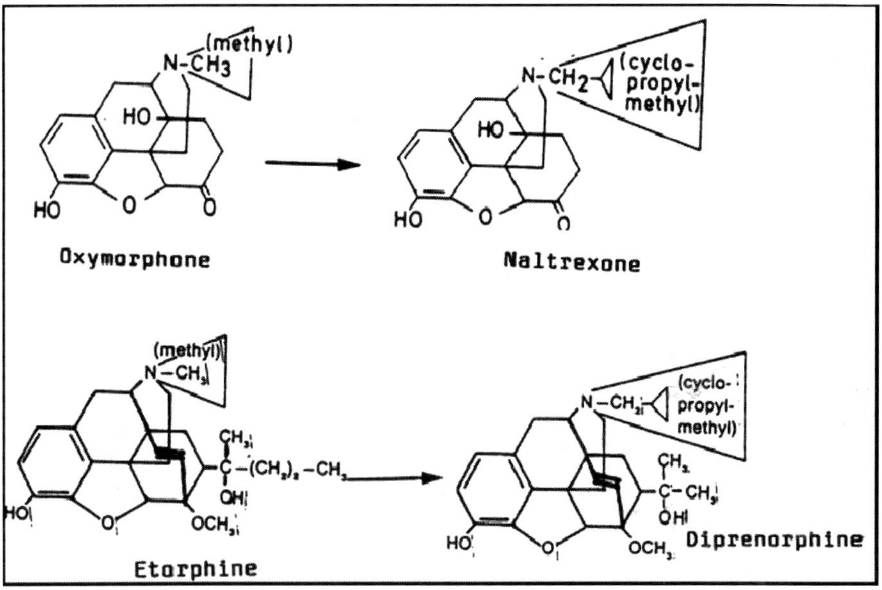

Figure II-15. Chemical structures of the pure agonists oxymorphone (Numorphane®) and etorphine (Immobilone®) and their derivatives naltrexone (Trexane®) and diprenorphine (Revivon®) respectively, both of which are pure opioid antagonists

neuron while, simultaneously, descending nerve fibers from the reticular system (the cortico- and reticulo-spinal tract) induce either a facilitation or an attenuation of pain transmission, which results in a modulation of pain impulses at the spinal level (Figure II-11). The course of pain transmission is to the contralateral side of the spinal cord where impulses already undergone a distinct separation. It is the paleospinothalamic pathway, consisting of nonmyelinated C-fibers, which mediate the excruciating, dull pain component, which is difficult to localize as it ends in the nonspecific nuclei of the medial thalamus [27]. En route, the paleospinothalamic tract sends off afferent fibers to the midbrain area, such as the periaqueductal grey matter and the reticular formation [28]. The pathway ends in intralaminar nuclei of the thalamus and the nucleus limitans, a patch of pigmented nerve cells border the mesencephalon (Figure II-16).

From there, subcortical pain pathways link with the pallidum, the alleged psychomotoric center that sends fibers to all areas of the brain hemisphere. The neospinothalamic pathway, in contrast, consists of myelinated $A\delta_2$-fibres, which transfer impulses to the nucleus ventrocaudalis-parvocellularis (N.v-c parvocellularis). From there pain sensations are projected to the postcentral gyrus, which enables the patient to localize the source of pain (Figure II-16). Both, the central grey matter and the pallidum are characterized by a dense accumulation of opiate binding sites [29, 28]. It is worth noting that nervous pathways transmitting the dull, chronic and less pinpointed pain components are more affected by opioids, while

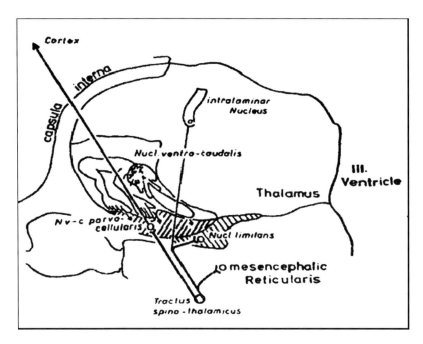

Figure II-16. The nucleus limitans, lying adjacent to the nucleus ventro-caudalis-parvocelluraris (N.v-c parvocellularis), is an important relay station in the mediation of nociceptive afferents to higher pain modulating and discriminating centers of the CNS, which is necessary for the nonspecific feeling of pain and is closely coupled with emotions

the neospinothalamic pathway conveys the sharp and well localized pain components which accompany any injury and are always the first to be perceived. The indefinable, dull, emotional component is perceived later, giving pain its negative character. This separation in pain pathways is of special importance. Impulses from the fast pathway usually antagonize the mediation of slow afferent impulses on all levels in the CNS: substantia gelatinosa and reticular formation, as well as the specific and the nonspecific projecting nuclei of the thalamus [30]. Opioid binding sites, as they are visualized with receptor-binding techniques, strikingly map the paleospinothalamic pain pathway (Figure II-17). Furthermore, there is a high density of opioid binding sites in various other parts of the brain [3, 17, 18, 31]:

1. The corpus striatum, being part of the limbic and the extrapyramidal motor system, is responsible for triggering opioid-induced muscular rigidity. It is not only the regulatory center for locomotion but it is also the center for the regulation of attention and perception.
2. The area postrema in the brain stem where opioids apparently induce respiratory depression, nausea and vomiting.
3. The caudal portion of the trigeminal nucleus being responsible for the transmission of painful afferences from the face and head.

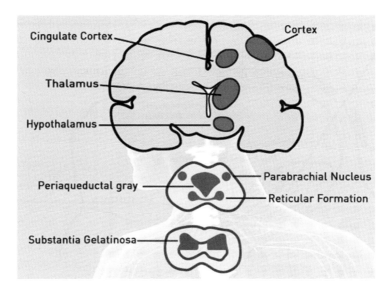

Figure II-17. The different areas within the central nervous where a dense accumulation of opioid receptors can be found

4. The nucleus solitary tract in the brain stern, which is the origin of the noradrenergic dorsal pathway bundle, which is in command of vigilance and the cough reflex.
5. The nuleus amygdala, being part of the limbic system, is in charge of the mediation of euphoria (or "kick") when opioids are used for other purposes than pain.
6. The locus coeruleus being the origin of the neurosympathetic system in the brain stem, regulates peripheral vasodilatation.
7. Lastly, a dense accumulation of opioid binding sites is found in the substantia gelatinosa at the dorsal horn of the spinal cord.
– Current thinking is that effective opioid analgesics work through stimulating mu (μ) receptors, which also produce euphoria.
– Euphoria is mediated by the actions of opiates at a cluster of brain areas that include the nucleus accumbens and ventral segmental area. Dopamine influx seems to cause subjective pleasure, or euphoria.
– Opioids may have a "disinhibiting" (inhibition of inhibitory neurons) effect that allows greater dopamine influx.

Because the main property of opioids is the blockade of nociceptive transmission in the mesencephalon (i.e. the nucleus limitans and the limbic system) the following effects can be observed:
1. No pain (analgesia), since any sensation is not identified as painful.
2. A lack of the negative emotional component of pain. On the contrary, euphoria may result and pain is no longer experienced as an emotional distress, even

though pain impulses are transmitted via the ventrocaudal-parvocellular nucleus to the postcentral cortex.

3. During the opioid-induced pain-free state, the site of pain, however, still can be localized. As a consequence pain has lost its negative character and is no longer experienced or perceived as uncomfortable and distressing.

REASONS FOR DIFFERENCE IN POTENCY OF OPIOIDS

In contrast to the analgesics that have a peripheral site of action (e.g. acetylsalicylic acid; ASA), opioids act at the relay station of nociceptive-propagating pathways at the synapse of nerve conduction. Within the nerve, pain impulses are transmitted as a change in electric conduction. And in order to guarantee maintenance of the nociceptive impulse, the excitatory impulse releases a neurotransmitter at the terminal nerve. Due to its chemical configuration, the transmitter fits exactly into a binding site at the opposite nerve ending resulting in an increase of excitability and a change in the electrical nerve conduction. Opioids have the property of binding to specific receptor sites at pre- and post terminal nerve endings resulting in an inhibition of a release of the excitatory neurotransmitter. The continuity of the impulse is interrupted, the nociceptive signal is no longer transmitted and thus can no longer be perceived as such (Figure II-11). Due to the difference in stereoconfiguration, opioids differ in their affinity (i.e. goodness of fit) at these binding sites (Figure II-18).

This explains why different opioids are characterized by a large variety in potency. In addition, opioids also differ in their intrinsic activity (i.e. the degree of conformational change of the receptor site) resulting in different intracellular effects. Taken together affinity and intrinsic activity results in the efficacy of a drug within the system (Figure II-19).

Thus, binding properties are reflected in varying analgesic potencies. Contrary, the intensity of binding with the receptor site (i.e. the intensity with which the opioid adheres to the binding site) is reflected in the duration of effects (Table II-6 and Figure II-20)[32, 14, 33]. For instance opioid analgesics such as sufentanil or lofentanil have an exceptional goodness of fit to the opioid receptor site, which results in high potency. On the other hand, the low dissociation coefficient from the receptor of buprenorphine or lofentanil is characterized by a long duration of action, while the high association coefficient demonstrates increase of affinity to the binding site.

Contrary to agonists, antagonists are able to displace an opioid from its receptor binding site and take up his position. Displacement is only possible because the antagonist has a greater affinity to the binding site. Therefore, affinity of an opioid antagonist is expressed in its antagonistic potency. Naloxone or naltrexone have a very high affinity to the receptor and easily displace an opioid whereas levallorphan is five times weaker (Figure II-21). In order to induce a similar antagonistic effect, a higher dose of levallorphan is necessary.

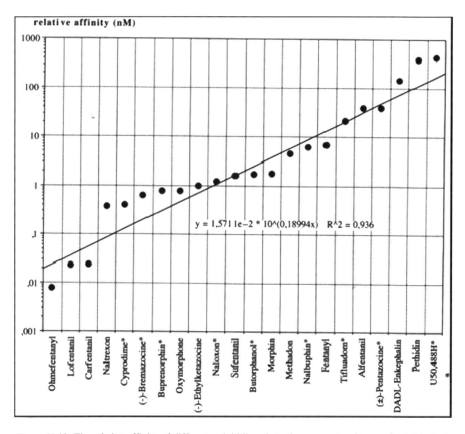

Figure II-18. The relative affinity of different opioid ligands to the μ-receptor site as reflected in their amount to displace a radioactive ligand. It can be seen that ligands with high potency (i.e. lofentanil, carfentanil) clinically also show high affinity while opioids with an asterix reflect antagonistic property at the μ-site

In order to induce increasing effects with opioids, the goodness of fit not only is a prerequisite. Of additional importance is the conformational change the receptor undergoes after binding, which is expressed in the "the intrinsic activity". An opioid must, therefore, not only fit to the receptor; it must also induce a chain reaction in the transmembrane receptor domain resulting in a net effect (Figure II-19). The reaction after opioid binding seems to depend on the side chain of the molecule. Thus it appears that one portion of the opioid molecule provides the binding to the receptor whereas another portion is responsible for the induction of a conformational change (i.e. intrinsic activity), which will either be of agonistic or antagonistic nature. In a sensitive and specific opiate-receptor assay, the guinea pig ileum with its dense accumulation of receptor binding sites, it was possible to demonstrate receptor affinity and pharmacological efficacy (Figure II-22).

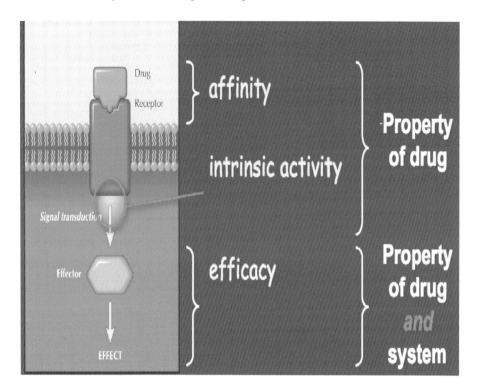

Figure II-19. Schematic drawing illustrating affinity and intrinsic activity of a ligand, both of which are necessary to induce an effect

This assumption is underlined by the effects induced by "pure" opioid antagonists such as naloxone or naltrexone, which also have a good fit with the receptor site, however when given on their own do not induce an analgesic effect. For instance, if naloxone is given by itself, the compound does not induce effects similar to its parent compound oxymorphone (Figure II-14). Also, in contrast to a potent opioid like fentanyl, the antagonist naloxone has a lower dissociation coefficient resulting in a shorter duration of action, which may result in a reoccurrence of an opioid-like effects such as respiratory depression. However, due to its high

Table II-6. Relative values of affinity and duration of action of different opioids, when compared to morphine ($= 1$).

	Morphine	Buprenorphine	Alfentanil	Fentanyl	Lofentanil
Association coefficient affinity	1	50	1	10	100
Dissociation coefficient (duration)	1	4	1/8	1/4	10
Potency of analgesia	1	30–40	40	125	1000

Source: Adapted from [33, 34, 35]

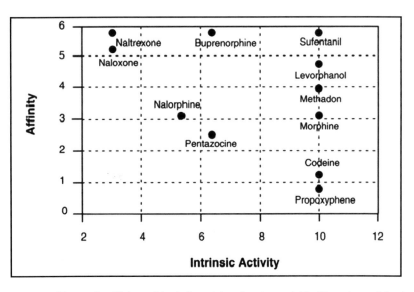

Figure II-20. Difference in affinity and intrinsic activity of various opioids. Note, that codeine has a similar intrinsic activity as sufentanil. However, due to the higher affinity of the latter the net analgesic potency is much larger

association coefficient (i.e. affinity), it induces a rapid displacement of the agonist and a reversal of all opioid effects.

On the other hand mixed agonist/antagonists, such as pentazocine, nalorphine, levallorphan, nalbuphine and butorphanol, demonstrate characteristics, which enable them to displace a pure agonist at the receptor site (antagonistic effect), but at the same time when administered by themselves, they induce opioid related effects such as analgesia and respiratory depression (agonistic effects; Table II-7). Such dual activity is only possible by means of their intrinsic activity at two distinct and different receptor sites: one the antagonistic activity at the μ- and its agonistic action art the κ-receptor site. And lastly, partial agonists like meptazinol and buprenorphine induce their analgesic potency via the μ-opioid receptor. Although having a high affinity, their analgesic ceiling effect at the higher dose range is due to a lesser intrinsic activity, resulting in a lesser net analgesic appearance than pure agonists. Such difference in the characteristic traits of opioids can be summarized as follows:

1. The affinity to the receptor (displacement properties or extrinsic activity)
2. The intensity of binding to the receptor (duration of effect)
3. The ability to change the conformation of the receptor (intrinsic activity)
4. The competitive potency (antagonism)
5. The degree of metabolism (duration of effect)

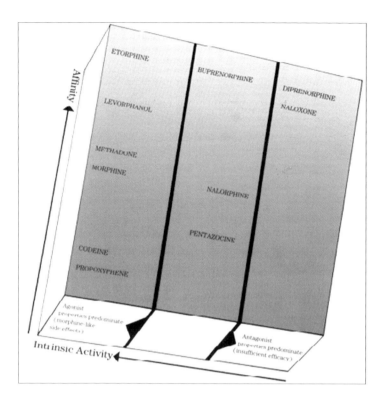

Figure II-21. The comparable degree of intrinsic and affinity of various opioids and their antagonists

Note the relatively high antagonistic potency of buprenorphine, however, is due to its high affinity to the receptor site resulting in the displacement of a ligand at the preoccupied receptor site.

Table II-7. Relative potencies of different mixed agonists/antagonists and partial agonists when compared to morphine (a pure agonist) and naloxone (a pure antagonist)

Generic name	Trade name	Antagonistic potency	Agonistic potency
Morphine	Morphine	0	1
Naloxone	Narcane	1	0
Butorphanol	Stadol	0.025	11
Nalbuphine	Nubain	0.4	0.8
Pentazocine	Talwin	0.04	0.4
Meptazinol	Meptid	0.02	0.25
Buprenorphine	Buprenex	0.5	30

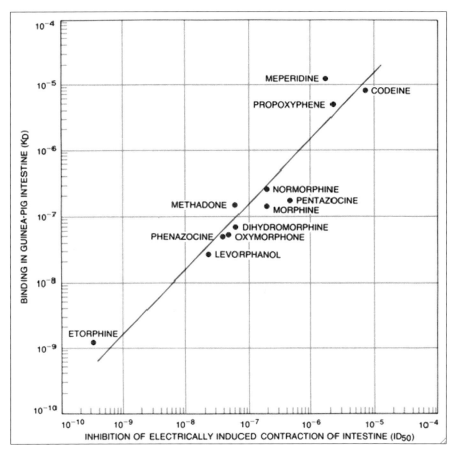

Figure II-22. Close correlation between pharmacologic potency of various opioid agonists in the guinea pig ileum (i.e. ID_{50} the concentration required to inhibit the contraction of the intestine by 50%) and their affinity for the opiate receptor site in the same tissue (i.e. KD, the concentration required to inhibit 50% of stereospecific binding of radioactive labeled naloxone)

INTRACELLULAR SIGNALING FOLLOWING OPIOID BINDING

Similarly like a hormone or other extracellular "first messengers" that bind to its receptor on a cell surface, a signal is transmitted or "transduced" to the cells interior, thus setting a series of events that produce a biological response. Such "events" include both chemical reactions and physical reactions like a conformational change in the protein molecules. The biological responses include cell differentiation, altered metabolism and cell growth and division.

There are three signaling pathways that share many of the same intracellular events. Each pathway is characterized by its receptor and by the cascade of intracellular events that lead to a biological response. Each receptor has an extracellular, transmembrane, and intracellular component and the binding of a ligand to the receptor represents the "primary message". The term "secondary messenger" is used for those mediators that diffuse from one part of the intracellular space to its spatially removed target. Among these secondary messengers are adenosine-3,-5-cyclic phosphate (c-AMP).

G-PROTEIN COUPLED RECEPTORS AND THE ADENYLATE CYCLASE SIGNALING SYSTEM, MEDIATORS OF OPIOID ACTION

Many integral membrane glycoprotein membranes share a seven transmembrane alpha-helix motif (Figure II-23). The ß-adrenergic receptor, whose natural ligands are epinephrine and norepinephrine, is an example of such receptors. Similarly in the opiate receptor, binding of a ligand presumably initiates a conformational change in the membrane protein that is transmitted to the cell interior. This physical reaction can then facilitate other physical or chemical reactions, which are conveyed to ion channels, resulting in a change of transmembrane ion flow. The transduction of the signals from external messengers, including opiate ligands involves intracellular heterotrimeric G-proteins, which are bound to the inner cell (plasma) membrane, a secondary messenger system, involving cyclic AMP, and a target response.

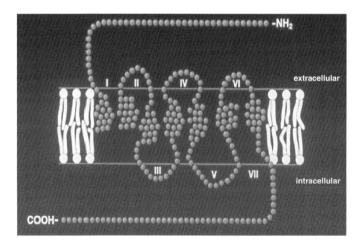

Figure II-23. Schematic serpentine model of the opioid receptor showing the sequence of the seven transmembrane domains as well as the extra- and intracellular peptide loops

SIGNIFICANCE OF THE HETEROTRIMERIC
G-PROTEINS IN INTRACELLULAR TRANSMISSION

As the name implies, these proteins are trimers, consisting of an α, β, and γ subunit. They are bound to the inner membrane and the subunit can bind the guanine nucleotides, GTP and GDP. G-proteins are involved in vision, smell, cognition, hormone secretion and muscle contraction in humans, and in mating in yeast. There are more than 100 receptors (not including odor receptors) that utilize G-proteins, and there are at least 20 members of the G-protein family, with each member having its characteristic α, β, and γ subunits. While the subunit is different for each G-protein, the ß/γ pair can be the same. However, all of the G-proteins share a similar structure. In regard to the opioid receptor, specifically the G-proteins transmit the signal from the intracellular part of the receptor to the effector. Adenylyl cyclase (AC), which is an inner membrane-bound enzyme, regulates the production of the secondary messenger, adenylyl cyclase. Other effectors that are G-protein-dependent include additional enzymes, like cyclic GMP phosphodiesterase, and transmembrane ion channels (Figure II-24).

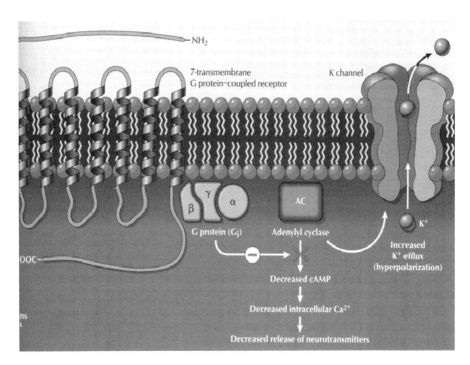

Figure II-24. Transmembrane changes following binding of an opioid to the external part of the receptor. By internal activation of secondary messengers, the close ion-channel is activated resulting in an increase of K^+-efflux

In its resting conformation, the G-protein consists of a complex of the three subunit chains and a GDP molecule bound to the alpha subunit. The alpha subunit is in close proximity to the intracellular part of the transmembrane receptor and, when a ligand binds to the receptor, the change in its conformation causes it to bind to the G-protein at the alpha subunit. This results in an exchange of bound GDP for GTP, which is more abundant in the cell than GDP. GTP causes a conformational change in the alpha subunit, thus "activating" it so that the alpha subunit dissociates from the β–γ pair. The alpha subunit diffuses along the membrane until it binds to an effector, thereby activating it. The alpha subunit is also a GTPase, so the signal transduction is regulated at this level by hydrolysis of GTP to GDP and inorganic phosphate. Such hydrolysis can occur spontaneously or upon interaction with a GTPase activating protein, "GAP". The GDP-alpha subunit complex then binds to the ß/γ complex to reform the original trimeric protein.

Since the stimulation of the external receptor can activate a number of G-proteins, signal amplification can occur. While this is a desired response in many instances, control at this level is needed to modulate it. G-proteins, then, are nano-switches when they turn on the effector by binding of the alpha subunit and turning it off when the GTP is hydrolyzed. The duration of production of secondary messenger, like cyclic AMP, is determined by the rate of hydrolysis. In this sense, the G-protein acts as a nano-timer.

Although there is controversy over the role of the ß/γ subunits in modulation of signals, it is likely that there are both inhibitory and stimulatory effects. If different receptors act on the same G-protein, or if different G-proteins act on the same effector, the potential exists for a "graded" response to an extracellular signal. If the same receptor acts on many G-proteins, or if one G-protein acts on many effectors, then there may be many simultaneous responses to the primary messenger.

Following binding the G-proteins activates the membrane-bound effector, adenylyl cyclase (AC). This enzyme catalyzes the synthesis of cyclic AMP resulting in the formation of ATP, cAMP and pyrophosphate.

Because this molecule is freely diffusing through the cytoplasm, it is a "secondary messenger" (Figure II-25). The reverse reaction, the formation of ATP from cAMP and pyrophosphate, is catalyzed by a specific phosphodiesterase. cAMP is involved in a number of physiologic processes. For the breakdown of glycogen, stimulation of the ß-adrenergic receptor involves activation of adenylyl cyclase and synthesis of cyclic AMP. The activity of cAMP-dependent protein kinase (cAPK) requires cAMP in order to phosphorylate Ser and Thr residues on other cellular proteins. Glycogen phosphorylase is activated by cAPK, making glucose-6-phosphate available for glycolysis.

Adenylyl cyclase activity is regulated at a number of levels, including modulation of GTPase activity of Ga, phosphodiesterase activity, and protein phosphatases. Inhibitory G proteins, Gi, are analogous to the stimulatory G proteins, Gs, except for the exchange of GTP by GDP by the α-subunit and the subsequent inhibitory action of Gia on adenylyl cyclase.

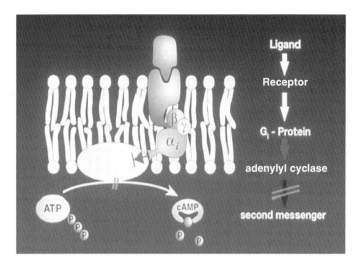

Figure II-25. Activation of the secondary messenger system following binding of a narcotic analgesic

Most of the activities in cells are controlled by kinases and phosphatases. The intracellular, C-terminal domains of many receptors have tyrosine kinase activity. Such receptors are usually monomers in their unliganded states, and contain only a single transmembrane segment. Ligand binding to these receptors stimulates tyrosine kinase catalytic activity in the intracellular domain of the receptor (Figure II-26), and such intracellular protein phosphorylation events are now well established as a means of transmembrane signal transduction. Structurally, though, it is unlikely that the signal from bound receptor to the kinase domain is mediated by a conformational change, as there is only a single transmembrane segment. Rather, it has been determined that ligand induced dimerization is the mechanism through which the receptor PTKs are activated. This dimerization brings the tyrosine kinase catalytic domain on each receptor into close enough arrangement so that each kinase can phosphorylate Tyr residues in the other's tyrosine kinase domain. Such activated catalytic domains can then phosphorylate tyrosines outside of the catalytic domains, which can then modify other intracytoplasmic proteins, either by phosphorylation or by other means.

All these changes are reversed with an overexpression of activation when an opioid is antagonized by a specific antagonist such as naloxone with activation of the excitatory NMDA-(N-methyl-D-aspartate) receptor, resulting in a rebound with an increase in transmission of stimuli (Figure II-27).

The next step in the signaling pathway involves activation of an inner membrane-bound monomeric G protein known as Ras, which initiates a series of kinase reactions that ultimately carry the signal to the transcriptional apparatus of the nucleus. Ras, being a G protein, is activated when its bound GDP in the resting state is replaced by GTP. It, too, has GTPase activity, but the half-life is too slow

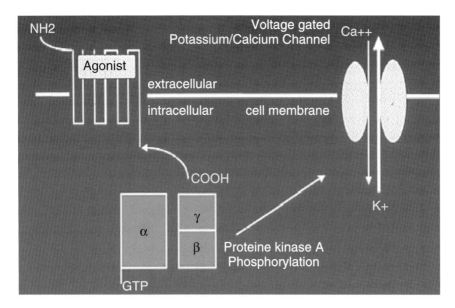

Figure II-26. Secondary intracellular phosphorylation of ion-channels by means of proteine kinase A (PKA) results in an increase of outflux of K^+ and a reduction of influx of Ca^{++}, inducing hyperpolarisation of the neuronal cell. As a consequence the cell no longer responds to incoming stimuli

to allow for effective regulation of a signal. Another GTPase activating protein, GAP, increases the rate of GTP hydrolysis by Ras. A "kinase cascade" ensues, involving Raf (a Ser/Thr kinase), MAP kinase (also known as MEK, which is both a Tyr kinase and Ser/Thr kinase, and a family of proteins known as MAPKs or ERKs.

DIFFERENCES IN CLINICAL EFFECTS OF VARIOUS OPIOIDS

Opioids induce a variety of clinical relevant effects, which can be subdivided in being advantageous and/or even detrimental. One of the major consequences following opioid administration is that of analgesia, or antinociception. And while NSAIDs induce their antiniociceptive effect via cyclooxygenase (COX) inhibition, local anesthetics selectively block ion-channels, thus inhibiting the transmission of nociceptive efferent to the higher pain modulating centers in the CNS. Contrary, opioids bind to those areas, which not only are involved in transduction but also in the modulation and identification of painful afferences. Although the majority of opioids are able to induce a maximal analgesic effect, the dosages necessary to induce such a result differ significantly. For instance, an opioid like sufentanil

G-protein coupled   **NMDA-receptor**
opioid-receptor   **ion channel**

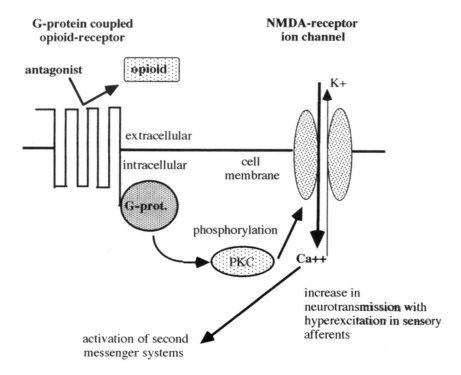

Figure II-27. Intracellular changes following displacement of the opioid from the receptor site by an antagonist. Via enzyme phosphorylation of phosphokinase C (PKC) the N-methyl-D-aspartate (NMDA) receptor is activated resulting in an increased inward shift of Ca^{++}-ions with an ensuing increase in neurotransmission of sensory afferents

needs a much lower dosage than the less potent opioid morphine. This is due to the higher affinity and intrinsic activity of sufentanil, suggesting that only a lesser portion of receptors needs to be occupied in order to induce the desired effect. However, a high analgesic potency necessarily does not reflect a better efficacy. This is because in certain painful conditions, some opioids are more efficacious than others. On the other hand, not all painful conditions, as the patient expresses them, can be treated successfully with an opioid. Therefore, before starting an opioid therapy it is mandatory to evaluate the kind of painful condition the patient has, use the specific opioids as indicated, and avoid those painful states where opioids are contraindicated or result in a lesser therapeutic effect. However, there is the general position:

> **In intense to severe, excruciating pain, opioids are the sole agents, which are able to induce sufficient analgesia**

OPIOID-REFRACTORY PAINFUL CONDITIONS

– **Pain from muscular dysfunction**. In patients who present pain of myofacial nature, opioids are contraindicated since they will not result in an alleviation of nociception. Due to muscle spasm or an increase in tension physical therapy presents the first defense line in the therapeutic approach. This is accompanied by the administration of a benzodiazepine, which induces a muscle relaxant effect and/or the injection of a corticoid together with a local anesthetic (0.5% bupivacaine) in so-called trigger points (Figure II-28). Trigger points are typical points which are sore and from which the pain radiates to referred areas. Such points can be felt as knots or bumps under the palpating finger, which can be moved over the underlying musculature.

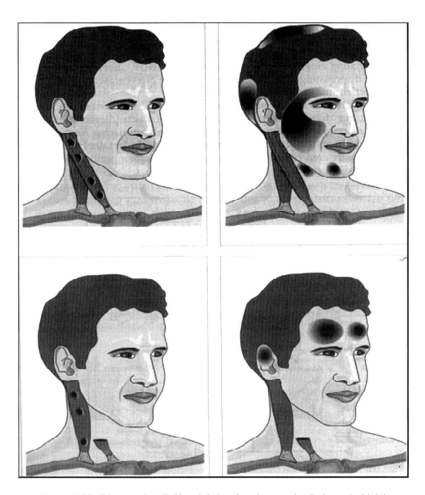

Figure II-28. Trigger points (left) and their referred areas of radiating pain (right)

Following the in injection of the local anesthetic the circulus vituosus of increased muscle tension and myofacial pain is interrupted. Local ischemia is alleviated and local accumulation of pain mediating substances is flushed out. A typical example is tension-type headache, which is the moist common type of headache. Originating from increased stress, it is accompanied by emotional factors and fear. Thus the painful condition can be considered of psychosomatic nature.

– **Pain of neurogenic or deafferentiation origin**, also termed as complex regional pain syndrome (CRPS), this type of pain is mostly seen after injury of peripheral nerves leading to spontaneous and paroxysmal discharges. Such pain typically is seen as post-herpetic pain, central pain after stroke, diabetic peripheral neuropathy, phantom limb pain, traumatic nerve avulsion, trigeminal neuralgia, lumbosacral plexopathy, all being circumscribed as neuropathic pain. It origi-nates proximal of the peripheral nociceptor (Figure II-29), and characteristically is due to a dysfunction or lesion of the peripheral nerve fibers and/or centrally located nervous structures. Typically this type of pain is accompanied by a sensory deficit: it is of a burning, shooting, stabbing, piercing, tearing or electric-shock-like, paroxysmal and vice-like nature. This pain is of paresthetic, hypo-or hyperesthetic quality often is refractory to any opioid therapy. The causes for such painful conditions may be quite different:

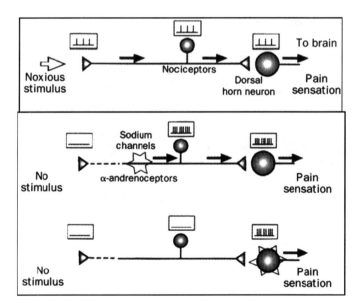

Figure II-29. Compared to a normal situation (top), there is spontaneous ectopic firing from increased sodium-channel activity after peripheral nerve injury (middle), which eventually results in central sensi-tization with stimulus independent pain (bottom). Modified from [36]

○ **Ectopic spontaneous discharges** originating from a lesioned or a cut nerve, this results in an upregulation of sodium-channels being the source of spontaneous discharge. Continuous nociceptive barrage later results in central sensitisation and "wind-up" (Figure II-29).

○ **Partial denervation with spontaneous discharge** of nerve activity is followed by an induced release of a nerve growth factor (NGF). Such release induces sprouting of fibers into adjacent afferent somatic nerve fibers resulting in an enlargement of the receptive field and an increased conduction of nociceptive impulses to higher pain centers (Figure II-30).

– **Imbalance or loss of central inhibitory modulation** within the spinal cord, due to a lesion of the descending inhibitory system, results in a decay of local inhibitory nerve cells within the spinal cord followed by an overdrive of incoming excitatory activity (Figure II-31). Such increase in the barrage of nociception is further conveyed to supraspinal pain centers resulting in sensitization.

– **Sympathically maintained pain** by means of a short cut of afferent, nociceptive and efferent sympathetic nerve fibers (Figure II-32). Such an emphatic sensory stimulation of sensorsy fibers by adjacent autonomic fibers is set off via sympathetic spinal ganglia, where IL-6 or the NGF induce a basket-like sprouting of sympathetic nerve fibers. By the release of noradrenalin spontaneous excitatory activity with noxious stimuli is initiated. Via the spinal ganglion pain can also be projected to corresponding areas of the skin (head zones), while through the excessive release of neurotransmitters, molecular changes, changes in gene expression within the spinal cord, and changes in the receptive fields of neurons in the perception of pain is initiated.

While opioids in such conditions often result in insufficient pain relief, therapeutically antidepressants, neuroleptics, antiarrhythmics and anticonvulsants are the agents of choice. Also, application of a transcutaneous patch with

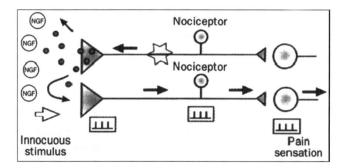

Figure II-30. Partial denervation results in spontaneous activity in injured afferents can produce peripheral sensitization in uninjured adjacent neurons via release of nerve growth factor (NGF). This is followed by an enlargement of painful areas with mechanical and thermal hyperalgesia. Modified from [36]

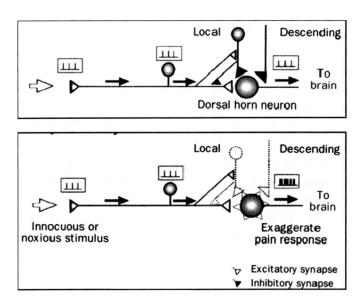

Figure II-31. Normally there is a balance between excitatory input from primary afferents and inhibitors input (locally and descending) at the spinal cord level. Nerve injury reduces inhibitory input with an increase in excitability in dorsal horn neurons. Primary efferents now evoke a much greater response and dorsal horn may fire spontaneously. Disinhibition of incoming nociceptive stimuli will result in subsequent "wind up". Modified from [36]

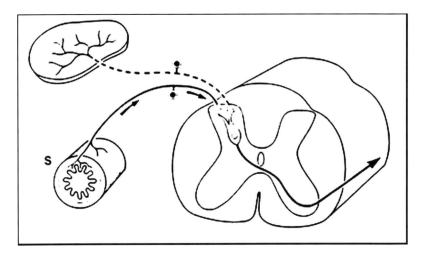

Figure II-32. Efferent mediation of pain via the spinal ganglion in sympathetically maintained nociception

the local anesthetic lidocaine (being a sodium-channel blocker!) is advocated. Other topical formulations with capscaicin or EMLA cream present additional therapeutic options for treatment of neuropathic pain. In addition, transcutaneous electrical stimulation (TENS) or even spinal cord stimulation (SCS) may present an alternative and effective strategy, resulting in the attenuation of pain. In the latter technique, analgesia is induced by the electrically induced release of endogenous opioids (enkephalins, endorphins, dynorphin) in the spinal cord and within the hypothalamus activating the descending serotoninergic and noradrengergic pathways.

– **Opioids in visceral painful condition**. Another type of pain, which cannot be treated sufficiently with an opioid, is visceral pain. Such a painful condition may arise from the intestine (e.g. the irritable bowel syndrome or IBS) or pain emerging from other internal organs such as the gall bladder, the urinary tract or pain following an appendectomy, cholecystectomy or hysterectomy (Figure II-33). Due to the participation of smooth muscles in such a condition a peripheral analgesic with a muscle relaxant effect can be of advantage. Because the sympathetic nervous system to a major part is involved in such a condition, therapeutic implications incorporate a ganglionic blocker, surgical sympathectomy, or intravenous conduction anesthesia with guanethidine.

– **Psychosomatic painful conditions**, if treated with an opioid, in the long run are bound to end in opioid resistance. Such a painful condition is mainly seen in the depressive patient or it may even be a premonitoring sign of schizophrenia. However, pain can also be part of a conversion-neurotic syndrome [37, 38], where aside from pain fear, phobia, and obsessive-compulsive symptoms are the dominant elements.

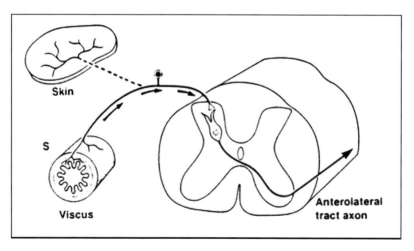

Figure II-33. Pain from the viscus being transferred spinally via the anterolateral tract to the supraspinal centers

Painful conditions being sensitive to opioids
All agonizing painful states, which are due to

- posttraumatic
- postoperative
- ischemic, or of
- tumor

origin, can be treated sufficiently with an opioid. The rational for the therapy
with a central analgesic is related to the fact, that the nociceptive impulses are
transmitted via specific pain afferents reaching supraspinal areas. By blockade of
specific receptor sites within the brain, opioids induce a reduction and/or result in
a total blockade of nociceptive impulses. Opioids therefore present the main line of
defense in all medium to severe painful conditions.

Opioid-Related Side Effects

OPIOID-INDUCED RESPIRATORY DEPRESSION

When using opioids one has to realize that this group of ligands, besides their
beneficial analgesic effect at the same time also induces a detrimental respiratory
depression. This is a mayor drawback when using opioids in acute pain and is
directly proportional to their analgesic potency. For instance a potent opioid such
as fentanyl already is able to induce respiratory depression in the lower dose range.
However, a less potent opioid like codeine or tramadol, even when given in dosages
higher than their therapeutic margin, will not induce a clinically relevant respiratory
depressive effect (Figure II-34). Because opioids given for alleviation of chronic
pain are given orally and in a controlled release formulation, there is no acute rise
in opioid plasma level, which otherwise would induce respiratory impairment. In
addition, chronic pain patients cannot be considered as being opioid naïve. Their
respiratory center already has developed some degree of habituation, being less
sensitive to the opioid agent.

Those opioid ligands, which inherit a lesser respiratory depressive effect,
however, are characterized by a comparable reduced analgesic potency. Also, a pure
μ-type ligand such as morphine, fentanyl or sufentanil is characterized by a dose-
related decrease in respiration until total apnea becomes apparent. Contrary, the
potent partial agonist buprenorphine with increasing doses demonstrates a ceiling
effect, which is seen at a dose of $2\,\mu g/kg$ (Figure II-35).

Typically, when administering high dosages of potent μ-type ligands such as
fentanyl or alfentanil, a time related sequence of effects on respiration can be
observed. The progression of respiratory depression is a characteristic trait, which
develops within seconds to minutes:

1. A reduction in respiratory rate (bradypnea) with a partial compensation of tidal
   volume.
2. A respiration, which is only kicked off by external stimuli, such as noise or pain.

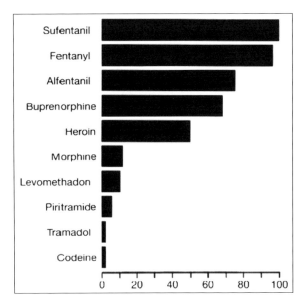

Figure II-34. Intensity of respiratory depression induced by different dosages of opioids achieving similar analgesic potency. Note, the higher the potency the more likely the agent will induce respiratory depression

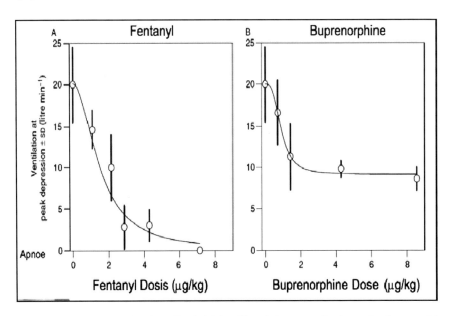

Figure II-35. Changes in tidal volume (liter/min) in subjects being exposed to increasing dosages of the pure μ-type ligand fentanyl and the partial agonist buprenorphine. Note, the ceiling effect in respiratory depression at higher doses of buprenorphine. Adapted from [22]

3. A short period where respiration is forgotten, originally termed in Europe as "oublie respiratoire", as it was observed in the early times of neuroleptanesthesia when using fentanyl together with a neuroleptic agent for the induction and maintenance of anesthesia. At this stage, however, the patient can be ordered to take deep breaths.
4. The total apnea, where in spite of any external stimuli or the command to breathe the patient spontaneously will not be able to take a deep breath. He needs immediate respiratory assistance.

This centrally-induced opioid-related respiratory depression is due to a blockade of the respiratory regulating centers within the brain stem (pons and medulla), resulting in a lesser sensitivity to an increase in arterial pCO_2 and/or a reduction of arterial pO_2 [39, 40]. In addition the activating reticular system (ARS), which descends down into the brain stem, acts as a regulatory pacemaker for the inspiratory center, by which respiratory depressive effect of opioids are affected. This is reflected in the clinics when in addition to an opioid a benzodiazepine is added, which by depressing vigilance, results in an immediate cessation of respiration [41].

Any opioid-induced respiratory depression instantaneously and effectively can be reversed by the administration of a specific opioid antagonist such as naloxone. Because of the higher affinity of the antagonist, naloxone displaces the agonist from the receptor site (competitive antagonism), and after binding respiratory depression is reversed and normal ventilation is instigated (Figure II-36).

Clinically, an opioid-related respiratory depression is reversed by *titrating* the dose of naloxone necessary to

• initiate a sufficient spontaneous respiration, however
• avoiding an acute abstinence syndrome with tachycardia and hypertension, and at the same time
• remaining a sufficient level of analgesia

During reversal one should consider the half-life of naloxone, which is between 20 and 30 min [42, 43]. Therefore "remorphinisation" with a reoccurrence of respiratory depression may appear if the half-life of the agonist is longer than the antagonist, or if high concentrations of the agonist are still circulating in the blood plasma [44]. Following successful reversal it therefore is mandatory to administer an additional dose of naloxone intramuscularly, which acts like a depot, or hook the patient up to a continuous intravenous drip of a naloxone solution, sufficient for long-term receptor occupation by the antagonist. All these procedures, however, do not replace the need for a continuous surveillance, which is necessary in order to detect any possible gradual development of respiratory impairment.

Respiratory depression can also be reversed by a mixed agonist/antagonist such as nalbuphine. Although being less potent than naloxone, it however is one of the mixed ligands having a sufficient antagonistic potency (Table II-8). At the same time the ligand has a 3-fold longer duration of action than

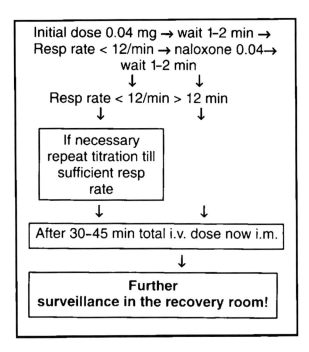

Initial dose 0.04 mg → wait 1-2 min →
Resp rate < 12/min → naloxone 0.04→
wait 1-2 min
↓   ↓
Resp rate < 12/min > 12 min
↓   ↓

If necessary
repeat titration till
sufficient resp
rate

↓   ↓

After 30–45 min total i.v. dose now i.m.

↓

**Further
surveillance in the recovery room!**

Figure II-36. Titration of opioid-related respiratory depression with naloxone until normal respiration activated

naloxone [47, 48], while the lesser antagonistic potency results in a more gradual and not in abrupt displacement, resulting in lesser sympathetic overdrive [49] (Figure II-37).

Another pure antagonist, nalmefene shows the longest duration of antagonism with up to 8 h of action [51]. Because of its high antagonistic potency (2.5-fold of naloxone) an acute abstinence syndrome can be induced if the necessary dose is not titrated to patients need [52].

Table II-8. Difference in analgesic and antagonistic potency of some mixed agonist/antagonists when compared to the pure agonist morphine (= 1) and the pure antagonist naloxone (= 1).

Agonist/Antagonist	Agonistic potency	Antagonistic potency
Butorphanol	11.0	0.025
Nalbuphine	0.8	0.4
Pentazocine	0.4	0.04
Levallorphane	1.0	0.2
Morphine	1	0
Naloxone	0	1

Adapted from [45, 46]

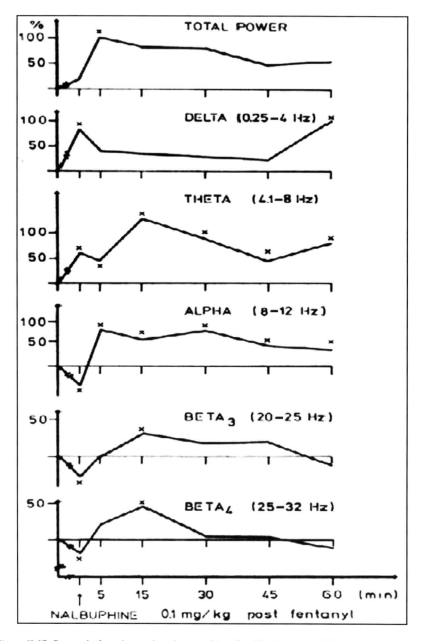

Figure II-37. Reversal of respiratory impairment with nalbuphine in patients following anesthesia with high dose fentanyl. Note the increase in the high frequency bands of the EEG (alpha, beta$_3$ and beta$_4$) reflecting increase in vigilance. Adapted from [50]

SIGNIFICANCE OF THE DIFFERENT
OPIOID RECEPTORS IN THE MEDIATION
OF RESPIRATORY DEPRESSION

It had been proposed that different receptor sites in the CNS mediate opioid-related analgesia and respiratory impairment [53]. Such difference has also been demonstrated for fentanyl-analogues in the animal [54], suggesting a clinical relevance for reversal of respiratory impairment, however at the same time maintaining antinociception. Such connotation was further corroborated by experimental data where the selective antagonist naloxonazine was able to reverse opioid induced analgesia, but not respiratory impairment. This led to the assumption that μ-opioid subreceptors are involved in the mediation of opioid-induced respiratory depression (i.e. μ_1 and μ_2) [55, 56]. Clinical data seem to underline this assumption, as low doses of sufentanil demonstrated a lesser respiratory depressive effect and a higher analgesic potency when compared to fentanyl. Such difference in action reportedly is due to a disparity in receptor affinity to μ-subsites, with a higher affinity to the μ_1- and a lesser affinity to the μ_2-receptor [57].

Other experiments, however, suggest that the co-binding of μ-selective ligands to the δ-receptor results in respiratory impairment. Subanalgesic doses of the δ-selective ligand D-Ala^2-D-Leu-Enkephalin, when co-administered with morphine, induced a potentiation of analgesia, while another δ-ligand D-Ala^2-Met-Enkephalinamid produced a reduction in analgesia [58]. Such δ-related differentiation in efficacy was also seen with the potent ligand sufentanil. There respiratory impairment was reversed while at the same time maintaining antinociception using the highly selective δ-antagonists naltrindol and naltribene respectively [59] (Figure II-38).

The implication of μ/δ-receptor interaction is further supported by receptor binding studies, where sufentanil demonstrates higher δ-selectivity than fentanyl (Table II-9).

Such putative interaction between μ- and δ-receptors is further corroborated when co-administering intrathecally a μ- and a δ-selective ligand resulted in a potentiation of effects [61]. From such data it can be concluded that a coupling mechanism between the μ- and δ-opioid receptor not only seems to result in an increase in analgesia, but at the same time also seems to cause respiratory depression. Such coupling mechanisms may result in a modulation to potentiation of effects whereby it is still uncertain whether both sites independently operate from each other or whether the δ-receptor only accentuates the effects induced by μ-binding.

VIGILANCE, LEADING PARAMETER
IN OPIOID-RELATED RESPIRATORY DEPRESSION

Besides a direct action of opioids on the sensitivity of the respiratory center to changes of arterial pO_2 and pCO_2, also centrally-induced sedative effects very likely influence respiration. Such sedative effects can be derived with the aid of the electroencephalogram where clinically different potent opioids qualitatively induce

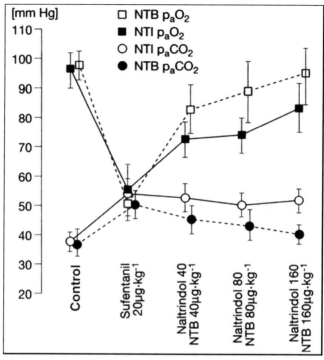

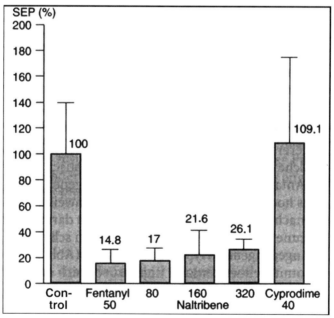

Table II-9. Affinity data (displacement constants in nmol/L, where a high concentration reflects low binding, and vice versa) of various opioid ligands with the three main opioid receptor sites μ, κ and δ in brain homogenates. Note the high affinity of sufentanil to the δ-subsite. Adapted from [11]

Opioid	^{3}H-D-Ala^2-Met-Phe^4-Gly-ol^2-Enkephalin (μ)	^{3}H-D-Ala^2-D-Leu^5-Enkephalin (δ)	^{3}H-Ethyl-ketocycla-zocine (κ)
Morphine	1.8 ± 0.26	90 ± 16	317 ± 68
Pethidine	385 ± 51	4345 ± 1183	5140 ± 789
Pentazocine	7.0 ± 1.8	106 ± 10	22.2 ± 4.1
Fentanyl	7.0 ± 0.83	151 ± 21	470 ± 68
Sufentanil	1.58 ± 0.38	23.4 ± 7.2	124 ± 11

a different in the EEG pattern. Since such EEG changes are dose-related, one is able to derive a dose-relationship. At the same time such EEG-changes reflect the bioavailability of centrally active agents acting on nervous structures of the CNS, depicting the effect-concentration site [62, 63]. Thus, following intravenous administration of an agent, it is not the plasma concentration, which is responsible for a centrally induced effect. More importantly, it is the actual concentration of the opioid at the receptor site, which is affected significantly by issues such as distribution of an agent, its lipophilicity, or the present brain perfusion.

Therefore vigilance changes can be considered as important aspects in an opioid-related respiratory impairment being derived in two relevant experiments:

1. Wakefulness by itself already is a fact resulting in sufficient respiration. This could be demonstrated nicely in volunteers where hyperventilation and the resultant hypocapnia resulted in a rhythmic respiratory pattern. If however, the same volunteers were asleep or in anesthesia, hypocapnia was followed by apnea [64].

2. In the animal laryngeal stimulation during anesthesia resulted in apnae, without, however, initiating a cough reflex. Being awake, a cough reflex without apnae was induced following laryngeal stimulation [65].

3. There is a close exponential correlation of the physiologic regulatory mechanism affecting respiration. This had been demonstrated after sufentanil application in the canine, whereby increasing dosages of a selective antagonist not only

Figure II-38. Dose-related reversal of sufentanil-induced hypercarbia and hypoxia with the two selective δ-antagonists naltrindol (NTI) and naltribene (NTB) respectively, in the canine. Due to the higher lipophilicity of naltribene being able to pass through the blood-brain barrier, there is a superior reversal effect. In spite of increasing doses of the antagonist there is a blockade of response to the electrically induced evoked potential, which is only reversed by the highly specific μ-antagonist cyprodime. Adapted from [60]

reversed the depressed respiratory drive but at the same time induced an increase of power in the high frequency beta band (13–30 Hz) of the EEG (Figure II-39), reflecting increase in vigilance [66].

4. Clinically such sedative related respiratory depression can also be derived in patients, when cumulative dosages of an opioid reach a point where the respiratory center "forgets" to respond adequately by initiating deep breaths (oublie respiratoire). This is seen in classical neuroleptanalgesia where the patient's vigilance can be increased to a point by external stimuli (e.g. pain, auditory stimuli) resulting in the initiation of an inspiratory effort [67].

From all these data it can be derived that the simultaneous binding of opioid within the activating reticular system (ARS) in the brain stem, vigilance is depressed, which secondarily affects the response of the respiratory center following hypercapnia. At such instances the overall mesencephalic reticular control mechanism is no longer able to adequately respond to a stimulus and only with an increase in vigilance there is an accelerated reactivity, being able to sufficiently respond to an increase in arterial pCO2. Since the reticular mechanism is coupled with reticulo-cortical afferences, such changes can be derived from cortical changes in the EEG. Such a "forgotten" reaction to sufficiently respond to a given stimulus [65] is also seen in the clinical environment when a benzodiazepine is given on-top of an opioid resulting in a further deterioration of respiratory drive. This is because a benzodiazepine depresses the reaction of the ARS, and the concomittant reduction in vigilance results in a lessened reaction to external stimuli, producing a clinically relevant suppression of respiration.

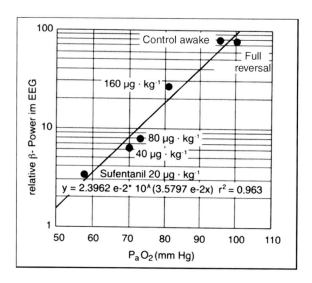

Figure II-39. Close linear correlation between increase in desynchronisation (beta activation) of cortical activities and rise in arterial pO_2 in the canine following sufentanil and the dose-related reversal by an antagonist. Adapted from [66]

REASONS FOR PROLONGATION OF OPIOID-RELATED RESPIRATORY DEPRESSION IN PATIENTS

In general prolongation of respiratory depression after opioid administration has to be expected when the following agents are coadministered:

1. All agents that inhibit the biotransformation of opioids such as contraceptives, anti-tumor agents, anti-arrhythmics, antidepressants, systemically administered antimycotics, neuroleptic drugs, and volatile anesthetics [68, 69, 70, 71, 72]. By inhibition of conjugation of glucoronide and oxidative dealkylation, the necessary metabolic pathways for degradation and termination of activity of most agents, a prolongation of action has to be expected.

2. All agents, which are able to displace the opioid from protein binding within the plasma, resulting in a higher portion of the pharmacologically active agent. Preparations such as cumarine derivatives, and phenylbutazone, which when coadminstered are prone to result in a prolongation of effects [73, 74, 75, 76].

3. In addition, hypoproteinemia and acidosis of the blood, both of which result in lesser protein binding, cause a higher concentration of non-bound opioid in the blood plasma. Such increase in plasma concentration now is able to bind to the receptor site with an increase of efficacy and a longer duration of action [77].

Following opioid-based anesthesia, several factors cause an overhang of opioid action, which may even result in a "re-morphinisation" and the re-occurrence of respiratory impairment:

1. The excessive intramuscular premedication with an opioid, which may act like a depot.

2. The premedication with a long-acting benzodiazepine, which is able to induce a reduction in vigilance lasting into the postoperative period.

3. The uncritical intraoperative use of high concentrations of a volatile anesthetic, which results in a lesser biodegradation of the opioid.

4. The intraoperative administration of fractional doses of an opioid, which results in an accumulation. Due to the fact that a portion of each dose of an intra-venously administered opioid is also taken up by peripheral sites (e.g. fatty tissue, musculature, skin, internal organs) there is an accumulation of the agent, which act like a depot. From there the drug later diffuses into the blood-stream, resulting in a prolongation of effects (Figure II-40).

5. An insufficient loading dose of the opioid, which may result in the necessity of re-administration of small amounts of the drug intraoperatively with consequent peripheral accumulation.

6. Long-term intravenous administration of an opioid by drip, resulting in the increase of the agent in the peripheral compartment with later recirculation into the blood stream.

7. The combination of opioids with different half-lifes, which may result in an unforeseen potentiation of effects.

8. Uncritical administration of bicarbonate resulting in alkalosis of the blood, which induces a faster release of the opioid from the peripheral compartment.

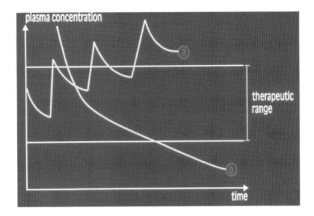

Figure II-40. Schematic drawing of repetitive administration of fractional doses of fentanyl (**a**). Contrary to one high loading dose (**b**), there is an accumulation of the opioid in the peripheral compartment resulting in a prolongation of effects into the postoperative period. Adapted from [67]

9. A non-corrected hypovolemia, which coincides with lesser protein binding of the agent and a higher portion of the free active compound.
10. Uncritical use of a selective antagonist such as naloxone, not considering that its half-life is shorter than the agonist, resulting in a later reoccurrence of respiratory impairment.

DIFFERENCE IN SEDATIVE-HYPNOTIC EFFECT OF OPIOIDS

The sedative effect of opioids goes in hand with their capability to induce sleep (lat. *hypnos*). Such an effect is mostly seen with the mixed agonist/antagonists, while morphine takes a medium position (Figure II-41). The hypno-sedative effect of opioids is useful in premedication and during postoperative analgesia, where a sedated status of the patient is advantageous. In contrast to a potent sedative nature of mixed agonist/antagonists, the pure μ-type ligand fentanyl is characterized by a very low sedative potency. When in the beginning of use of neuroleptic analgesia for anesthesia, fentanyl was used together with the neuroleptic agent droperidol, often patients reported of intraoperative "awareness". Although being an obligatory part of anesthesia, sleep, was not sufficiently maintained throughout the whole procedure. Therefore in order to guarantee a sufficient level of sleep in patients receiving a fentanyl-based anesthetic technique, an additional hypnotic (propofol), a benzodiazepine (midazolam), a neuroleptic agent (i.e. dehydrobenzperidol), or a volatile anesthetic (sevoflurane, desflurane, or enflurane) has to be given on-top the opioid. Nowadays the problem of awareness again has gained much attention [78], since the technique of total intravenous anesthesia (TIVA) with remifentanil and

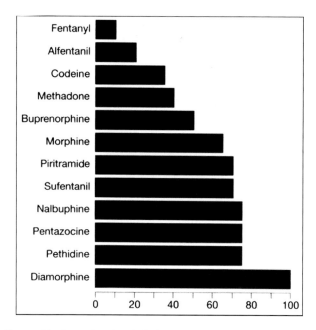

Figure II-41. Comparable hypnotic, sleep-inducing capacity of various opioid agents. Adapted from [84]

propofol, completely omitting nitrous oxide (N_2O), often results in an insufficient level of sleep with awareness.

Typically pure κ-ligands such as bremacozine and tifluadom (Table II-3), which in comparison to morphine have a 2-fold analgesic potency [79, 80], do not induce a respiratory depressive effect [81]. Their lack in respiratory impairment is due to the selective binding in deep layers of the cortex [19, 82], where in comparison to the brain-stem, a more than 50% higher concentration of κ-binding sites is found [3, 83]. Their predominant sedative effect is due to centripetal fibers descending down from deep layers of the cortex to the thalamus, thus decreasing the nociceptive input [20].

Although having the advantage of an increased sedative effect combined with the lack in respiratory impairment, clinically, the use of κ-ligands had to be abandoned. This is because of their intense dysphoric side effects, which lasts for several hours. In addition, their analgesic potency, in comparison to pure μ-ligands is much lower. Therefore such agents cannot be regarded as suitable for intraoperative use, where an intense nociceptive barrage can only be blocked by a potent μ-opioid. Only the mixed agonist/antagonists (e.g. nalbuphine, butorphanol), which exert their analgesic action through binding at the κ-site, currently are in clinical use mainly for postoperative analgesia [85, 86]. This is because cumulative dosages, contrary to a typical μ-ligand like morphine, result in a ceiling effect for respiratory depression (Figure II-42). In addition, because of their wide margin of safety, high dosages

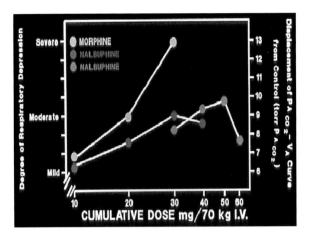

Figure II-42. Ceiling effect of respiratory depression following cumulative doses of the mixed agonist/antagonist nalbuphine. In contrast to morphine, at a certain dose there is no further increase in the degree of respiratory impairment. Adapted from [89]

have been advocated in balanced anesthesia where the opioid resulted in an up to 70% reduction in MAC (minimal alveolar concentration) of the volatile agent [87, 88].

DIFFERENCE IN THE HYPNOSEDATIVE AND ANALGESIC EFFECT OF POTENT OPIOIDS

Opioids in general induce a dose-related hyposedative component, which is mirrored in the electroencephalogram by an increase of activity in the slow δ- with concomitant decrease of power in the fast β-domain. However, when giving a large bolus dose of fentanyl (7–10 μg/kg body weight) alfentanil (50 μg/kg body weight) morphine (3–10 mg/kg body weight) or sufentanil (2–3 μg/kg body weight) an immediate dominance of delta-waves in the EEG becomes evident, being accompanied by sleep. For instance, such effects clinically are seen when high-dose opioid anesthesia is used in cardiac patients for the induction of anesthesia. Such a sleep-inducing effect is due to a short-term blockade of all afferences being switched in the activating reticular system (ARS) of the mesencephalon. Aside from a blockade within the nucleus limitans a deep level of analgesia is initiated [90]. Such a "narcotic component", with dominance of delta-activity in the EEG, and contrary to equi-analgesic doses of fentanyl, it is more apparent after sufentanil [91], which makes this agent more suitable for the induction of cardiac patients (Figure II-43).

Following induction with a potent μ-ligand such as fentanyl or sufentanil the initial "narcotic component" later transforms into a "pure analgesic component". This is because the opioid is redistributed, which results in a lesser concentration within the CNS and a lesser binding in areas within the ARS. At this stage there is a

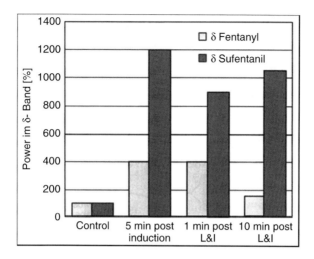

Figure II-43. Difference in the hynosedative effects of sufentanil and fentanyl following intravenous administration of equi-analgesic doses in cardiac patients undergoing laryngoscopy and intubation (L & I). Note, a pronounced delta activation after injection and a lesser arousal reaction induced by laryngoscopy and intubation, which in the sufentanil group reflected in a lesser decline of power in the slow delta-domain of the EEG. Adapted from [92]

dominance in the α-band (7–13 Hz) of the EEG, which is stable, not being affected by any nociceptive stimuli [93, 94]. Clinically, such an effect has been described for the precursor of fentanyl, the opioid phenoperidine [95] and for fentanyl [96]. After a period of 10–15 min the deep narcotic component changes into a sedative state, which is stable and cannot be reversed to desynchronization by any nociceptive stimulus. During such "analgesic state" the patient again is able to respond to verbal commands, while at the same time having a deep analgesic level (Figure II-44).

Without the addition of nitrous oxide, such patients are awake, however, nociceptive afferents are not able to modulate the ARS, the endotracheal tube is tolerated while at the same time nociception is only sensed as a touch. Such phenomena are due to afferents ascending along the spinothalamic tract, which directly ascend to the postcentral cortical area by which the impulse can be localized. Collaterals, which ascend through the nucleus limitans within the limbic system and convey nociception, are sufficiently blocked by the opioid and the patient does not perceive pain (Figure II-45).

The opioid receptor system bordering the fourth cerebral ventricle and the under-lying activating reticular system is the relevant anatomical structure in mediating sedation. Selective perfusion of increasing concentrations of the opioid fentanyl in the awake canine induced a dose-related enlargement of slow-wave high amplitude delta-activity within the EEG, characterized by a sleep-like behavior (Figure II-46).

This effect was reversed by the levo-isomer of naloxone inducing an arousal reaction. It, however, was not reversible by the dextro-isomer of the antag-onist [98]. The physiological significance of opioid receptors in the control of

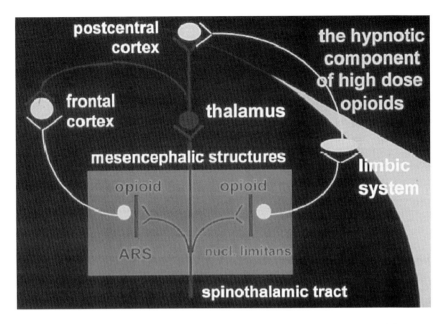

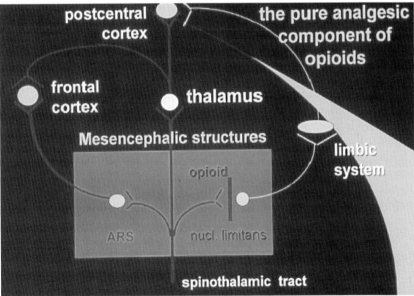

Figure II-44. Schematic drawing of the "narcotic and the analgesic components" of potent μ-opioids when being administered in high dosages. (ARS = activation reticular system). Modified from [97]

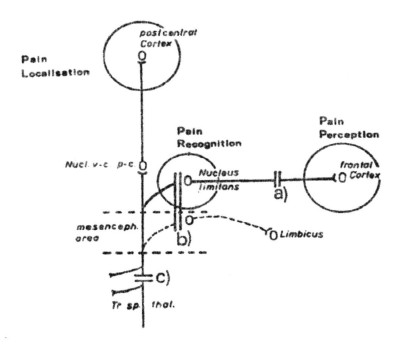

Figure II-45. The nucleus limitans bordering the mesencephalon and the thalamic area, is an important relay station within the CNS, a necessary component for the mediation of identifying a stimulus as being painful and where the input receives its negative, throbbing component

vigilance is also reflected in the high density of opioid binding sites in the mesencephalon [99]. Physiologically this is mirrored by an arousal reaction following intense acoustic or a nociceptive stimulus, both of which induce a reversal from the low frequency delta- to high frequency beta-activity in the EEG (Figure II-47).

In summary, it is concluded that opioids primarily affect the limbic system, the specific site for inducing the negative component of nociception. Lastly such assumption is underlined by the result from Mc Kenzie and coworkers in the animal where the opioids morphine and pethidine were not able to sufficiently block any pain related nervous transmission from the mesencephalon to the higher cortical areas [100]. In contrast, both ligands were able to block nociceptive transmission from the mesencephalon to hippocampal areas of the limbic system, the part of the CNS, which is responsible for the identification of pain, causing the negative, grief, stinging and an intense emotional feeling associated with pain (Figure II-48).

Such differences in pain modulation were corroborated in patients undergoing stereotactic, painful stimulation within specific areas of the CNS [101]. Nociceptive afferents of the spinothalamic tract end in the nucleus ventrocaudalis parvo-cellularis

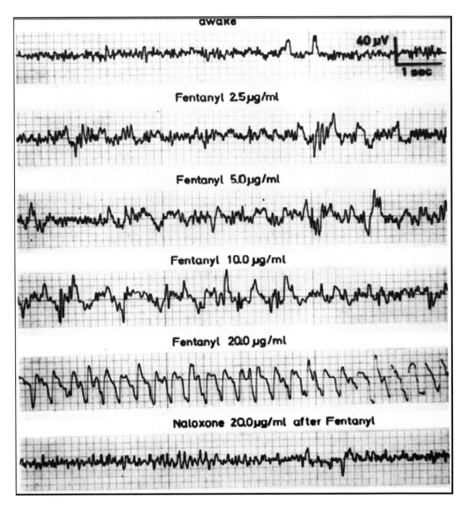

Figure II-46. Selective perfusion of increasing doses of fentanyl through the fourth cerebral ventricle of the awake canine. Note, the direct sedative (delta-synchronisation in the EEG) effect via the underlying ARS. This effect is mediated through opioid receptors located on the floor of the ventricle, since it was reversible with naloxone (desynchronisation with beta activation in the EEG). Adapted from [98]

thalami, from where they further ascend to different cortical areas. Since these nuclei reflect a specific somatotopic differentiation, electrical stimulation within this area induced painful sensations in different parts of the body. Decoding of painful afferents was only possible when the stimulating electrode was placed within the nucleus limitans, where collaterals of the spinothalamic tract switch to the limbic system. There stimulation induced a less well-localized, however, intense unspecific displeasure [102].

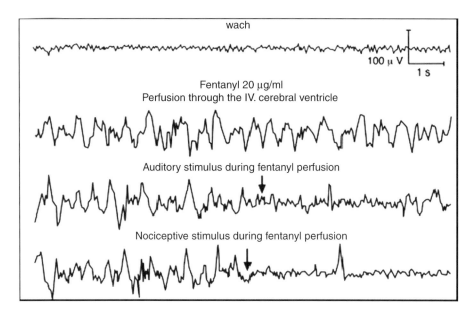

Figure II-47. Selective perfusion of the fourth cerebral ventricle with fentanyl in the canine results in the initiation of slow, high amplitude EEG-waves in the cortex. Auditory or nociceptive stimuli are able to reverse this pattern to a high frequency configuration pinpointing to the lesser sedative component of fentanyl. Adapted from [98]

POTENTIAL EPILEPTOGENIC POTENCY OF OPIOIDS

Following the administration of high dosages of opioids with different potency, epileptogenic activities in the EEG with tonic-clonic seizures can be induced in the animal. Pethidine (meperidine), morphine, alfentanil, fentanyl and sufentanil when administered in doses above 20, 180, 5, 4 and 4 mg/kg body weight respectively, induced epileptogenic discharges [103]. Because such massive dosages are never used in anesthesia or for analgesia in acute or chronic pain, epileptogenic effects, although being cited in the literature after fentanyl [104, 105] and sufentanil [106] are of insignificant nature. This is because the clinical picture resembles tonic-clonic seizures, however, in the EEG no such discharges could be derived [107]. Therefore, those high doses of opioids, which induced epileptogenic activity in the rat [108] or the canine [103] are far off from therapeutic range. Thus, in general, an epileptogenic activity of opioids can be canceled out. One exception is the use of high dosages of pethidine (meperidine), where the metabolic product norpethidine is a potent epileptogenic compound, which especially in the newborn is able to induce epileptogenic activity [109]. The cause for the few observations of a pseudo-epileptogenic activity of opioids when being administered within the therapeutic range very likely is due to a desinhibition of the cortical motor center within the CNS, as this phenomenon was observed during the induction of anesthesia or following a decline in plasma concentration. Such assumption is underlined by

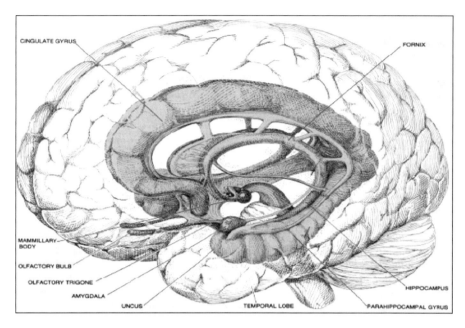

Figure II-48. Two main components of painful afferents: localization of nociception (cortical area) and the initiation of the negative component (i.e. the limbic system within the mesencephalon). Opioids mainly modify the latter area

"epileptogenic activity" during the induction of anesthesia with the pure hypnotic etomidate, where desinhibition of the motor cortex activity was the cause of cortical discharges [110].

THE ANTITUSSIVE ACTION OF OPIOIDS (BLOCKADE OF COUGH REFLEX)

Each cough involves a complex reflex arc beginning with the stimulation of sensory nerves that function as cough receptors. There is evidence, primarily clinical, that the sensory limb of the reflex exists in and outside of the lower respiratory tract. Although myelinated, rapidly adapting pulmonary stretch receptors (RARs), also known as irritant receptors, are the most likely type of sensory nerve that stimulates the cough center in the brain, afferent C-fibers and slowly adapting pulmonary stretch receptors (SARs) also may modulate cough. RARS, C-fibers, and SARs have been identified in the distal esophageal mucosa; however, studies have not been performed to determine whether they can participate in the cough reflex. Although gastroesophageal reflux disease can potentially stimulate the afferent limb of the cough reflex by irritating the upper respiratory tract without aspiration and by irritating the lower respiratory tract by micro- or macroaspiration, there is evidence that strongly suggests that reflux commonly provokes cough by stimulating an esophageal-bronchial reflex. Each involuntary cough involves a complex reflex arch beginning with the stimulation of sensory nerves in the airway epithelium that function as "cough receptors." Efferent impulses from these receptors are conducted by means of the vagus nerve to the "cough center" in the brain stem. Because cough can be voluntarily suppressed, controlled, or initiated, there also can be afferent input from the cerebral cortex. The function of this "cough center" is to receive these impulses and produce a cough by activating efferent nervous pathways to the diaphragm and laryngeal, thoracic, and abdominal musculature. The possibility that there might be afferent input other than the vagus nerve and cerebral cortex was based on clinical observations described in case reports and a few animal studies [111].

Histologic studies of the respiratory tract in both animals and humans have revealed sensory nerve endings within the basal layer of the epithelium and between epithelial cells of the larynx, trachea, and bronchi [111]. These nerve endings are thought to be cough receptors. They contain neuropeptides, such as substance P and calcitonin-gene related peptide (CGRP), which mediate neurogenic inflammatory events in the airways. These sensory nerve endings have been found to be most numerous in the posterior wall of the trachea, at branching points of large airways, and less numerous in the more distal, smaller airways. None have been found beyond terminal bronchioles.

It is not known for certain which type of afferent nerve mediates cough. A model that summarizes the current understanding of cough is schematically depicted in the figure. It shows the myelinated, rapidly adapting pulmonary stretch receptors (RARs), also referred to as irritant receptors, as the most likely type of sensory nerve that stimulates the cough center in the brain. Both mechanical and chemical stimulation of RARs have been shown experimentally to cause cough. Another type of sensory nerve in the airways, C-fibers, may also participate in regulating cough. They are unmyelinated, vagal afferent fibers that may be activated by the same triggers as RARs. Their activation releases neuropeptides locally that may secondarily stimulate cough by activating RAR nerves. However; impulses transmitted by C-fibers alone probably do not stimulate cough, because experimental evidence has shown that they inhibit cough centrally in the brain. A third type of sensory nerve, the slowly adapting pulmonary stretch receptors (SARs), may modulate cough. Although these nerves do not directly respond to chemical and mechanical triggers, they do appear to be activated by the deep breath of a cough and may enhance cough by making the expiratory effort more forceful. In addition to mechanical and chemical stimuli, cough has been caused in animals by thermal and electrical provocation. The sites most sensitive to all stimuli are the larynx, trachea, and cannulae of the larger airways.

Outside of the lower respiratory tract, cough receptors have been demonstrated histologically only in the hypopharynx [111]. However, it has been inferred from clinical studies that sensory nerve endings subserving the cough reflex via the vagus nerve probably exist in the extemal auditory canals and eardrums, hypopharynx, pericardium, stomach, and esophagus, because stimulation of these sites has been reported to cause cough [111]. Based on the fact that cough can be voluntarily initiated, postponed, and/or suppressed, this provides evidence that there also can be afferent input from the cerebral cortex. In addition to directly stimulating cough by carrying impulses from cough receptors to the cough center, vagal afferents may indirectly provoke cough by another mechanism. They may stimulate neurotransmitter release or mucus secretion from airway submucosal glands that, in turn, stimulate the cough reflex [111].

The existence of a discrete central cough center is controversial. What is known is that afferent pathways first relay impulses to an area in or near the nucleus tractus solitarius. These impulses then are integrated into a coordinated cough response in the medulla oblongata of the brain stem, probably separate from the medullary centers, which control breathing. Although electrical stimulation studies of different areas in the medulla have evoked cough in animals, suggesting that the cough center is diffusely located [111] a discrete cough center still may exist, because these electrical stimulations may have activated afferent pathways of the cough reflex.

The motor outputs from the cough center are in the ventral respiratory group, with the nucleus retro-ambigualis sending impulses via motoneurons to the respiratory skeletal muscles and the nucleus ambiguus sending impulses to the larynx and bronchial tree. More specifically, the efferent impulses of the cough reflex are transmitted from the medulla to the expiratory musculature, through the phrenic nerve and other spinal motor nerves, and to the larynx through the recurrent laryngeal branches of the vagus nerves (Figure II-49).

Vagal efferents also innervate the tracheobronchial tree and mediate bronchoconstriction [111]. Although stimulation of cough and bronchoconstriction can be experimentally separated using nonpermeant anions to stimulate cough without bronchoconstriction, these two phenomena normally are activated simultaneously to facilitate the most effective cough. Bronchoconstriction may improve clearance of secretions by narrowing the cross-sectional area of the airways, thereby increasing the velocity of air leaving the patients lower respiratory tract during the expiratory phase of coughing [111]. Experimentally, it has been shown in animals that the efferent pathways of the cough reflex are anatomically distinct and separate from the efferent pathways of normal spontaneous ventilation.

Blockade of the cough reflex arch by means of opioids, known as the antitussive action, refers to the fact that they suppress this protective reflex. This is of benefit during anesthesia and/or in patients being artificially ventilated in the intensive care unit (ICU) because it results in the tolerance of an endotracheal tube. However, the antitussive potency differs significantly among the various opioids (Figure II-50).

The action is not related to a specific receptor site, because a stereoselective action of opioids in regard to their antitussive effect could not be demonstrated. In addition, reversal with the selective antagonist naloxone is less selective [112]. The mode of action is a blockade of the cough center within the brainstem. Three of the most commonly used suppressors of the cough reflex are hydrocodone, codeine and hydromorphone. All of them are characterized by low analgesic potency, they

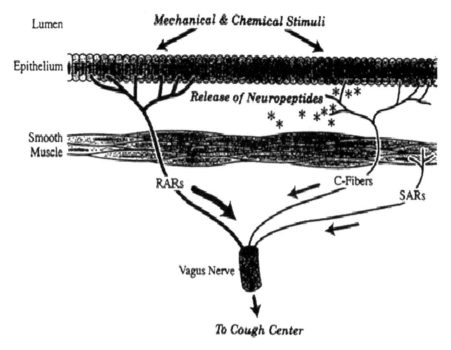

Figure II-49. Model for afferent limb of cough reflex in airways. Myelinated. rapidly adapting pulmonary stretch receptors (RARs) and unmyelinated C-fibers are sensory nerves that participate in the afferent limb of the cough reflex. Mechanical and chemical stimuli activate sensory nerve enelings in the epithelial layer. RARs appear to be the main type of sensory nerve stimulating cough centrally. Although C-fibers may inhibit cough centrally, neuropeptides released in the periphery upon stimulation of C-fibers may indirectly stimulate cough by activating RARs. Slowly adapting pulmonary stretch receptors (SARs) do not respond to irritant stimuli that initiate cough but may enhance cough centrally by making expiratory muscular effort more forceful

demonstrate a negligible dependence liability, and they are common components in DOC (drugs over the counter) cough medicine.

A similar antitussive potency, however, is also seen with the more potent opioids such as diamorphine, fentanyl or sufentanil. The latter are used in an opioid-based anesthetic regimen or in ICU patients who are in need of ventilatory support. When a potent opioid such as sufentanil is used, the patient is adapted much easier to the respiratory cycle of the ventilator resulting in lesser doses of additional sedative agents. Morphine in this regard has a much weaker antitussive activity while pethidine (meperidine) and all mixed agonist/antagonists are characterized by a negligible antitussive action (Figure II-50). It can be summarized that potent opioids also inherit a marked antitussive effect, while weak opioids and especially the mixed opioid analgesics are unable to sufficiently suppress the cough reflex.

During the induction of anesthesia, while injecting an intravenous bolus dose of a potent opioid such as fentanyl or sufentanil, often a cough reflex is initiated. Such

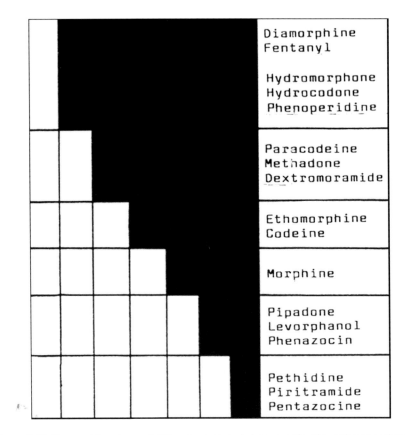

Figure II-50. Comparable potency of different opioids to induce an antitussive action at equianalgesic doses

a reflex is induced by an increasing rate of binding of the ligand at the target site. While lower dosages first induce a stimulatory effect, later when sufficient receptor sites are occupied, this results in inhibition of the cough reflex.

DEPENDENCE LIABILITY OF OPIOIDS – PHARMACOLOGICAL PRINCIPLES OF ADDICTION

Dependence or addictive liability (how addictive a drug is likely to be) depends upon how quickly the drug enters/leaves the brain. Also, it is directly proportional to the analgesic potency and it depends on the opioid receptor sites with which the ligand interacts. For instance, members of mixed agonist/antagonists (i.e. nalbuphine, pentazocine, butorphanbol) demonstrate a predominant interaction with the κ-opioid receptor, which is characterized by a low dependence liability (Figure II-51). In addition, development of dependence also is related to the speed

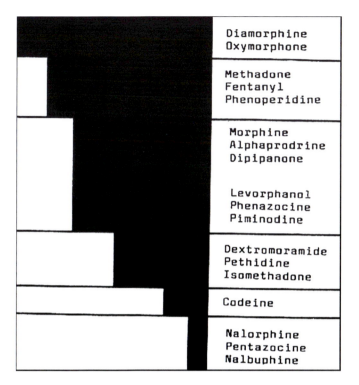

Diamorphine
Oxymorphone

Methadone
Fentanyl
Phenoperidine

Morphine
Alphaprodrine
Dipipanone

Levorphanol
Phenazocine
Piminodine

Dextromoramide
Pethidine
Isomethadone

Codeine

Nalorphine
Pentazocine
Nalbuphine

Figure II-51. Difference in dependence liability of commonly used opioids

of dissociation, i.e how fast the ligand leaves the binding site. For instance, an opioid like buprenorphine is characterized by a low dissociation constant reflecting long binding to the receptor, a long duration of action and a slow separation from the receptor. The definition of addiction is based in two different terms:

1. *Physiological dependence* produced by repeated drug-taking that is characterized by a *withdrawal syndrome*, when drug is removed (e.g. alcohol, opiates).
2. *Psychological dependence* produced by repeated drug taking that is characterized by obsessions and compulsive drug-seeking behaviors; results in a detrimental impairment in physical, mental or social functioning.

There are five classes of abused psychoactive drugs

1. *Opioids* produce a dream-like state; effects include: analgesic (reduction in pain), hypnotic (sleep inducing), euphoria (sense of happiness or ecstasy) using morphine, heroin, or the cough suppressant codeine.
2. *Depressants* produce feelings of relaxation/sedation and a dream-like state, anxiolytic (anxiety-reducing) and hypnotic effects; reduce central nervous system activity. Members of the class are alcohol, barbiturates, and benzodiazepines.
3. *Stimulants* increase alertness, arousal, and elevated mood; activate central nervous system (sympathomimetic = mimic the activation of the sympathetic

nervous system). Members of this class are cocaine, amphetamines, nicotine, caffeine.

4. *Psychedelics* produce distortions of perception and an altered sense of reality. Typical representatives are LSD, psilocybine, mescaline, MDMA (ecstasy), and PCP (phencyclidine).

5. *Marijuana with one of its major active ingredient THC* produces feelings of well-being and sense of acuity (sharpness). It also can produce feelings of relaxation.

Also, it is recognized, that opioids, which demonstrate a fast onset of action or due to their galenical preparation (injection, smoking) result in an immediate high plasma concentration, followed by an instantaneous receptor binding, results in a "kick" with an euphoric feeling. Such preparations therefore are more prone to induce a behavior pattern of abuse. Therefore addictive liability or how addictive a drug is likely to be, depends upon how quickly the drug enters/leaves the brain (Table II-10).

Most importantly, the tendency of opioids to result in an abuse is very much linked to the fact of why and when the opioid is ingested. For instance, an opioid taken only for the mere pleasure will rapidly result in the development of dependency. Contrarily, if an opioid is taken for the attenuation of pain, the likelihood to develop an abuse behavior is very low.

Aberrant drug related behavior has to be suggested when the following signs of abuse are obvious: in physical examination. A routine physical examination can elucidate common complications of heroin use or assist in diagnosing opioid dependence. Chronic intravenous use can be confirmed by the presence of "track" marks, which are callouses that follow the course of a subcutaneous vein. These are caused by repeated injections into adjacent sites over an accessible vein. Tracks are often found in easily accessible body areas, such as the backs of the hands, antecubital fossae, on the legs, or in the neck. Signs of recent injection may be found in unusual places in patients attempting to hide their sites of injection. A thorough examination for tracks or recent injection sites should include looking between the

Table II-10. Factors that influence how quickly a drug will enter the brain

1. Chemical structure: How fatty is the drug (i.e. its lipophilicity)? Does the drug have nutrients that our brain uses?

2. How fast does the drug cross the blood brain barrier (BBB) Lipophilic drugs (i.e. heroin, fentanyl) cross the BBB much faster than hydrophilic agents (i.e., morphine); they mimic nutrients our brain needs and can "slip" through transporters in the BBB.

3. Route of administration: Is the drug entering directly into the blood stream or is it entering first into the stomach? The routes of administration increase the likelihood that a drug enters the blood stream whereby it increases the addictive liability of the drug. Intravenous injection > smoking/snorting > sublingual application > inhalation via nostrils and lungs because they have abundant blood capillaries and more blood supply under the tongue and the lung respectively.

fingers and toes, under the fingernails and toenails, in the axillae, breast veins, and the dorsal vein of the penis.

One complication of drug use that can be found on examination is nasal septal perforation from repeated intranasal insufflation (especially when cocaine is mixed with heroin and snorted). A heart murmur may indicate subacute bacterial endocarditis, a complication of intravenous injection without using good sterile technique. Posterior cervical lymphadenopathy may suggest early viral infection, especially with HIV. Hepatic enlargement may indicate acute hepatitis; a small, hard liver is consistent with chronic viral hepatitis due to hepatitis B or C virus, which are common among injection drug users who share needles.

Signs of opioid intoxication may include pinpoint pupils, drowsiness, slurred speech, and impaired cognition. Signs of acute opioid withdrawal syndrome include watering eyes, runny nose, yawning, muscle twitching, hyperactive bowel sounds, and piloerection. On the other hand the following behaviors are more suggestive of an addiction disorder:

- Selling prescription drugs
- Prescription forgery
- Stealing or "borrowing" drugs from others
- Injecting oral formulations
- Obtaining prescription drugs from nonmedical sources
- Concurrent abuse of alcohol or illicit drugs
- Multiple dose escalations or other non-compliance with therapy despite warnings
- Multiple episodes of prescription "loss"
- Repeatedly seeking prescriptions from other clinicians or from emergency rooms without informing the prescriber or after warnings to desist
- Evidence of deterioration in the ability to function at work, in the family, or socially that appear to be related to drug use
- Repeated resistance to changes in therapy despite clear evidence of adverse physical or psychological effects from the drug

The following behavior pattern is less suggestive of an addiction disorder.

- Aggressive complaining about the need for more drugs.
- Drug hoarding during periods of reduced symptoms.
- Requesting specific drugs.
- Openly acquiring similar drugs from other medical sources.
- Unsanctioned dose escalation or other noncompliance with therapy on one or two occasions.
- Unapproved use of the drug to treat another symptom.
- Reporting psychic effects not intended by the clinician.
- Resistance to a change in therapy associated with "tolerable" adverse effects with expressions of anxiety related to the return of severe symptoms. And while addiction is characterized by a compulsive drug-using and drug-seeking behavior that interferes with normal functioning and causes use of the drug despite increasingly damaging consequences, there are different mechanisms from dependence

as addicts can experience intense cravings for drugs even years after sobriety (after body set-points, etc. should have adjusted back to normal).

The nervous pathways involved in the development of dependence is the mesolimbic-dopaminergic reward system, where direct activation (i.e. cocaine, nicotine, alcohol) or inhibition of the inhibitory GABAergic neurons in the ventral tegmental area (VTA) directly project to dopaminergic neurons in the nucleus accumbens (i.e. opioids such as heroin) results in an increased release of dopamine in the nucleus accumbens and stimulation of the prefrontal area resulting in euphoria. On the other hand, insufficient release of dopamine in this area results in dysphoria, which is seen in abstinence (Figure II-52).

NEUROBIOLOGICAL CHANGES WITH ADDICTION

In the acute phase, opioids inhibit adenylyl cyclase and cAMP. Over time, the downstream transcription factor (CREB) is activated which increases adenlyly cyclase production (Figure II-53).

Chronic opioid use leads to upregulation of cAMP and CREB, directing to tolerance, dependence and withdrawal symptoms. The significance of intracellular changes in CREB is supported by data in mice without CREB, which are less likely to develop addiction. Also, recent research has also implicated an opioid peptide, dynorphin, in this pathway. Besides initial changes in CREB, chronic administration of an opioid results in the induced increased formation of peptides syntheses FosB within the nucleus accumbens. Such overexpression of ΔFosB increases the sensitivity to cocaine and opioids resulting in an increased likelihood of relapse.

In general an opioid-related dependency has to be distinguished from a dependency of the barbiturate-, alcohol- or cocaine-type. This is because they all result in different psychopathological and withdrawal symptoms. The latter is a set of physiological reactions that occur in response to removal of a drug following repeated treatment; often (although not always), the reactions are opposite those produced by the drug itself. In the beginning it is the pleasure seeking behavior that results in repetitive drug administration until finally, the drugs of abuse that produce physical dependence (e.g., opiates or alcohol), results in the avoidance of the unpleasant withdrawal syndrome can contribute to repeated drug-taking (Figure II-54).

OPIOIDS INDUCING NAUSEA AND EMESIS

The main physiological consequence of nausea and emesis is the removal of toxins, which is an important protective reflex mechanism being induced during food intoxication. It however, is also seen after radiation or chemotherapy, after the administration of an opioid-based anesthetic regimen or during long-term therapy for alleviation of chronic pain. About 20% of all patients experience nausea and/or emesis after opioid anesthesia. The cause of such reaction is a stimulation of the chemoreceptor

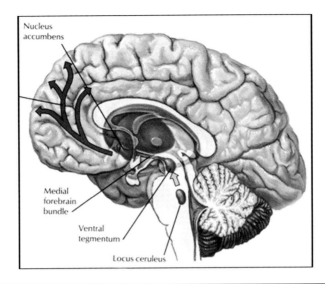

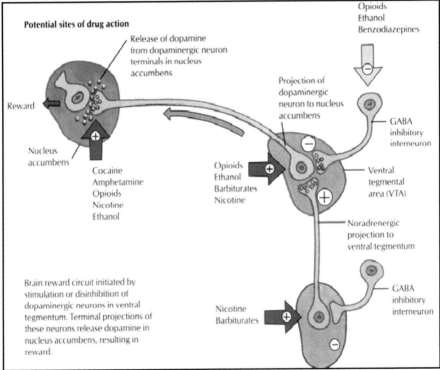

Figure II-52. The dopaminergic rewarding system within the brain, where activation by addictive drugs results in a seeking behavior pattern either directly by reuptake inhibition (i.e. cocaine) or indirectly by disinhibition of the inhibitory GABAergic pathway (i.e. opioid). Mostly all abused drugs increase dopamine levels in the nucleus accumbens

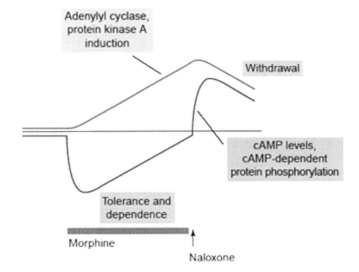

Figure II-53. Biochemical changes induced during addiction and the development of tolerance, which is followed by withdrawal when an antagonist is administered or by lack in maintenance dosages

trigger zone (CTZ), which lies in close vicinity to the emetic center, bordering the fourth cerebral ventricle, above the area postrema (Figure II-55). This area is richly supplied with dopaminergic, histaminergic, serotonergic (5-HT$_3$), and cholinergic receptor sites, being the origin of metabolic or drug induced vomiting [113].

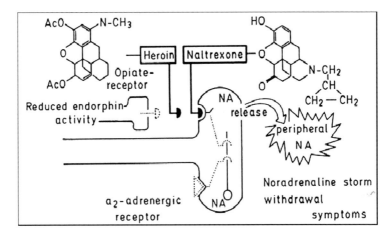

Figure II-54. Schematic representation of an acute abstinence syndrome with an accompanying norepinephrine storm induced by a decline in sufficient opioid binding or by application of an antagonist in the addict. Note the close interaction with the α_2-agonist, where clonidine exerts its mode of action by reducing withdrawal symptoms

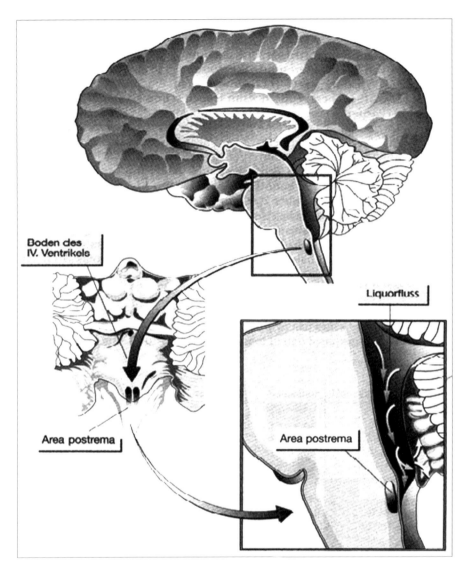

Figure II-55. The area postrema at the border of the fourth cerebral ventricle with its chemoreceptors, inducing opioid-related nausea and vomiting

Contrary to the other areas within the CNS, the CTZ is characterized by leaking capillaries (windowed capillaries), through which opioids as well as toxins can disseminate. Such anatomical difference indicates that this area does not contain the usual blood-brain barrier (BBB). Being located within the dorsal part of the activating reticular formation (ARS), all visual, cortical and limbic efferences, as well as efferences of nearby nuclei of the vasomotor center and the center for salivation and respiratory control are switched, resulting in a controlled succession during vomiting. Once the vomiting center is stimulated by any of the efferent stimuli, a coordinated sequence of events is commenced:

- Stop of rhythmical contractions of the stomach, followed by an accumulation of food in the abdomen, resulting in.
- Retroperistaltic action.
- Contraction of the cardia with increase of pressure in the stomach.
- Due to the coordinated contractions of diaphragm, intercostal muscles and the rectus abdominis muscle, food is being expelled forcefully via the opened orifice of the stomach, the dilated esophagus and the opened glottis.

Because the CTZ shows a dense accumulation of serotonin receptors, the serotonin-antagonist ondansetron (Zofran®) is able to induce an antiemetic effect [114, 115]. Other agents, which are given for reversal of emesis, are metoclopramide, and/or the neuroleptic agents haloperidol, triflupromazine, or alizapride-HCl, all of which interact through direct binding with the dopaminergic D_2-receptor. Another antiemetic is diphenhydramine, which exerts its action via binding at the cholinergic and histaminergic receptors (Figure II-56).

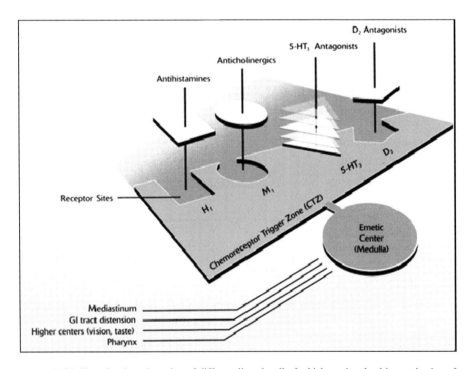

Figure II-56. Site of antiemetic action of different ligands, all of which are involved in a reduction of post-operative nausea and vomiting (PONV)

Postoperative nausea and emesis (PONV), however, still present a problem specifically related to anesthesia. In a large survey with over 2000 patients and using multivariance analysis, the following main risk factors for PONV were identified:

- Female sex
- Young age
- History of PONV/motion sickness
- Nonsmoking status
- Long duration of anesthesia

Each 30 min increase in duration increases PONV risk by 60%, and a baseline risk of 10% is increased to 16% after 30 min [116]. The type of operation, the addition of nitrous oxide (N_2O), high age and/or the addition of an opioid to the anesthetic regimen, in comparison to the above risk factors, had a lesser impact on the incidence on PONV [117, 118].

Commonly the key strategic antiemetic agents for reducing patients PONV are as follows (Figure II-56):

1. *Serotonin (5-HT$_3$)-Receptor Antagonist*

   The 5-HT$_3$-receptor antagonists are used for both the prevention and treatment of PONV and have a low side-effect profile. They are given toward the end of surgery for greatest efficacy, and are more effective in preventing vomiting than in preventing nausea. Dolasetron, granisetron, and ondansetron all have favorable side-effect profiles. No evidence has revealed differences in efficacy and safety among the 5-HT$_3$-receptor antagonists used for the prophylaxis of PONV. A recent study demonstrated the equivalent efficacy and safety of granisetron and ondansetron when these agents were used in combination antiemetic therapy. In this study, low-dose granisetron (0.1 mg) plus dexamethasone 8 mg was found to be not inferior to ondansetron 4 mg plus dexamethasone 8 mg in patients undergoing abdominal hysterectomy with general anesthesia. The combinations prevented vomiting in 94% and 97% of patients, respectively, in the first 2 h after tracheal extubation, and in 83% and 87% of patients, respectively, in the 24 h after extubation.

2. *Dexamethasone*

   Dexamethasone has been found to be effective for the management of PONV and their proposed mechanism of action is that of membrane stabilization and inhibition of inflammation. Use of this agent is controversial because of its alleged association with delayed wound healing. It has a slow onset but a prolonged duration of action, and therefore it is advised that dexamethasone be administered upon induction of anesthesia. The most commonly used dose for adults is 8–10 mg i.v. Smaller doses of 2.5–5 mg have also been used and found to be as effective. Based on a quantitative, systematic review of the data, no adverse side effects, especially delayed wound healing, have been noted following a single antiemetic dose of dexamethasone [119].

3. *Droperidol*

   The neuroleptic drug droperidol, a butyrephenone derivative, is widely used for PONV prophylaxis and is comparable with ondansetron as a prophylactic antiemetic. Similar to haloperidol it acts as a dopamine antgonist at the CTZ and the area postrema. For greatest efficacy, droperidol is administered at the end of surgery or concomitantly with morphine via patient-controlled analgesia systems. The use of low doses (0.625–1.25 mg) of droperidol has not been associated with the typical side effects of higher doses of this drug (hypotension, extrapyramidal symptoms, sedation, akathisia, dysphoria). In 2001, the Food and Drug Administration began requiring that droperidol labeling include a "black box" warning stating that the drug may cause death or life-threatening events resulting from QTc prolongation and the possibility of life-threatening *torsades de pointes*. The labeling requirement was based on 10 reported cases associated with droperidol use (at doses of 1.25 mg) during its approximately 30 years on the market [120]. However, no case reports in peer-reviewed journals have linked droperidol with QTc prolongation, cardiac arrhythmias, or death at the doses used for the management of PONV. Also, in a randomized, double-blind, placebo controlled trial, droperidol was not associated with a significant increase in the QTc interval in comparison with saline solution [121]. In another recent study, droperidol did not increase the QTc interval any more than did ondansetron [122].

4. *Other Antiemetics*

   Transdermal scopolamine (Transderm Scop® 1.5 mg), an antimuscarinic ganet, works by blocking the cholinergic receptor. It has an antiemetic effect when applied the evening before surgery or 4 h before the end of anesthesia preventing the patient from post-discharge nausea, vomiting and retching.

   The phenothiazines, promethazine, and prochlorperazine act both as D_2- and the H_1-receptor antagonist. They also inhibit histamine receptors and possibly cholinergic receptors in the gut. Both have been shown to be effective antiemetics when administered intravenously at the end of surgery. All three drugs may cause sedation, dry mouth, and dizziness.

   Metoclopramide is benzamide that blocks D_2-receptors both centrally and peripherally in the gastrointestinal tract increasing gastric emptying.

   The antihistamines, especially diphenhydramine act on both the CTZ and the vestibular pathways of the inner ear. At higher doses however, they can prolong general anesthesia and recovery times.

   Consensus guidelines agree that patients at high or moderate risk for PONV are most likely to benefit from prophylaxis. Patients at low risk for PONV are usually not candidates for prophylaxis unless their condition may be compromised by the medical sequelae or vomiting. Those at moderate risk for PONV should receive antiemetic monotherapy or combination therapy. Those at high risk should receive combination therapy with two or three antiemetics from different classes. Drugs with different mechanisms of action can be combined for optimal efficacy. For example, the $5-HT_3$-receptor antagonists (more effective against vomiting) can be combined with droperidol (more effective against nausea).

5. *Multimodal Approach*

A multimodal approach that incorporates both baseline risk reduction and antiemetic therapy should be adopted for PONV prophylaxis. A recent prospective, double blind, randomized, controlled trial compared three strategies for the prevention of PONV in patients undergoing laparoscopic cholecystectomy: (1) a multimodal approach using ondansetron, droperidol, and total intravenous anesthesia (TIVA) with propofol; (2) a combination of ondansetron and droperidol, with isoflurane and nitrous oxide-based anesthesia; and (3) TIVA with propofol alone. The complete response rate was higher in the multimodal group (90%) than in the combination group (63%) or TIVA-only group (66%), as was the degree of patient satisfaction.

6. *Rescue medication in PONV*

Nausea and vomiting may persist in some patients after they leave the postanesthesia care unit (PACU). After medication and mechanical causes of PONV have been excluded, rescue therapy with antiemetics can be initiated. For patients who received no prophylaxis, low-dose therapy with $5\text{-}HT_3$-receptor antagonists may be initiated. Consensus guidelines also recommend low-dose therapy with a $5\text{-}HT_3$-receptor antagonist for patients in whom dexamethasone prophylaxis has failed. For patients in whom initial $5\text{-}HT_3$-receptor antagonist prophylaxis has failed, a $5\text{-}HT_3$-receptor antagonist rescue therapy should not be given within the first 6 h after surgery. Similarly, patients in whom prophylactic combination therapy with a $5\text{-}HT_3$-receptor antagonist plus dexamethasone has failed should be treated with an antiemetic from a different class. As a general guideline, patients who experience PONV within 6 h after surgery should be treated with an antiemetic other than the one used for prophylaxis. For the treatment of patients who experience PONV > 6 h after surgery, drugs from the prophylactic antiemetic regimen may be repeated, except for dexamethasone and transdermal scopolamine, which have a longer duration of action. Also, propofol may be used in small doses (20 mg as needed) for the treatment of PONV in a supervised environment. The preliminary results of a recent analysis support the recommendation that a rescue antiemetic should be from a class other than that of the original antiemetic agent [123]. This analysis of a previous trial reported that in patients who failed prophylaxis with ondansetron or droperidol, promethazine was significantly more effective in controlling PONV than the original agent. Dimenhydrinate was also more effective than droperidol in patients who failed prophylaxis with droperidol.

In summary, the first step in the management of PONV is to identify surgical patients at high or moderate risk for PONV, then reduce baseline risk factors in these patients. Combination antiemetic therapy is recommended for patients at high risk for PONV for patients at moderate risk, monotherapy or combination therapy may be considered. A multi modal approach for the prevention of PONV including the use of antimetics with different mode of action, hydration and TIVA with propofol has been shown to be most effective. Patients who have not received prophylaxis and experience PONV can be treated with a low dose of a

5-HT$_3$-receptor antagonist. In patients who fail prophylaxis treatment with an antiemetic, another agent than the one used for prophylaxis is recommended.

OPIOIDS AND MUSCULAR RIGIDITY

Opioids can induce muscular rigidity, which is due to an increased tone of the striatal muscle. Especially, the muscles of the thoracic cage and of the abdomen show this rigidity, a phenomenon, which is observed after the bolus injection of a potent opioid, such as the fentanyl series (i.e. fentanyl, sufentanil, alfentanil and remifentanil; Figure II-57).

Increase in muscle tone is directly correlated to the μ-receptor interaction, because mixed agonist/antagonists and highly selective μ-opioid antagonists (i.e. CTAP), but not κ-(e.g. nor-binaltorphine) nor δ-antagonists (e.g. naltrindole) were able to reverse such muscular rigidity [124, 125]. In addition, administration of the selective antagonist methylnaltrexone in the nucleus raphe pontis was able to reverse increased muscle tone after alfentanil in the animal [126] suggesting this nucleus is an additional important site of action of opioids to induce rigidity.

Clinically this rigidity is a disadvantage because it results in an insufficient ventilation of the patients and is characterized by the following features [127, 128]:

• It appears shortly after intravenous injection of a potent opioid.
• It can be induced especially in the elderly patient population.
• It is potentiated by nitrous oxide (N$_2$O).
• It is more likely to develop in patients with Parkinson's disease.

The anatomical correlate by which opioids induce muscular rigidity is the striatum, and, being part of the basal ganglion system, it has the task to control locomotion (Figure II-58). Within the striatum there is a dense accumulation of opioid binding sites, which interact with dopaminergic D$_2$-receptors. Similar as in Parkinson's disease, there is a reduction in the dopamine level with an ensuing imbalance of the cholinergic transmitter system, both of which are in balance with each other and a necessary prerequisite for the control of muscle tone [129]. While in Parkinson's disease, increased muscle tone is induced by decrease of dopaminergic neurons in the striatum, opioid-induced rigidity is due to an enhanced degradation of the transmitter dopamine resulting in a functional deficit of a sufficient level in the nigro-striatal pathway [130]. The exact mode of action of opioids to reduce dopamine level within the nigrostriatal system and induce muscular rigidity, very likely is induced by inhibition of tyrosine hydroxylase, the necessary enzyme for the synthesis of dopamine [131]. Due to the interconnection with the inhibitory gabaminergic system, output of GABA in the pallidum declines (Figure II-58). This, in turn, causes an overactivity of cholinergic neurons projecting to thalamic neurons. From here the area 6a of the cortical premotor center is activated and the corticospinal tract leads efferents to the anterior horn of the spinal cord [132].

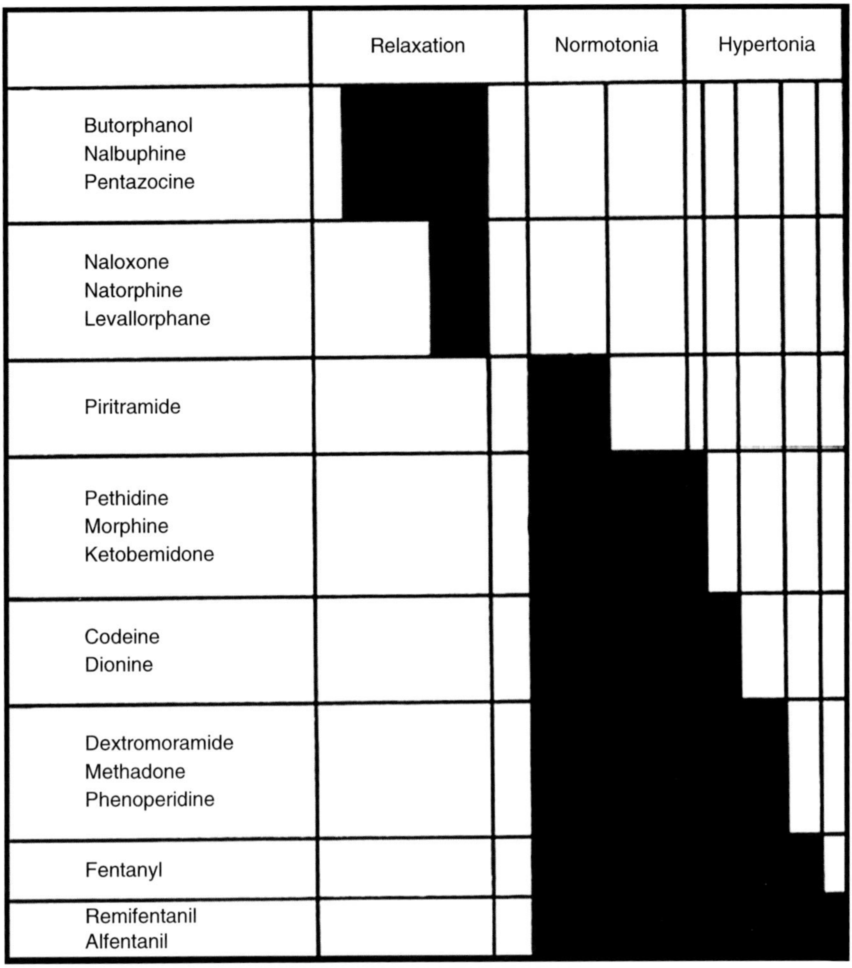

	Relaxation	Normotonia	Hypertonia
Butorphanol Nalbuphine Pentazocine			
Naloxone Natorphine Levallorphane			
Piritramide			
Pethidine Morphine Ketobemidone			
Codeine Dionine			
Dextromoramide Methadone Phenoperidine			
Fentanyl			
Remifentanil Alfentanil			

Figure II-57. Tendency of different opioids to induce truncal muscular rigidity

Although opioids do not directly affect muscle tone, rigidity rapidly can be reversed by the injection of a competitive or non-competitive muscle relaxant [133]. Although the increased efferent output at the neuromuscular junction is not reduced, muscle relaxants induce their action by inhibiting the binding of acetylcholine at the motor endplate (Figure II-59).

Because the gabaminergic system in the putamen is involved in the mediation of opioid-induced muscular rigidity, any increase in gabaminergic transmission can also ease this side effect. Such a notion has been supported by results, where a benzodiazepine reduced the increased muscle tone, an effect that could be reversed by the specific benzodiazepine antagonist flumazenil [125]. In addition,

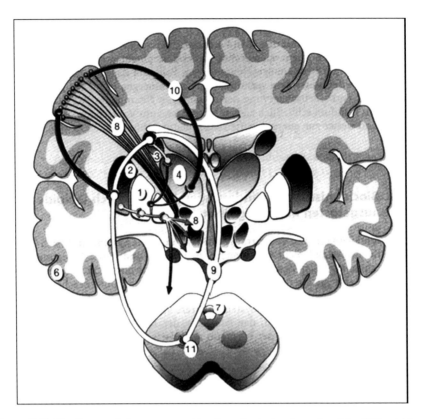

Figure II-58. Significance of the neurotransmitter dopamine in basal ganglia of the CNS, which are involved in the regulation of muscle tone 1 = pallidum externum; 2 = putamen; 3 = nucleus caudatus; 4 = thalamus; 5 = hypothalamus; 6 = lobus parietalis; 7 = central grey; 8 = corticospinal tract; 9 = inhibitory dopaminergic pathway; 10 = thalamo-cortical neurons; 11 = substantia nigra

since neighboring α_2-receptors interact with the substantia nigra, opioid-related rigidity could be attenuated by the additional administration of the α_2-agonist dexmedetomidine [135].

THE PUPILLARY EFFECT OF OPIOIDS

The miotic action of opioids on the pupil is an easily recognizable and quantifiable effect in man. The neural pathways responsible for regulating pupil size are reasonably well defined. Yet, the mechanisms behind this and related effects of opioids on the eye in humans and laboratory animals have just begun to be explored.

Opioid-induced miosis in the human, dog and rabbit is thought to be mediated through the central nervous system. This action is a specific opioid effect as demonstrated by its antagonism by naloxone. Theories have been advanced suggesting

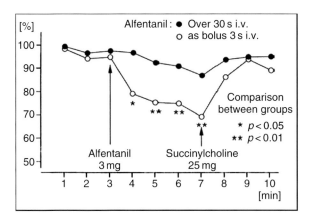

Figure II-59. Alfentanil-induced truncal rigidity in patients following induction of anesthesia. In comparison to the rapid bolus injection of the drug, slow injection over a period of 2 min resulted in a significant lesser reduction of thoracic compliance. The increase in truncal rigidity was instantly reversed by a low dose (25 mg/70 kg body weight) of the fast acting muscle relaxant succinylcholine. Adapted from [134]

that morphine produces its effects by direct stimulation of the Edinger-Westphal (preganglionic parasympathetic) nucleus [181]. An alternative view has been postulated that morphine depresses cortical centers, which normally inhibit the Edinger-Westphal nucleus. Others have suggested that miosis is caused by stimulation of opioid receptors located on the iris sphincter, although this opinion seems to be in the minority.

The exact site, or sites, of action within the CNS, which are responsible for opioid-induced miosis remain obscure. It is generally accepted, however, that sympathetic innervation is not essential, the miotic effect being entirely dependent on the integrity of the parasympathetic system. For example, Lee and Wang [182] have shown that dogs with a sectioned oculomotor nerve fail to show miosis even with a 30 fold increase in the dose of morphine. In contrast, dogs show normal responses following sympathectomy. While local application of a muscarinic antagonist (scopolamine) that blocks the pupil sphincter completely abolishes the pupillary effects of morphine in the rabbit, application of a sympathetic neuronal blocker (guanethidine) or of an alpha-adrenergic antagonist (phentolamine) that block the pupil dilator had no effect in those experiments. Thus, pharmacologic dissection of the autonomic innervation of the pupil suggests that opioid-induced miosis is mediated solely through the parasympathetic system.

Other CNS structures may also be involved in opioid-induced miosis. Lee and Wang [182] have shown that removal of the cerebral hemispheres potentiates the miotic action of morphine in the dog. They interpreted this effect as being a reflection of the loss of tonic inhibition originating in the occipital lobes. The latter are known to play a regulatory role in pupillary function, particularly with respect to the near-response (accommodation, convergence and miosis) and, hence, their removal might be expected to alter the pupillary response to drugs. The same authors also observed that acute or chronic optic nerve section did not alter the miotic response to morphine in dogs.

In humans, it was shown that morphine produced a dose-related miosis under conditions of low ambient light. Taken together, these findings suggest that morphine may cause miosis through more than one mechanism. The main neural structures, which are thought to regulate pupillary size are found in the midbrain, mainly the pretectal area and the Edinger-Westphal nucleus of the oculomotor complex. Because neuronal unit activity in the Edinger-Westphal nucleus has been shown to correlate with light-induced pupillary constriction. Opioids therefore depress or abolish spontaneous and light-induced firing of pupilloconstrictor neurons in the pretectal area, while the opposite effect is observed in the Edinger-Westphal nucleus where a marked increase in spontaneous firing rate resulting in madriasis. It is because of this increase in activity that certain animal species (rat, cat, monkey) demonstrate an opioid-induced mydriasis.

In addition, the brain stem region regulating pupil size is known to have multiple inputs, including the cortex and midbrain, and several others can be assumed to exist. Depression by morphine of tonic inhibitory input trom the cortex may partially account for the miosis observed by Lee and Wang [182]. These findings suggest that opioids may act directly on the neurons subserving the parasympathetic light reflex. Also, in contrast to other workers, morphine has no local action on the iris. For example, Lee and Wang [182] could not produce miosis by injecting 20% of an effective systemic dose of morphine (1 mg) directly into the anterior chamber of the eye in dogs. Although opioid binding sites have been found in the retina of the rat, cow, toad and skate, opioids injected into the anterior chamber may stimulate retinal receptors in some species, causing miosis via reflex parasympathetic output.

OPIOIDS AND GASTROINTESTINAL INHIBITION (CONSTIPATION)

Following oral ingestion, but also after the systemic administration, opioids also bind to selective receptors located within the intestinal tract. The physiological significance of peripherally located opioid binding sites within the intestine is that of regulation of the propulsive transit. The intestine with a total surface of nearly $400\,m^2$ is an underestimated important anatomical site as it has a high accumulation of neuronal tissue, which has been termed the enteral nervous system (ENS), which acts like a second brain. Since there is a close interconnection of the ENS with the CNS via the vagus nerve, regular impulses to and from the ENS are being exchanged. Anatomically the intestine is surrounded by two separate syncytial, net-like nervous structures. One is the myentericus plexus (Auerbach) located between the longitudinal and the circulatory muscle fibers (Figure II-60). The second is the submucosal Meissner plexus, located between circulatory and the submucosal muscle fibers.

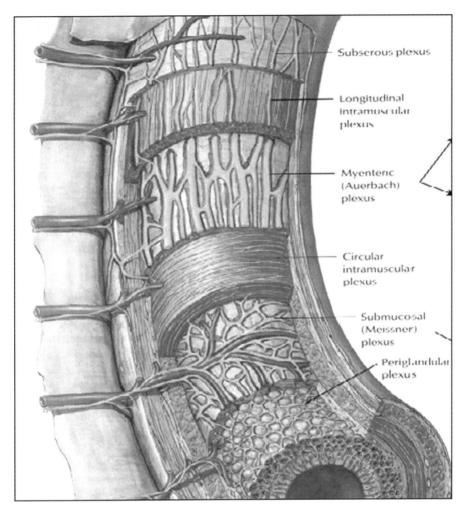

Subserous plexus

Longitudinal
intramuscular
plexus

Myenteric
(Auerbach)
plexus

Circular
intramuscular
plexus

Submucosal
(Meissner)
plexus

Periglandular
plexus

Figure II-60. The two different nervous plexus surrounding the intestinal tract, the myenteric and the submucosal plexus, necessary parts in the propulsive transit and the regulation of digestion

Within the Auerbach plexus of the intestinal tract, there is a balance between the cholinergic and enkephalinergic neurons: Binding of systemically applied opioids to enkaphalinergic receptor sites results in an inhibition of transit followed by constipation. Contrarily, cholinesterase inhibitors induce an accumulation of acetylcholine at ACh-receptors with an increase in motility and an enhancement of transit. Presently, however, not very much is known of the long-term effect of central analgesics on opioid-receptors within the myenteric plexus, and if opioid ligands induce only a constipating effect, whether they also depress the immune system in the intestine or result in a distress the neuroregulatory and endocrine function.

CLINICAL RELEVANCE OF OPIOID-INDUCED CONSTIPATION

While analgesia, respiratory depression, bradycardia, antitussive action and miosis all are centrally induced opioid effects, the most relevant peripheral opiod action is that of constipation [109] [136]. This is most relevant in patients with chronic pain taking an opioid for its attenuation. Being one of the major side effects, it often results in the necessity to take a laxative on a routine basis. The cause for such constipation is the constriction of the pylorus resulting in a delay in emptying of the stomach [137]. However, most important, opioids induce a constriction of the small intestine resulting in a delay of the propulsive transit. Because selective opioid binding sites are mainly located in the small intestine, opioids inhibit the release of local acetylcholine [136, 137, 138], followed by a concomitant loss of coordinated propulsive movements of the gut. A constipating effect of opioids on the large intestine is of significantly lesser degree, because this part of the intestinal tract contributes to a much lesser extent to the overall constipating effect. This is because continuous propulsive movements are not seen on this area, and contrary to the small intestine, the percentage of enkephalinergic neurons is significantly lower [139, 140]. In addition, enkephalin derivatives are able to inhibit transit in the small while at the same time increasing contractions in the large intestine [141]. Systemically μ-selective applied opioids therefore primarily interact with enkephalinergic neurons in the antrum, the duodenum, and the small intestine, all of which results in a delay of transit [142, 143, 144, 145]. The constipating effect of an opioid can be reversed by a selective peripheral acting antagonists such as methylnaltrexone [146, 147] or alvimopane [148].

Opioids, which interact primarily with the κ-opioid receptor induce a lesser constipating effect [148, 149], while δ-selective ligands induce no effect on gastrointestinal transit [150].

Comparable to a ketamine- or a volatile anesthetic based regimen, an opioid-based anesthesia results in a longer delay of gastrointestinal emptying in the postoperative period [151, 152] (Figure II-61). This, however, is clinically of little significance, as the potential constipating effect does not last longer than 48 h after anesthesia.

OPIOIDS AND THE CARDIOVASCULAR SYSTEM

Contrarily to many other anesthetics, opioids in general do not depress the cardiovascular system. This is also reflected in the higher therapeutic range (LD_{50}/ED_{50}) being derived in the animal (Table II-11). Such data can also be conveyed to the human, since a wide therapeutic margin of safety is directly correlated with a lack in cardiovascular impairment.

While carfentanil, with a potency twice that of sufentanil, is solely used in veterinary medicine for the immobilization of wild animals [153], lofentanil (20-fold potency of fentanyl), due to its intensive receptor binding, is characterized by a duration of action of 24 h [154]. Both fentanyl derivates are not in clinical

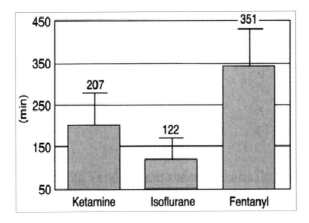

Figure II-61. Different postoperative gastrointestinal transit times (min) in patients after a fentanyl-, a ketamine-, and an isoflurane-based anesthesia regimen respectively. Note the significant longer delay of gastrointestinal transit in the fentanyl-based technique. Adapted from [151]

Table II-11. Margin of safety of different opioid ligands in comparison to barbiturates and the hypnotic etomidate

Pharmacological agent	Therapeutic margin of safety LD_{50}/ED_{50}
Tramadol	3
Pentazocine	4
Thiopental	8
Pethidine	6
Methohexital	11
Ketamine	11
Methadone	12
Meptazinol	18
Etomidate	32
Butorphanol	45
Morphine	71
Dextromoramide	105
Lofentanil	112
Fentanyl	277
Nalbuphine	1034
Alfentanil	1080
Buprenorphine	7933
Carfentanil	10.000
Sufentanil	26.716
Remifentanil	33.000

use, because the high potency and the intense receptor binding would be difficult to handle in patients. From the table, however, it is obvious that the higher the selectivity to the receptor site, and the higher the potency, the lesser the amount of cardiovascular depression [33, 35, 103, 155, 156, 157].

Following the injection of potent opioids, bradycardia is the most prominent cardiovascular effect seen in patients. This is due to a direct central stimulation of the nucleus nervi vagi and a typical effect of μ-ligands. Thereafter, a reduction of the sympathetic drive is initiated resulting in an overexpression of parasympathetic activity. Also, a direct peripheral negative inotropic activity with a potentiation of acetylcholine release at the sinus node of the heart is discussed [158]. The increase in vagal tone and the reduction of sympathetic drive on the peripheral vasculature results in a decline of mean arterial pressure. A reduction of sympathetic tone on vessel tone and a reduction of resistance is also termed as "pooling" of circulating blood volume. Such a reduction of peripheral resistance in certain cases may be of benefit for the patient, as it is accompanied by a reduction in afterload of the heart [159, 160]. Bradycardia, the reduced peripheral resistance (i.e. afterload of heart) as well as the pooling effect with a reduction of preload of the heart, can be of benefit for a patient with myocardial infarction. This is because those three variables are major determinants in myocardial oxygen consumption (MVO_2) [160, 161]. It, however, should be noted that the sympatholytic action with pooling of blood volume induced by potent opioids might demask a previously compensated hypovolemic condition in a patient resulting in significant hypotension. For instance, in patients with multiple trauma a reduced dose of the opioid should be given, either diluted or slowly injected while measuring blood pressure continuously. In general, however, especially in polytraumatized patients, opioids are of benefit, as they reduce the stress-related release of hormones and particularly of angiotensin II, maintaining the effect of circulating catecholamines on the vasculature.

Opioid-related bradycardia with an accompanying hypotension can rapidly be reversed with increasing doses of the vagolytic agent atropine (0.25–05–1.0 mg/kg body weight). The incidence and the severity of such a drop in blood pressure cannot be foreseen. It is related to the autonomic basal tone of the patient and the dose of the injected potent μ-ligand (Figure II-62).

Depending on the product, the autonomic basal tone of, and the applied dosages to the patient, either parasympathetic (inhibitory) and/or a sympathetic (excitatory) symptoms are induced (Table II-12). Such clinical effects can be diminished by atropine, an α-blocker (e.g. phenoxybenzamine), a ß-blocker (e.g. propranolol), and a ganglionic blocker (e.g. hexamethonium) respectively [103].

The stimulatory effects of opioids can also be explained in the laboratory where stimulation of cyclic AMP formation, phosphinoside hydrolysis, and the elevation of intracellular calcium, resulting from mobilization of calcium stores and by stimulating influx, which leads to an increased neurotransmitter release and neurotransmission [163]. Thus, at the cellular level these changes may underlie the opioid stimulatory effect. In addition, such stimulation is also discussed as playing a part in the development of tolerance to opioid drugs [164].

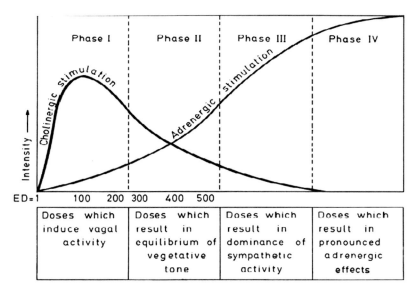

Figure II-62. The effect of increasing doses (mg/kg body weight) of potent opioids on the cardiovascular system of the canine, where low amounts result in parasympathetic activation, and high to massive doses induce an increase of sympathetic drive. Adapted from [103]

In opioid-based anesthesia, vagal- or sympathetic-induced side effects can be reduced or eliminated by the following techniques:

1. The preliminary administration of atropine (up to 1 mg/kg body weight).
2. The simultaneous administration of a volatile anesthetic (N_2O, enflurane, desflurane, sevoflurane).
3. The simultaneous use of a neuroleptic agent (e.g. droperidol, haloperidol).
4. The simultaneous use of a benzodiazepine (e.g. diazepam, midazolam, lorazepam).
5. The simultaneous use of a hypnotic (e.g. barbiturate, etomidate, propofol).

Table II-12. The main inhibitory (parasympathetic) and excitatory (sympathetic) effects induced by different doses of opioids

Dominant sympathetic drive	Dominant parasympathetic drive
Hypertonia	Bradycardia
Tachycardia	Hypotonia
Hyperglycemia	Emesis
Hyperlactemia	Sweating
Acrocyanosis	Salivation
Scleral injection	Bronchospasm
Reddening of the face	Sphincter spasm
Antidiuresis	Miosis

Adapted from [103, 162]

All these agents induce a depression of CNS activity in different areas of the central nervous system, which results in equilibrium of the autonomic nervous system discharge, thus, reducing the overshoot of sympathetic and/or parasympathetic tone (Figure II-63).

Mixed agonist/antagonists, when given in dosages above the therapeutic range, induce a cardiostimulatory sympathomimetic effect, which purportedly is induced via stimulation of σ-receptor sites [165]. As a result, tachycardia, an increase in peripheral vascular resistance, and an increase in pulmonary artery pressure are induced (Table II-13), all of which increase myocardial oxygen consumption (MVO2). Therefore agonist/antagonists should not be given above their therapeutic range in patients with MI or with a preexistent cardiovascular disease [166].

A malfunction at the atrio-ventricular node in the myocardium, followed by prolongation of the P–Q interval is a phenomenon, which can be induced in patients demonstrating a preexisting abnormal conduction system in the heart. Such prolongation manifests itself especially when potent opioids are being administered (fentanyl, sufentanil), whereby the opioid-induced acetylcholine release induces a stimulation of vagal activity. Thus, patients already having a prolongation of P–Q time or who present a sick-sinus syndrome, extreme bradycardia has to be anticipated, which could result in concomitant cardiac arrest. In order to prevent such a scenario, the opioid should not be given as a bolus, but rather as a diluted solution. In addition, the solution should be injected slowly over a long period of time

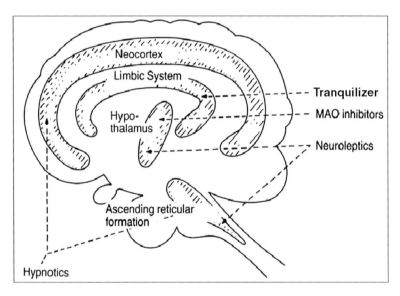

Figure II-63. Site of action of different pharmacological agents in the CNS to potentiate opioid action. Neuroleptics block afferents from entering the ascending reticular formation, which increase vigilance; tranquillizers protect the hippocampus from an excitatory activation, while barbiturates, hypnotics and volatile anesthetics primarily block the cerebral cortex from arousal

Table II-13. Different cardiovascular effects of μ-ligands, mixed agonist/antagonists, and partial agonists resulting in a decrease (⇓) or an increase (⇑)

Opioid	Blood pressure	Heart rate	Pulmonary artery pressure
Morphine	⇓	⇓ to 0	⇓ to 0
Buprenorphine	⇓	⇓ to 0	0
Butorphanol	⇑ to 0	0	⇑
Pentazocine	⇑	⇑	⇑
Meptazinol	(⇑)	(⇑)	⇑
Nalbuphine	0	⇓ to 0	0
Fentanyl	⇓	⇓	0
Sufentanil	⇓	⇓	0

Adapted from [166, 167, 168]

of at least 2 min. If, however, extreme bradycardia is recognized on the monitor, atropine is the agent of choice (0.5–1.0 mg/kg body weight) for rapid reversal. In very extreme cases, the antiarrythmic agent metaproterenol may become necessary, as it is able to increase atrio-ventricular conduction.

High doses of methadone or its derivative α-levoacetylmethadol (LAAM) may result in life threatening *torsades de points* with the potential of ensuing ventricular fibrillation. Predisposing factors for the development of such a situation are a prolongation of atrio-ventricular conduction time, hypopotassemia, and/or the simultaneous intake of agents, which inhibit metabolism of the opioid (e.g. tricyclic antidepressants, imidazol derivatives, antimalaria agents, or antihistaminics).

A direct negative inotropic effect on the myocardium has been demonstrated in the isolated papillary muscle and in the Langendorff preparation of the heart for a variety of opioids [169, 170]. Such direct effects, however, are not of clinical significance, because such a depression is only evident in concentrations above the therapeutic range. In addition, compensatory cardiovascular and the autonomic regulatory mechanisms come into play when an opioid is given to a subject.

Following the intravenous injection of pethidine (meperidine, USP), hypotonia and syncope may result. Because of the atropine-like molecular structure of this agent, tachycardia, as well as reflex bradycardia can be observed [171]. For the reason of these potential side effects pethidine should not be given to patients with myocardial infarction [109].

In addition, it is observed that in a shock-like situation, due to the release of endogenous opioids (enkephalins, endorphins), the additional administration of an exogenous opioid results in an additional occupation of opioid binding sites within the myocardium. This aspect is followed by a negative inotropic effect with an unfavorable consequence on hemodynamics [172].

Some experimental work has postulated a putative direct negative inotropic effect of N_2O in an opioid-based anesthetic regimen [173]. Since this is mainly seen when N_2O is given in concentrations above 50% with a resultant drop in FIO_2, this very

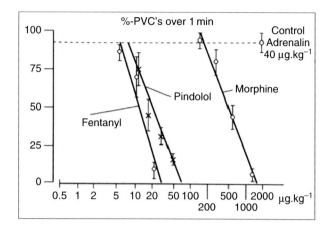

Figure II-64. Antiarrythmic effect of fentanyl and morphine in comparison to the ß-blocker pindolol. Both agents dose-dependently reduce adrenaline-induced ventricular extrasystoles. Adapted from [180] PVC-premature ventricular countraction

likely is due to an insufficient myocardial oxygen supply. In addition, high concentrations of N_2O have a direct vasodilatory effect, resulting in a reduction of venous return to the heart and a drop in blood pressure [174]. It therefore is advocated that in patients receiving opioid anesthesia with a preexisting cardiovascular disease, the optimal concentration in FIO_2 should be around 0.5.

Opioids also have been demonstrated to induce an anti-arrhythmic effect. This has been shown in the animal for meptazinol [175] and in experimental coronary artery occlusion, using fentanyl, sufentanil and carfentanil respectively [176, 177, 178] (Figure II-64). The reason for such an antifibrillatory effect seems to be due to the increase in vagal tone [179].

References

1. Dhawan, B.N., et al., *International union of pharmacology. XII. Classification of opioid receptors.* Pharmacol Rev, 1996, **48**: pp. 567–592.
2. Ling, G.S.F., et al., *Separation of opioid analgesia from respiratory depression: evidence of different receptor mechanism.* J Pharmacol Exp Ther, 1985, **232**: pp. 149–155.
3. Della Bella, D., F. Casacci, and A. Sassi, *Opiate receptors: different ligand affinity in various brain regions.* Adv Biochem Psychopharmacol, 1978, **18**: pp. 271–277.
4. Pan, Y.X., et al., *Identification and characterization of three new alternative spliced mu-opioid receptors.* Mol Pharmacol, 1999, **56**: pp. 396–403.
5. Martin, W.R., et al., *The effects of morphine and nalorphine-like drugs in the non-dependant and morphine-dependant chronic spinal dog.* J Pharmacol Exp Ther, 1976, **197**: pp. 517–532.

6. Gorman, A.L., K.J. Elliott, and C.E. Inturrisi, *The D- and the L-isomers of methadone bind to the non-competitive site on the NMDA receptor in the rat forebrain and spinal cord.* Neurosci Lett, 1997, **223**: pp. 5–8.

7. Quiding, H., et al., *Plasma concentrations of codeine and its metabolite morphine, after single and repeated oral administration.* Eur J Clin Pharmacol, 1986, **30**: pp. 673–677.

8. Rossi, G.C., et al., *Novel receptor mechanisms for heroin and morphine-6ß-glucoronide analgesia.* Neurosci Lett, 1996, **216**: pp. 1–4.

9. Ross, F.B. and M.T. Smith, *The intrinsic antinociceptive effects of oxycodone appear to be k-opioid receptor mediated.* Pain, 1997, **73**: pp. 151–157.

10. Ebert, B., S. Andersen, and P. Krogsgrad-Karsen, *Ketobemidone, methadone and pethidine are non-comptitve N-methyl-D-aspartate (NMDA) antagonists in the rat cortex and spinal cord.* Neurosci Lett, 1995, **187**: pp. 165–168.

11. Magnan, J., et al., *The binding spectrum of narcotic analgesic drugs with different agonist and antagonist properties.* Naunyn-Schmiedebergs Arch Pharmacol, 1982, **319**: pp. 197–205.

12. Corbett, D., S.J. Paterson, and H.W. Kosterlitz, *Selectivity of ligands for opioid receptors*, in *Opioids I. Handbook of Experimental Pharmacology*, A. Herz, Editor, 1993, Springer: Berlin, Heidelberg, New York. pp. 645–680.

13. Schmidt, W.K., et al., *Nalbuphine.* Drug Alcohol Depend, 1985. **14**: pp. 339–362.

14. Meert, T.F., et al., *Comparison between epidural fentanyl, sufentanil, carfentanil, lofentanil and alfentanil in rats: analgesia and other in vivo effects.* Eur J Aneasth, 1988, **5**: pp. 313–321.

15. Kögel, B., et al., *Interaction of μ-opioid receptor agonists and antagonists with the analgesic effect of buprenorphine in mice.* Eur J Pain, 2005, **9**: pp. 599–611.

16. Engelberger, T., et al., *In vitro and ex vivo reversibility of the opioid receptor binding of buprenorphine*, in *Pain in Europe IV*, 2003, Prague, European Federation of the International Association for the Study of Pain Chapters: Czek Republik.

17. Pert, P.B. and S.H. Snyder, *Opiate receptor: demonstration in nervous tissue.* Science, 1973, **179**: pp. 1011–1014.

18. Wood, P.L., *Multiple opiate receptors: support for unique mu, delta and kappa sites.* Neuropharmacology, 1982, **21**: pp. 487–497.

19. Foote, R.W. and R. Maurer, *Autoradiographic localization of opiate k-receptors in the guinea pig brain.* Eur J Pharmacol, 1982, **85**: pp. 99–103.

20. Goodman, R.R. and S.H. Snyder, *Autoradiographic localization of kappa opiate receptors to deep layers of the cerebral cortex may explain unique sedative and analgesic effects.* Life Sci, 1982, **31**: pp. 1291–1294.

21. Kosterlitz, H.W. and S.J. Paterson, *Characterization of opioid receptors in nervous tissue.* Proc R Soc Lond, 1980, **210**: pp. 113–122.

22. Dahan, A., et al., *Buprenorphine causes ceiling effect in respiratory depression but not in analgesic effect.* Anesthesiology, 2003, **99**: p. A1530.

23. Walsh, S.L. and T. Eissenberg, *The clinical pharmacology of buprenorphine: extrapolating from the laboratory to the clinic.* Drug Alcohol Depend, 2003, **70**: pp. S13–S27.

24. Walsh, S.L., K.L. Preston, and M.L. Stitzer, *Clinical pharmacology of buprenorphine: ceiling effects at high doses.* Clin Pharmacol Ther, 1994, **55**: pp. 569–580.

25. Terenius, L., *Specific uptake of narcotic analgesics by subcellular fractions of the guinea pig ileum.* Acta Pharmacol Toxicol, 1972, **31**: p. 50.

26. Kosterlitz, H.W. and A.A. Waterfield, *In vitro models in the study of structure-activity relationships of narcotic analgesics.* Ann Rev Pharmacol, 1975, **15**: pp. 29–47.

27. Hassler, R., *Über die antagonistischen Systeme der Schmerzempfindung und des Schmerzgefühls im peripheren und zentralen Nervensystem*, in *Pentazocin im Spiegel de Entwöhnung*, S. Kubicki and G.A. Neuhaus, Editors, 1976, Springer: Berlin, Heidelberg, New York. pp. 1–17.

28. Simantov, R., A.M. Snowman, and S.H. Snyder, *A morphine-like factor "enkephalin" in rat brain: subcellular localization*. Brain Res, 1976, **107**: pp. 650–655.

29. Hong, J.S., et al., *Determination of methionine enkephalin in discrete regions of rat brain*. Brain Res, 1977, **134**: p. 383.

30. Melzack, R. and P.C. Wall, *Pain mechanisms: a new theory*. Science, 1965, **150**: p. 971.

31. Snyder, S.H., D.C. U'Prichard, and D.A. Greenberg, *Neurotransmitter receptor binding in the brain*, in *Psychopharmacology: A Generation of Progress*, M.A. Lipton, A. DiMascio, and K.F. Killam, Editors, 1978, Raven: New York. pp. 361–370.

32. Pazos, A. and J. Florez, *Interaction of naloxone with mu- and delta-opioid agonists on respiration of rats*. Eur J Pharmacol, 1983, **87**: pp. 309–314.

33. Leysen, J.E., W. Gommeren, and C.J.E. Niemegeers, *3H-sufentanil, a superior ligand for the mu-opiate receptor: binding properties and regional distribution in rat brain and spinal cord*. Eur J Pharmacol, 1983, **87**: pp. 209–225.

34. Niemegeers, C.J.E. and P.A.J. Janssen, *Alfentanil (R 39 209) – a particularly short-acting narcotic analgesic in rats*. Drug Dev Res, 1981, **1**: pp. 83–88.

35. Van Bever, W.F.M., et al., *N-4-substituted 1-(2arylethyl)-4-piperidinyl-N-phenylpropanamides, a novel series of extremely potenet analgesics with unusually high safety margin*. Drug Res/Arzneimittelforsch, 1978, **26**: pp. 1548–1551.

36. Woolf, C.J. and R.J. Mannion, *Neuropathic pain: aetiology, symptoms, mechanisms, and management*. Lancet, 1999, **353**: pp. 1959–1964.

37. Pilowsky, J., *Current views on the role of psychiatrists in the management of the chronic pain*, in *The Therapy of Pain*, N. Swerdlow, Editor, 1981, MTI Press: Lancaster.

38. Pinsky, J.J., *Psychodynamics and psychotherapy in the treatment of patients with chronic pain*, in *Chronic Pain*, B.L. Crue, Editor, 1978, Spectrum: New York.

39. Ngai, S.H., *The effects of morphine and meperidine on the central respiratory mechanisms in the cat: the action of levallorphan in antagonizing these effects*. J Pharmacol Exp Ther, 1961, **131**: pp. 91–102.

40. Florez, J. and A. Mediavilla, *Respiratory and cardiovascular effects of met-enkephalin applied to the ventral surface of the brain stem*. Brain Res, 1978, **138**: pp. 585–590.

41. Freye, E. and E. Hartung, *Fentanyl in the fourth cerebral ventricle causes respiratory depression in the anesthetized but not in the awake dog*. Acta Anesthesiol Scand, 1981, **25**: pp. 171–173.

42. Ngai, S.H., et al., *Pharmacokinetics of naloxone in rats and man. Basis for its potency and short duration of action*. Anesthesiology, 1976, **44**: p. 44.

43. Freye, E., E. Hartung, and S. Kalibe, *Prevention of late fentanyl-induced respiratory depression after the injection of the opiate antagonists naltrexone and S-20682 as compared to naloxone*. Br J Anaesth, 1983, **55**: pp. 71–77.

44. Stoeckel, H., J.H. Hengstmann, and J. Schüttler, *Pharmacokinetics of fentanyl as a possible explanation for recurrence of respiratory depression*. Br J Anaesth, 1979, **51**: p. 741.

45. Houde, R.W., *Analgesic effectiveness of the narcotic agonist-antagonists*. Brit J Clin Pharmacol, 1979, **7**: pp. 297S–308S.

46. Freye, E., *Opioid agonists, antagonists and mixed narcotic analgesics: their use in postoperative and chronic pain management*. Drugs of Today, 1989, **25**: pp. 741–754.

47. Magruder, M.R., R.D. DeLaney, and C.A. DiFazio, *Reversal of narcotic-induced respiratory depression with nalbuphine hydrochloride.* Anesthesiol Rev, 1982, **9**: pp. 34–37.

48. Freye, E., L. Azevedo, and E. Hartung, *Reversal of fentanyl-related respiratory depression with nalbuphine; effects on the CO2-response curve of man.* Acta Anaesth Belg, 1985, **36**: pp. 365–374.

49. Bailey, P.L., et al., *Antagonism of postoperative opioid-induced respiratory depression: nalbuphine versus naloxone.* Anesth Analg, 1987, **66**: pp. 1109–1114.

50. Freye, E., E. Hartung, and M. Segeth, *Nalbuphine reverses fentanyl-related EEG changes in man.* Acta Anaesth Belg, 1984, **35**: pp. 25–36.

51. Gal, T.J. and C.A. DiFazio, *Prolonged antagonism of opioid action with intravenous nalmefene in man.* Anesthesiology, 1986, **64**: pp. 175–180.

52. Moore, L.R., et al., *Antagonism of fentanyl-induced respiratory depression with nalmefene.* Meth Find Expt Clin Pharmacol, 1990, **12**(1): pp. 29–35.

53. Smith, T.W., et al., *Enkephalins: isolation, distribution and function,* in *Opiates and Endogenous Opioid Peptides,* 1976, Elsevier: Amsterdam.

54. Yeadon, M. and I. Kitchen, *Multiple opioid receptors mediate the respiratory depressant effect of fentanyl-like drugs in the rat.* Gen Pharmac, 1990, **21**: pp. 655–664.

55. Pasternak, G.W. and P.J. Wood, *Minireview: multiple mu opiate receptors.* Life Sci, 1986, **38**: pp. 1889–1898.

56. Pasternak, G.W., *Multiple morphine and enkephalin receptors and the relief of pain.* JAMA, 1988, **259**: pp. 1362–1367.

57. Bailey, P.L., et al., *Differences in magnitude and duration of opioid induced respiratory depression and analgesia with fentanyl and sufentanil.* Anesth Analg, 1990, **70**: pp. 8–15.

58. Vaught, J.L., R.B. Rothman, and T.C. Westfall, *Mu and delta receptors: their role in analgesia and in the differential effects of opioid peptides on analgesia.* Life Sci, 1982, **30**: pp. 1443–1455.

59. Freye, E., M. Schnitzler, and G. Schenk, *Opioid-induced respiratory depression and analgesia may be mediated by different subreceptors.* Pharm Res, 1991, **8**: pp. 196–199.

60. Freye, E., L. Latasch, and P.S. Portoghese, *The delta receptor is envolved in sufentanil-induced respiratory depression.* Eur J Anaesthesiol, 1992, **9**: pp. 457–462.

61. He, L. and N. Lee, *Delta opid receptor enhancement of mu opioid receptor-induced antinociception in spinal cord.* J Pharmacol Expt Ther, 1998, **285**: pp. 1181–1186.

62. Egan, T.D., et al., *The pharmacokinetics and pharmacodynamics of GI87084B.* Anesthesiology, 1992, **77**(3A): p. A369.

63. Hughes, M.A., P.S.A. Glass, and J.R. Jacobs, *Context-sensitive half-time in multicompartment pharmacokinetic models for intravenous anesthetic drugs.* Anesthesiology, 1992, **76**: pp. 334–341.

64. Fink, B.R., *Influence of cerebral activity in wakefulness on regulation of breathing.* J Appl Physiol, 1961, **16**: pp. 15–23.

65. Sullivan, C.E., et al., *Waking and ventilatory responses to laryngeal stimulation in sleeping dogs.* J Appl Physiol, 1978, **45**: pp. 681–688.

66. Latasch, L. and R. Christ, *Respiratory safety,* in *Transdermal Fentanyl,* K. Lehmann and D. Zech, Editors, 1991, Springer: Berlin, Heidelberg, New York, Tokyo. pp. 149–157.

67. De Castro, J., *Association des analgésiques centraux et des neuroleptiques en cours d'intervention,* in *Les analgésiques et la douleur. Influences pharmacologiques diverses exercées sur morphiniques,* G. Vourch, et al., Editors, 1971, Masson: Paris. pp. 185–194, 383–403.

68. Maurer, P.M. and R.R. Bartkowski, *Drug interactions of clinical significance with opioid analgesics.* Drug Safety, 1993, **8**: pp. 30–48.

69. Sifton, D.W., *Drug interaction and side effects index™*, in 42 ed. Physicians Desk Reference (*PDR*), M. Trelewicz, Editor, 1988, Medical Economics Company Inc: Oradell, New York pp. 1–787.

70. Lehmann, K.A., et al., *Biotransformation von fentanyl. II. Akute Arzneimittelinteraktion – Untersuchungen bei Ratte und Mensch.* Anaesthesist, 1982, **31**: pp. 221–227.

71. Harper, M.H., et al., *The magnitude and the duration of respiratory depression produced by fentanyl and fentanyl plus droperidol in man.* J Pharmacol Exp Ther, 1976, **199**: pp. 464–455.

72. Becker, C.E., et al., *A quick guide to common drug interaction*, in *Patient Care*, J. Bigelow, Editor, 1974, Miller & Fink: Philadelphia. pp. 1–32.

73. Gibaldi, M. and D. Perrier, *Pharmacokinetics*, 1975, Marcel Dekker: New York.

74. Elstrom, J., *Plasma protein binding of phenytoin after cholecystectomy and neurosurgical operations.* Acta neur scand, 1977, **55**: p. 455.

75. MacClain, D.A. and C.C.J. Hug, *Intravenous fentanyl kinetics.* Clin Pharmacol Ther, 1980, **28**: p. 106.

76. Olson, G.D., W.M. Bennett, and G.A. Porter, *Morphine and phenytoin binding to human plasma protein in renal and hepatic failure.* Clin Pharmacol Ther, 1975, **17**: p. 677.

77. Corall, I.M., A.R. Moore, and L. Strunin, *Plasma concentrations of fentanyl in normal surgical patients and those with severe renal and hepatic disease.* Br J Anaesth, 1980, **52**: p. 101.

78. Ekman, A., et al., *Reduction in the incidence of awareness using BIS monitoring.* Acta Anaesth Scand, 2004, **48**: pp. 20–26.

79. Römer, D., et al., *Bremazocine: a potent, long-acting opiate kappa-agonist.* Life Sci, 1980, **27**: pp. 971–978.

80. Freye, E., E. Hartung, and G.K. Schenk, *Tifluadom (KC-5103) induces suppression and latency changes of somatosensory-evoked potentials which are reversed by opioid antagonists.* Life Sci, 1983, **33**: pp. 537–540.

81. Freye, E., E. Hartung, and G.K. Schenk, *Bremazocine: an opiate which induces sedation and analgesia but no respiratory depression.* Anesth Analg, 1983, **62**: pp. 483–488.

82. Wevers, A., et al., *Cellular distribution of the mRNA for the k-opiod receptor in the human neocortex: a non-isotopic in situ hybridization study.* Neurosci Let, 1995, **195**: pp. 1–4.

83. Pfeiffer, A., et al., *Opiate receptor binding sites in human brain.* Brain Res, 1982, **248**: pp. 87–96.

84. De Castro, J. and P. Viars, *Utilisation pratique des analgesiques centraux en anesthesie et reanimation.* Ars Med, 1968, **23**: pp. 1–228.

85. Wermeling, D.P., et al., *Patient-controlled analgesia using butorphanol for postoperative pain control: an open label study*, in *Butorphanol Tartrate: Research Advances in Multiple Clinical Settings*, C.E. Rosow, Editor, 1986, S. Karger: Basel, Paris, London, New York, Singapore, Sydney. pp. 31–39.

86. Freye, E., F. Ciramelli, and A. Fournell, *Nalbuphine versus pentazocine in postoperative pain after orthopedic surgery.* Schmerz-Pain-Douleur, 1986, **3**: pp. 101–105.

87. Murphy, M.R. and C.C. Hug, *The enflurane sparing effect of morphine, butorphanol, and nalbuphine.* Anesthesiology, 1982, **57**: pp. 489–492.

88. Dumas, P.A. *MAC reduction of enflurane and isoflurane and postoperative findings with nalbuphine HCl and fentanyl: A retrospective study*, in *VII World Congress of Anaesthesiologists*. 1984, Exerpta Medica: Manila/Philippines, Amsterdam.

89. Romagnoli, A. and A.S. Keats, *Ceiling effect for respiratory depression by nalbuphine*. Clin Pharmacol Ther, 1980, **27**: pp. 478–485.

90. Kubicki, S. and R. Stölzel, *The "narcotic" component of fentanyl. L'anesthese vigile et subvigile*. Ars Med, 1970, **1**: p. 37.

91. Kugler, J., et al., *Die hypnotische Wirkung von Fentanyl und Sufentanil*. Anaesthesist, 1977, **26**: pp. 343–348.

92. Freye, E. and E. Hartung, *Kardiovaskuläre und zentralnervöse Effekte unter Fentanyl versus Sufentanil bei der Intubation herzchirurgischer Patienten*. Anästhesie Aktuell, 1993, **9**: pp. 3–14.

93. Nilsson, E. and D.H. Ingvar, *EEG findings in neuroleptanalgesia*. Acta Anaesth Scand, 1967, **11**: pp. 121–127.

94. Kubicki, S.T., G. Freund, and M. Schoppenhorst, *Fentanyl und Sufentanil im elektroenezephalographischen Vergleich*. Anaesthesist, 1977, **26**: pp. 333–342.

95. Ingvar, D.H. and E. Nilsson, *Central nervous effects of neuroleptanalgesia as induced by haloperidol and phenoperidine*. Acta Anaesth Scand, 1961, **5**: pp. 85–88.

96. Kubicki, S. and Z. P., *EEG-Veränderungen durch Neuroleptanalgesie*. Anästh Wiederbelebg, 1966, **9**: pp. 44–49.

97. Kubicki, S., and P. Zodeck, *Exzitatorische und inhibitorische Phänomene am Zentralnervensystem, verursacht durch Fentanyl*, in *Neue Klinische Aspekte der Neuroleptanalgesie*, W.F. Henschel, Editor, 1970, Schattauer: Stuttgart, New York. pp. 21–30.

98. Freye, E. and J.O. Arndt, *Perfusion of the fourth cerebral ventricle with fentanyl induces naloxone reversible hypotension, bradycardia, baroreflex depression and sleep in unanaesthetized dogs*. Naunyn-Schmiedebergs Arch Pharmacol, 1979, **307**: pp. 123–128.

99. Kuhar, M.J., C.B. Pert, and S.H. Snyder, *Regional distribution of opiate receptor binding in monkey and human brain*. Nature, 1973, **245**: pp. 447–450.

100. Mc Kenzie, J.S. and N.R. Beechy, *The effects of morphine and pethidine on somatic evoked responses in the midbrain of the cat, and their relevance to analgesia*. Electroenceph Clin Neurophysiol, 1962, **14**: pp. 501–519.

101. Hassler, R., *Wechselwirkungen zwischen dem System der schnellen Schmerzempfindung und dem des langsamen, nachhaltigen Schmerzgefühl*. Arch Klin Chir, 1976, **342**: p. 47.

102. Hassler, R., *Über die Zweiteilung der Schmerzempfindung und des Schmerzgefühl*, in *Schmerz*, J. R., et al., Editors, 1972, Thieme: Stuttgart. p. 105.

103. De Castro, J., et al., *Comparative study of cardiovascular, neurological, and metabolic side effects of eight narcotics in dogs*. Acta Anaesth Belg, 1979, **30**: pp. 5–99.

104. Goroszeniuk, I., A. Malagosia, and R.M. Jones, *Genralized grand mal seizure after recovery from uncomplicated fentanyl-etomidate anesthesia*. Anesth Analg, 1986, **65**: pp. 979–981.

105. Hoten, A.O., *Another case of grand mal seizure after fentanyl aministration*. Anesthesiology, 1983, **60**: pp. 387–388.

106. Brian, S.E. and A.B. Seifen, *Tonic-clonic activity after sufentanil*. Anesth Analg, 1987, **66**: p. 481.

107. Scott, J.C. and F.H. Sarnquist, *Seizure-like movements during fentanyl infusion with absence of seizure activity in a simultaneous EEG recording*. Anesthesiology, 1983, **62**: pp. 812–814.

108. Carlsson, C., et al., *The effects of high-dose fentanyl on cerebral circulation and metabolism in rats.* Anesthesiology, 1982, **57**: pp. 375–380.
109. Jaffe, J.H. and W.R. Martin, *Opioid analgesics and antagonists*, in *The Pharmacological Basis of Therapeutics*, A.G. Gilman, et al., Editors, 1993, McGraw Hill: New York. pp. 485–531.
110. Kugler, J., A. Doenicke, and M. Laub, *Das Elektroenzephalogramm nach Etomidate.* Anaesthesiol Wiederbeleb, 1977, **106**: pp. 31–47.
111. Irwin, R.S., *Cough*, in *Diagnose and Treatment of Symptoms of the Respiratory Tract*, R.S. Irwin, F.J. Curley, and R.F. Grossman, Editors, 1997, Futura Publishing Company: New York. pp. 1–54.
112. Chau, T.T., F.E. Carter, and L.S. Harris, ^3H-codeine binding in the guinea pig lower brain stem. Pharmacology, 1982, **25**: pp. 12–17.
113. Borrison, H.L. and S.C. Wang, *Physiology and pharmacology of vomiting.* Pharmacol Rev, 1953, **5**: pp. 192–230.
114. Scuderi, P., et al., *Treatment of postoperative nausea and vomiting after outpatient surgery with the 5-HT3 antagonist ondansetron.* Anesthesiology, 1993, **78**(1): pp. 15–20.
115. McKenzie, R., et al., *Comparison of ondansetron versus placebo to prevent postoperative nausea and vomiting in women undergoing ambulatory gynecologic surgery.* Anesthesiology, 1993, **78**(1): pp. 21–28.
116. Gan, T.J., et al., *Coinsensus guidelines for managing postoperative nausea and vomiting.* Anesth Analg, 2003, **97**: pp. 62–71.
117. Apfel, C.C., et al., *Postoperatives Erbrechen – Ein Score zur Voraussage des Erbrechensrisikos nach Inhalationsanästhesien.* Anaesthesist, 1998, **47**: pp. 732–740.
118. Sneyed, J.R., et al., *A meta-analysis of nausea and vomiting following maintenance of anaesthesia with propofol or inhational agents.* Eur J Anaesth, 1998, **15**: pp. 433–445.
119. Heinz, I., B. Walder, and M.R. Tramler, *Dexamethasone for the prevention of postoperative nausea and emesis- A quantitative systemic review.* Anesth Analg, 2000, **90**: pp. 186–194.
120. Habib, A.S. and T.J. Gan, *Food and drug admistration black box warning on the perioperative use of deoperidol: a review of the cases.* Anesth Analg, 2003, **96**: pp. 1377–1379.
121. White, P.F., et al., *Effect of low-dose droperidol on the QT interval during and after general anesthesia: a placebo-controlled study.* Anesthesiology, 2005, **102**: pp. 1101–1105.
122. Charbit, B., et al., *Prolongation of QTc interval after postoperative nausea and vomiting treatment by droperidol or ondansetron.* Anesthesiology, 2005, **102**: pp. 1094–1100.
123. Habib, A.S. and T.J. Gan, *The effectiveness of rescue antiemetics after failure of prophylaxis with ondansetron or droperidol: a preliminary report.* J Clin Anesth, 2005, **17**: pp. 62–65.
124. Havemann, U., L. Turski, and K. Kuschinsky, *Role of opioid receptors in the substantia nigra in morphine-induced muscular rigidity.* Life Sci, 1982, **31**: pp. 2319–2322.
125. Paakkari, P. and G. Feuerstein, *Antagonism of dermorphin-induced catalepsy with naloxone, TRH-analog CG3703 and the benzodiazepine antagonist, Ro 15-1788.* Neuropharmacology, 1988, **27**(10): pp. 1007–1012.
126. Amalric, M., et al., *"Catatonia" produced by alfentanil is reversed by methylnaloxonium microinjections into the brain.* Brain Res, 1986, **386**: pp. 287–295.

127. Freund, F.G., et al., *Abdominal muscular rigidity induced by morphine and nitrous oxide*. Anesthesiology, 1973, **38**: p. 358.

128. Sokoll, M.D., J.L. Hoyt, and S.D. Georgids, *Studies in muscular rigidity, nitrous oxide and narcotic analgesic agents*. Anesth Analg, 1972, **51**: p. 16.

129. Freye, E. and K. Kuschinsky, *The effect of fentanyl and droperidol on the dopamine metabolism of the rat striatum*. Pharmacology, 1976, **14**: pp. 1–7.

130. Kuschinsky, K. and O. Hornykiewicz, *Morphine katalepsy in the rat: relation to striatal dopamine metabolism*. Eur J Pharmacol, 1972, **19**: p. 119.

131. Freye, E., *Tyrosine hydroxylation in the rat striatum after fentanyl and droperidol in vivo*. Expt Brain Res, 1976, **26**: pp. 541–545.

132. Kelly, P.H. and K.E. Moore, *Decrease of neocortical choline acetyltransferase after lesion of the globus pallidum in the rat*. Exp Neurol, 1978, **61**: pp. 479–483.

133. Jaffe, T.B. and F.M. Ramsey, *Attenuation of fentanyl-induced truncal rigidity*. Anesthesiology, 1983, **58**: p. 562.

134. Freye, E., E. Hartung, and R. Buhl, *Die Lungencompliance wird durch die rasche Injektion von Alfentanil beeinträchtigt*. Anaesthesist, 1986, **35**: pp. 543–546.

135. Weinger, M.B., I.S. Segal, and M. Maze, *Dexemedetomidine, acting through central alpha2-adrenoceptors, prevents opiate-induced muscle rigidity in the rat*. Anesthesiology, 1991, **71**: pp. 242–249.

136. Kromer, W., *Gastrointestinal effects of opioids*, in *Opioids II*, A. Herz, Editor, 1993, Springer: Berlin, Heidelberg, New York. pp. 163–190.

137. Champion, S.E., et al., *Naloxone and morphine inhibit gastric emptying of solids*. Can J Physiol Pharmacol, 1982, **60**: pp. 732–734.

138. Dingledine, R. and A. Goldstein, *Effect of synaptic transmission blockade on morphine action in the guinea pig myenteric plexus*. J Pharmacol Exp Ther, 1976, **196**: pp. 97–106.

139. Polak, J.M., et al., *Enkephalin-like immunoreactivity in the human gastrointestinal tract*. Lancet, 1977, **1**: pp. 972–974.

140. Dashwood, M.R., et al., *Autoradiographic localisation of opiate receptors in rat small intestine*. Eur J Pharmacol, 1985, **107**: p. 267.

141. Wienbeck, M. and M.M. Körner, *Influence of opiates on colonic motility*. Clin Res Rev, 1981, **1**: pp. 199–204.

142. Ward, S.J. and A.E. Takemori, *Relative involvement of mu, kappa, and delta receptor mechanisms of opiate-mediated antinociception in mice*. J Pharmacol Exp Ther, 1983, **22**: pp. 525–530.

143. Manara, L., et al., *Inhibition of gastrointestinal transit by morphine in rats results primarely from direct drug action on gut opioid sites*. J Pharmacol Exp Ther, 1986, **237**: pp. 945–949.

144. Vater, M. and A.R. Aitkenhead, *Effect of morphine on gastric emptying*. Anaesthesia, 1985, **40**: pp. 81–82.

145. Park, G.R. and D.A. Weir, *A comparison of the effect of oral controlled release morphine and intramuscular morphine on gastric emptying*. Anaesthesia, 1985, **39**: pp. 645–648.

146. Yuan, C.S., et al., *Methylnaltrexone prevents morphine-induced delay on oral-cecal transit time without affecting analgesia: a double-blind randomized placebo-controlled trial*. Clin Pharmacol Ther, 1996, **59**: pp. 469–475.

147. Yuan, C.S. and J.F. Foss, *Oral methylnaltrexone for opioid-induced constipation*. JAMA, 2000, **284**: pp. 1383–1384.

148. Liberto, J.G., et al., *Effects of ADL 8-2698, a peripherally restricted mu opioid anntagost, on gut motility in methadone and LAAM-dependent patients with opioid-induced constipation. A dose-ranging study.* Drug Alcohol Depend, 2001, **63**: p. s91.

149. Wong, C.L., *The effects of morphine and nalbuphine on intestinal transit in mice.* Meth and Find Exptl Clin Pharmacol, 1984, **6**: pp. 685–689.

150. Shook, J.E., et al., *Peptide opioid antagonist seperates peripheral and central opioid antitransit effects.* J Pharmacol Exp Ther, 1987, **243**: pp. 492–500.

151. Freye, E. and V. Knüfermann, *Die gastro-coekale Transitzeit nach Fentanyl/Midazolam- im Vergleich zur Enfluran- und Ketamin/Midazolam-Narkose.* Anaesthesist, 1991, **40, Suppl 2**: p. S 264.

152. Freye, E. and V. Knüfermann, *Keine Hemmung der intestinalen Motilität nach Ketamin-/Midazolamnarkose.* Anaesthesist, 1994, **43**: pp. 87–91.

153. De Vos, V., *Immobilization of free-ranging wild animals using a new drug.* Vet Rec, 1978, **103**: pp. 64–68.

154. Cookson, R.F., *Carfentanil and lofentanil.* Clin & Anaesthesiol, 1983, **1**: pp. 156–158.

155. Niemegeers, C.J.E., et al., *Sufentanil, a very potent and extremely safe intravenous morphine-like compound in mice, rats and dogs.* Drug Res/Arzneimittelforsch, 1976, **216**: pp. 1551–1556.

156. Janssen, P.A.J., *The development of new synthetic narcotics*, in *Opioids in Anesthesia*, F.G. Estafanous, Editor, 1984, Butterworth: Boston. pp. 37–44.

157. Meert, T.F., *Pharmacotherapy of opioids: present and future developments.* Pharm World Sci, 1996, **18**: pp. 1–15.

158. Freye, E., *Hämodynamische Wirkungen hoher Dosen von Fenanyl, Meperidine und Naloxon beim Hund*, in *Probleme der intravenösen Anästhesie, 6. Bremer Neuroleptanalgesie-Symposium*, W. Henschel, Editor, 1976, Peri-Med Dr. med. Straube: Erlangen. pp. 109–124.

159. Freye, E., *Cardiovascular effects of high doses of fentanyl, meperidine and naloxone in dogs.* Anesth Analg, 1974, **53**: pp. 40–47.

160. Lappas, D.G., et al., *Filling pressures of the heart and pulmonary circulation of the patient with coronary artery disease after large doses of morphine.* Anesthesiology, 1975, **42**: p. 153.

161. Braunwald, E., *Control of myocardial oxygen consumption.* Am J Cardiol, 1971, **27**: p. 416.

162. De Castro, J. and P. Viars, *Utilisation pratique des analgésiques centraux en anesthésie et réanimation.* Ars Med, 1968, **23**: pp. 74–74.

163. Sarne, Y. and M. Gafni, *Determinants of the stimulatory opioid effect on transmitter release and possible cellular mechanisms: overview and original results.* Brain Res, 996, **722**: pp. 203–206.

164. Harrison, C., D. Smart, and D.G. Lambert, *Stimulatory effects of opioids.* Br J Anaesth, 1998, **81**: pp. 20–28.

165. Kaiser, C., M.J. Pontecorvo, and R.E. Mewshaw, *Sigma receptor ligands: function and activity.* Neurotransmissions, 1991, **7**(1): pp. 1–5.

166. Zola, E.M. and D.C. MacLeod, *Comparative effects and analgesic efficacy of the agonist-antagonist opioids.* Drug Intell Clin Pharm, 1983, **17**: pp. 411–417.

167. Boldt, J., et al., *Meptazinol, ein neuartiges Analgetikum.* Anaesthesist, 1987, **36**: pp. 622–628.

168. De Castro, J., S. Andrieu, and J. Boogaerts, *Buprenorphine. A review of its pharmacological properties and therapeutical uses*, in *New Drug Series*, J. De Castro, Editor. Vol. 1, 1982, Antwerpen: Kluwer NVM & ISA. p. 180.

169. Strauer, B.E., *Contractile responses to morphine, piritramid and fentanyl: a comparative study of effects on the isolated myocardium*. Anesthesiology, 1972, **37**: p. 304.

170. Vargish, T., et al., *Myocardial opiate receptor activity is stereospecific, independent of muscarinic receptor antagonism, and may play a role in depressing myocardial function*. Surgery, 1987, **102**: pp. 171–177.

171. De Castro, J., P. Viars, and J.C.L. Leleu, *Utilisation de la pentazocine comme analgesique pour le traitement des douleurs post-operatoires. Etude comparative entre le pethidine, la piritramide et la pentazocine*, in *Utilisation de la pentazocine en Anesthesie et Reanimation*, J. De Castro, Editor, 1969, Ars Medici: Bruxelles. pp. 99–109.

172. Vargish, T., et al., *Hemodynamic changes following corticosteroid and naloxone infusion in dogs subjected to hypovolemic shock without resuscitation*. Life Sci, 1983, **33**: pp. 489–493.

173. Michaels, I., J.R. Trout, and P.G. Barash, *Nitrous oxide as an adjunct to narcotic anesthesia*, in *Opioids in Anesthesa*, F.G. Estafanous, Editor, 1984, Butterworth: Boston, London, Sydney, Durban, Toronto. pp. 256–260.

174. Michaels, I. and P.C. Barash, *Does nitrous oxide or a reduced FI02 alter the hemodanymic function during high dose sufentanil anesthesia?* Anesth Analg, 1983, **62**: p. 275.

175. Craemer, J.E., M.B. Maltz, and A.J. Camm, *The antiarrhythmic effect of meptazinol*. Eur Heart J, 1985, **6**: pp. 717–718.

176. Freye, E., *Effects of high doses of fentanyl on myocardial infarction and cardiogenic shock in the dog*. Resuscitation, 1975, **3**: pp. 105–113.

177. Hess, L., et al., *The antifibrillatory effect of fentanyl, sufentanil, and carfentanbil in the acute phase of local myocardial ischemia in the dog*. Acta Cardiol, 1989, **150**: pp. 303–311.

178. Saini, V., et al., *Antifibrillatory action of the narcotic agent fentanyl*. Am Heart J, 1988, **115**: pp. 508–514.

179. DeSilva, R.A., R.L. Verrier, and B. Lown, *Protective effect of the vagotonic action of morphine sulfate on ventricular vulnerability*. Cardiovasc Res, 1978, **12**: pp. 167–181.

180. Freye, E., G. Avril, and E. Hartung, *Les effets anti-arrythmiques des opiaces. Comparison avec un beta-bloqueur chez le chien*. Cah d'Anesthesiol, 1981, **29**: pp. 591–598.

181. Sharpe, L.G. and W.B. Pickworth, *Opposite pupillary effects in the cat and the dog after microinjection of morphine, normorphine and clonioline in the Edinger–Westphal nucleus*. Brain Res Bull, 1985, **15**: pp. 329–333.

182. Lee, H.K. and S.C. Wang, *Mechanism of morphine – induced miosis in the dog*. J. Pharmacol Expt Ther. 1975, **192**: pp. 415–431.

Part III

Opioids, an Integrative Part in Perioperative Medicine

No other area in medicine has been affected by the use of opioids more than their application in anesthesia. Their use for the induction and maintenance of anesthesia has led to an increase in safety, especially since other anesthetic agents are characterized by a pronounced cardiovascular depressive effect. Such depression is seen with the use of barbiturates (i.e. methohexital, thiopental), high doses of hypnotics (i.e. etomidate, propofol), as well as all volatile agents (halothane, enflurane, isoflurane, desflurane, sevoflurane).

Intraoperative Use of Opioids for Anesthesia

Currently, opioids are the cornerstone in anesthesia (Figure III-1), whether it is in classical neuroleptic analgesia, using the butyrophenone droperidol or in a balanced type of anesthesia, where in addition to the analgesic low concentrations of a volatile agent are added for a sufficient depth of unconsciousness. Also, opioids are used in total intravenous anesthesia (TIVA), where no volatile agent is utilized and only an opioid with a short duration of action (e.g. remifentanil) and a hypnotic (preferably propofol) are employed for the maintenance of anesthesia.

The development of intravenous anesthesia with opioids was initially slow, has been erratic with long periods of stagnation, especially when volatile anesthetics, in particular ethrane and chloroform were the agents of choice. Due to their obvious side effects, especially the necessary high concentration needed to induce a sufficient level of analgesia, the slow onset of action, and long overhang of effects, led to the proposal to use an intravenous anesthetic agent for induction and maintenance of anesthesia.

Hexobarbital was the first drug to make intravenous anesthesia popular. It was synthesized by Krop and Taub from Bayer company in Elberfeld/Germany and was first used by Weese and Scharff in 1932. Shortly thereafter thiopental was synthesized and originally employed as the sole anesthetic given in intermittent dosages together with nitrous oxide and oxygen (Figure III-2). Potentiation of anesthesia with unconsciousness and concomitant attenuation of reactions of the autonomic nervous system at that time were considered sufficient to cover all parts in anesthetic practice.

However, similar to high concentrations of gaseous volatile anesthetics, side effects such as a significant cardiovascular depression and a delayed awakening were still

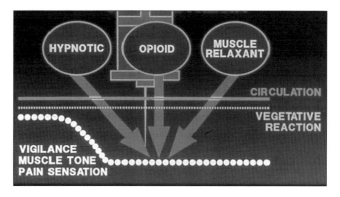

Figure III-1. The three major components in anesthesia where the opioid is the main component resulting in a beneficial stabilization of the cardiovascular system and a preservation of autonomic functions

evident. In order to minimize these side effects, another technique was introduced into the field of anesthesia when Gray ands Geddes from Liverpool/England propagated their *"Relaxant Anaesthesia"* in 1959 [1]. With this technique, high doses of a muscle relaxant were given followed by artificial hyperventilation and a $paCO_2$ between 20 and 25 mmHg with resulting respiratory alkalosis. In retrospect, this type of anesthesia may have worked because hyperventilation induced the concomitant release of endogenous opioids resulting in an alleviation of nociception. As this was followed by an increase in the level of analgesia, all other components of anesthesia (i.e. unconsciousness, analgesia and autonomic stabilization) were of lesser significance

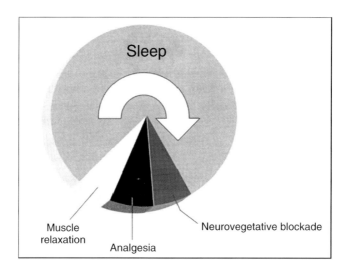

Figure III-2. Classical potentiation of anesthesia with intermittent dosages of a barbiturate, where unconsciousness (sleep) dominates the technique

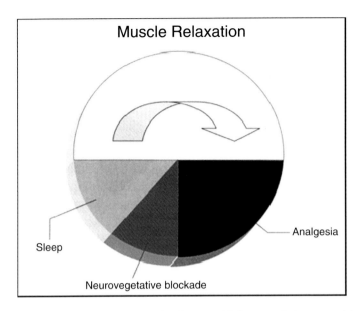

Figure III-3. Dominance of high dose muscle relaxants with hyperventilation as used in *Relaxant Anesthesia*

(Figure III-3). Due to the insufficient depth of analgesia and the hypocapnia-related reduction in cerebral perfusion, this was detrimental for the elderly patient population, which in addition to the simultaneous hyperventilation-related reduction in cardiac stroke volume, induced hypotensive episodes. Also, an overhang of muscle relaxant effects made a reversal necessary, which by itself was disadvantageous.

Thereafter, another component of anesthesia, i.e. blockade of the autonomic nervous system, became the target of a new anesthetic technique, called "*Neuroplegia*". Originally introduced by Laborit and Huegenard from France as a lytic cocktail in 1948, it first contained hyocine with morphine and later chlorpromazine plus hydergine. These agents were given together with the opioid pethidine (meperidine, USP). The cocktail was used in "*hibernation artificielle*" or artificial sleep for hypothermia in anesthesia, and for sedation in acute psychosis [2]. Following the synthesis of newer and more potent neuroleptic agents derived from the butyrophenones, the advantages of a complete neuroplegia with a stable autonomic nervous system became obvious. First, and most of all, the dose of the narcotic agent pethidine could be reduced. Secondly, any disturbance from a stimulated autonomic nervous system emerging during aggressive surgery, was eliminated. Thirdly, the patient was protected from stressful reaction resulting in a psychological indifference to the environment. This is because neuroleptic agents block subcortical centers such as the thalamus, the reticular activating system (RAS) and the limbic system (Figure III-4). However, since neuroleptic drugs also block the dopaminergic transmitter system, an imbalance in the dopaminergic-cholinergic equilibrium in the striatum and parts

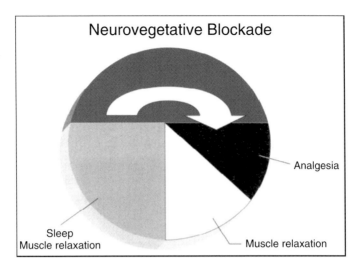

Figure III-4. Dominance of neurolepsia with potent neuroleptic agents, being the dominant part in anesthesia

of the extrapyramidal system became clinically noticeable. This often resulted in constipation, drowsiness, vision changes, and dry mouth, specifically in the postoperative period. More importantly, imbalance was accompanied by other severe side effects such as restlessness, muscle stiffness, weakness, difficulty in speaking, loss of balance, mask-like facial expression, trembling or shaking, dizziness, lip smacking or other uncontrolled movements of the head or the extremities. Intraoperatively, a concomitant blockade of α-receptors on the blood vessels often induced intense hypotensive episodes, which in conjunction with a vasodilatory agent, the use of MAO-agents, or hypovolemia, resulted in a severe drop of blood pressure with an ensuing cardiac arrest. Another disadvantage was the slow onset and the long duration of action of up to 12 h, which made fine adjustment to the anesthetic course and to surgery procedures impossible.

It was only with the synthesis of highly potent narcotics of the piperidine series by Janssen Pharmaceutical in Beerse/Belgium that neuroleptanalgesia (NLA) were successfully introduced into clinical practice whereby the analgesic component became the dominant part in the anesthetic regimen (Figure III-5). Based on the original work by De Castro and Mundeleer in 1959 [3], the opioids dextromoramide and phenoperidine (i.e., forerunners of fentanyl) were used for analgesia. Given together with the neuroleptic agent haloperidol or droperidol (50fold potency of chlorpromazine), analgesia became the dominant part in the anesthetic routine. This quickly spread all over the world as neuroleptanalgesia or the acronym NLA, being the ancestor of TIVA. De Castro put the emphasis on a deeper and reliable form of analgesia, which he recognized as the fundamental part of a sucessfull anesthetic course. The neuroleptic drug haloperidol and the synthetic opioid phenoperidine, a piperidine derivative, provided him with the means of removing surgical pain and

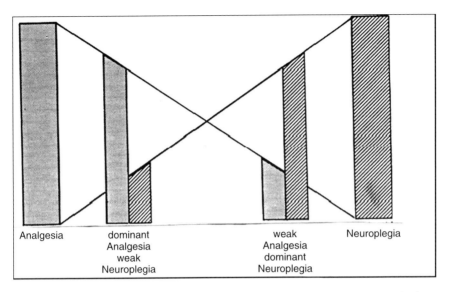

Figure III-5. The gradual development of anesthesia evolving away from neurolepsia to a dominance of analgesia

stress. They were the building blocks enabling him to develop this technique in anesthesia whereby neurolepsis and analgesia could be induced in a controllable manner filling the gaps in the Laborits cocktail.

The advantages of this new technique were obvious: a deep state of analgesia with unmatched cardiovascular stability and due to the butyrophenone agent, a stable neurovegetative system and a psychic indifference to the environment. Molecular redesign of existing compounds soon led to the development of other narcotic agents such as fentanyl, alfentanil and sufentanil, which allowed a greater and more specific use of opioid analgesics in clinical anesthesia. The rapid onset and short duration of action made these agents very suitable in those situations where rapid suppression of reflex responses is required (e.g., perioperative supplementation, during stressful surgical moments) or where longer acting compounds are less appropriate such as in short surgical procedures. The high specificity and potency of sufentanil provided deeper analgesia and a more complete stress protection than existing narcotics (Figure III-6), without increasing postoperative depression. Especially these characteristics made sufentanil beneficial in situations where complete stress protection is required, as in major procedures such as in cardiac surgery, major abdominal surgery or vascular surgery of the greater vessels.

The course of action in classical neuroleptanalgesia (NLA) was as follows:

1. Premedication with a fixed mixture of fentanyl and droperidol (Thalamonal® 0.25/05 per ml).
2. Use of separate injection of fentanyl as the analgesic agent and droperidol as the neuroleptic drug.

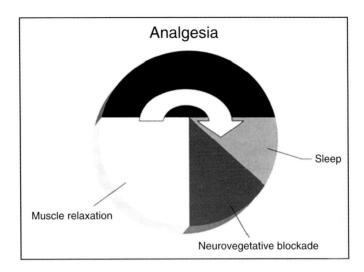

Figure III-6. Classical neuroleptanalgesia with dominance of analgesia, using the potent opioid fentanyl plus the neuroleptic droperidol, or a benzodiazepine (midazolam, flunitrazepam, which then is termed ataractanalgesia), together with low concentrations of a volatile anesthetic (N₂O, enflurane, desflurane, sevoflurane) to assure a sufficient sedative-hypnotic state

3. Priming with a competitive muscle relaxant (2 mg alcuronium, or 0.75 mg vecuronium)
4. Initial i.v. injection of droperidol 15–20 mg/70 kg body weight; this was followed by
5. Intravenous injection of 5–10 μg/kg body weight of fentanyl.
6. Induction of anesthesia by intravenous injection of a hynoptic (i.e. etomidate, propofol) or a barbiturate (i.e. methohexitone or hexobarbitone) followed by
7. Injection of an induction dose of a muscle relaxant
8. Ventilation by mask with pure oxygen for 2–3 min
9. Laryngoscopy and intubation
10. Ventilatory support using nitrous oxide/oxygen (FiO₂ 0.5)
11. For maintenance of analgesia, whenever necessary (i.e. rise in blood pressure and/or heart rate) sweating, movement of limbs) i.v. injection of an additional dose of fentanyl (0.05–0.2 μg/kg body weight).
12. Whenever necessary, reinjection of a muscle relaxant.
13. At end of operation, ventilation with pure oxygen until spontaneous respiratory drive occurs and recovery of protective reflexes, followed by extubation.
14. Postoperative analgesia with a peripheral acting analgesic in combination with a long acting opioid (i.e. morphine, oxymorphone, hydromorphone; see chapter on postoperative analgesia).

In order to increase the margin of safety in anesthesia, De Castro and coworkers developed another technique, which put all emphasis on the analgesic component. This was termed as *"anesthésie analgesique sequentielle"* or "Sequential Analgesia"

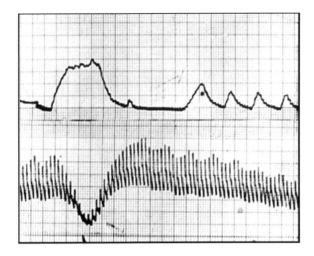

Figure III-7. Representative example in a patient undergoing anesthesia with high dose fentanyl (20 μg/kg body weight). Increase in intrapulmonary pressure (upper tracing) is followed by a reduction in arterial pressure (lower tracing)

[4], where high dosages of the opioid (50–100 μg/kg body weight of fentanyl) together with a muscle relaxant were used for maintenance of anesthesia, while the patient was ventilated either with air or oxygen. No additional anesthetic such as a volatile agent, a neuroleptic or a benzodiazepine was added (Figure III-8). The advantages of the sole use of fentanyl are:

1. A reactive autonomic nervous and cardiovascular system being able to compensate blood loss.
2. A remarkable cardiovascular stability even during aggressive surgical procedures.
3. A positive Valsalva-maneuver (increase of intrapulmonary pressure > 40 cm H_2O with a drop of blood pressure), reflecting a reactive autonomic nervous system (Figure III-7),
4. In case of hypercapnia an increase in blood pressure
5. Head down position results in compensatory vasoconstriction of the lower extremities.
6. An opioid-related bradycardia can immediately be reversed by the vagolytic agent atropine
7. Pressure on the eye ball evokes an oculocardiac reflex.

However, due to the respiratory depressive effects of the opioid an antagonist has to be given in sequence, at the end of anesthesia. Due to the short half-life of 20–30 min of the specific opioid antagonist naloxone, the patient had to be supervised in order to detect any possible later deterioration in respiration. Also, the antagonist had to be titrated to effect in order not to induce an "acute abstinence syndrome" with tachycardia and hypertension [5]. Because of lack of a long acting opioid antagonist and the need for postoperative surveillance, this technique has not gained wide

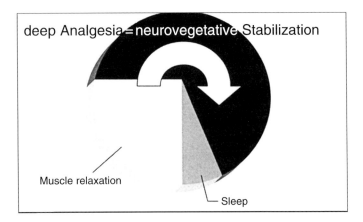

Figure III-8. Schematic presentation of sequential analgesia, where the respiratory depressive effects of the potent opioid fentanyl are reversed by an antagonist at the end of surgery

acceptance. Only in open-heart surgery, high-dose opioid anesthesia with either fentanyl or sufentanil is being used, and the patient ventilated postoperatively, being under close surveillance in the intermediate care unit.

Another anesthetic regimen, using high doses of vitamin B_1 (thiamine) was termed "*thiamine algosynaptolysis*" (Figure III-9). This is because high doses of up to 50 mg/kg body weight results in a cholinergic and an adrenergic blockade at synapses [6]. Such blockade was able to protect the autonomic nervous system from nociceptive afferents [7]. Also, the use of an additional muscle relaxant is obsolete because during regular physiological muscle innervation minute concentrations of thiamine are being released at the motor end-plate, whereby massive exogenous doses induce a muscle relaxant effect. In addition, high doses of thiamine induce an intense sedative effect, thus reducing the need for an additional hypnotic. The potential benefits of high dose thiamine anesthesia are:

1. Use of a natural, non-synthetic compound.
2. Thiamine plays an important part in the mitochondrial metabolic Krebs-cycle, resulting in the formation of high energy substrates, which activate myocardial contractile force [8].
3. Thiamine is a cheap compound, easy to be synthesized.
4. There is no need for an additional muscle relaxant during operation.
5. Due to synaptic blockade there is a vasodilatatory effect, which is followed by moderate hypotension. As a consequence there is reduced bleeding within the surgical field resulting in optimal operating conditions.

Aside from thiamine, the opioid fentanyl is given for analgesia resulting in preferable operating conditions [9].

However, due to the drawback of a long-lasting duration of thiamine, the lack of a potential antagonist and the potentially massive drop in blood pressure in latent hypovolemia, this technique has not gained wide acceptance.

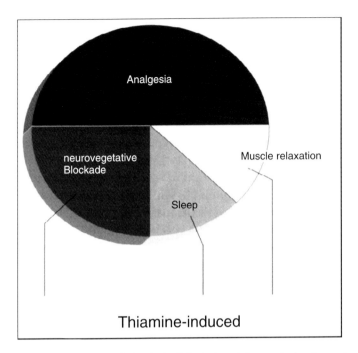

Figure III-9. Effects of high doses of vitamin B₁ (thiamine) used for anesthesia where only an opioid is needed for analgesia

During use of all these different techniques it became obvious that a potent opioid is a mandatory part in an anesthetic regimen, because an intensive nociceptive barrage, which needs to be blocked sufficiently, always accompanies operation. In addition, opioids do not have any detrimental effects on organ function while at the same time protecting the organism from stress-related consequences. Such demands are reflected in the therapeutic margin of safety (Table III-1), which mirrors the ratio of a dose necessary to induce analgesia and the dose resulting in cardiovascular depression.

The therapeutic margin of safety is of clinical significance because any side effects arising from the cardiovascular system are minimal. Also, preclinical as well as clinical data suggest that with higher affinity and stereoselectivity of an opioid to the receptor site, there is an increase of therapeutic safety [16, 17, 18, 19].

In summary, there are several reasons why an opioid should be incorporated into the anesthetic routine:

1. Volatile anesthetics and especially barbiturates, when given in high concentrations, depress the cardiovascular system (narrow therapeutic index).
2. Neuroleptic agents such as droperidol, but also sedatives (i.e., diazepam, midazolam) are not able to block nociceptive afferents.
3. The surgical procedure *per se* is a painful process. It therefore is only rational to administer agents, which selectively inhibit the increase in nociceptive afferents.

Table III-1. Therapeutic margin of safety of different opioids when compared to other intra-venous and/or volatile anesthetic agents. With higher receptor selectivity of the opioid, there is an increase in therapeutic safety

Anesthetic/analgesic compound	Therapeutic margin of safety (LD_{50}/ED_{50})
Halothane	1–3
Enflurane	2–3
Isoflurane	2–5
Tramadol	3
Pentazocine	4
Thiopental sodium	6
Pethidine	4–7
Methohexital	11
Ketamine	11
Methadone	12
Meptazinol	18
Etomidate	32
Phenoperidine	39
Butorphanol	45
Morphine	70–90
Lofentanil	112
Fentanyl	270–400
Nalbuphine	1034
Alfentanil	1080
Buprenorphine	7933
Carfentanil	10.000
Sufentanil	26.716
Remifentanil	33.000

Adapted from [10, 11, 12, 13, 14, 15]

4. Potent opioids are characterized by a wide therapeutic margin of safety.
5. Opioids are given intravenously. They represent the cornerstone in total intra-venous anesthesia (TIVA).
6. Ecologically opioids are superior to volatile agents, as they do not pollute the environment.
7. Selective antagonists can reverse the effects of opioids.
8. There is an abundant knowledge on opioid action and their specific receptor sites within the central nervous system.
9. Opioids do not depress internal organ function.
10. Malignant hyperthermia, contrary to volatile anesthesia, is not induced by opioids.
11. There is less postoperative pain after an opioid-based anesthesia when compared to a volatile anesthetic regimen.
12. Use of opioids for anesthesia results in a beneficial cost/benefit.

The aim of modern anesthesia is to induce analgesia, unconsciousness and muscle relaxation with agents having a selective profile, which do not depress the cardio-vascular and induce stabilization within the autonomic nervous system during operation. Present knowledge suggests that only opioids, when given alone or in combination with other anesthetics, are able to sufficiently fulfill such demands.

POTENTIATION OF OPIOID-BASED ANESTHESIA

A sufficient blockade of reflex mechanisms is already obvious during the induction of anesthesia when the maneuver of laryngoscopy and intubation results in an intense nociceptive stimulus. This is followed by defense mechanisms with an activation of the sympathetic nervous system, and a stimulation of the cardiovascular system with tachycardia and hypertension. It therefore is mandatory to block such reflex mechanisms by using an opioid for induction of anesthesia (e.g., fentanyl 0.2–0.5 mg/70 kg body weight, alfentanil 2–3 mg/70 kg body weight or remifentanil 0.5 mg/70 kg body weight) together with the hypnotic (i.e., etomidate, propofol, or a barbiturate). This results in stabilization of the cardiovascular system and a reduction in the dose of the hypnotic, which is necessary to induce unconsciousness for the induction of anesthesia. Such stabilization not only is reflected in blood pressure and heart rate but also in the stress-related plasma level of epinephrine and norepinephrine (Figure III-10).

In order to prevent a possible persistence of respiratory depression, and avoid the potential side effect such as nausea and emesis in the postoperative period, however, at the same time maintain a sufficient depth of anesthesia; there are several possibilities how to potentiate opioid-related analgesia. Also, a particular patient population has to be recognized, which demonstrates an opioid resistance. Medical history reveals an abuse of narcotics, of alcohol, shows a heavy nicotine dependency, or a regular benzodiazepine intake. Different techniques are capable to potentiate an opioid-based anesthesia:

Use of Hypnotics

All hypnosedative agents such as phenobarbital, methohexital etomidate, chlomethiazol, or propofol, when given together with an opioid, result in a potentiation and prolongation of opioid effects. The hazard of a prolongation, however, cannot be foreseen. In this regard, propofol seems to be the most suitable agent, because it is rapidly metabolized in the liver, resulting in a short duration of action. This is the major reason why this agent is preferred in total intravenous anesthesia (TIVA) [21, 22, 23].

Use of Neuroleptics (Butyrophenones)

Among the class of neuroleptics available for anesthesia, the agent droperidol when administered in low dosages (5–10 mg/70 kg body weight) is the preferred drug when given together with an opioid. This is because it has an antiarrythmic action, increases peripheral perfusion by means of an α-blockade and is a potent antiemetic with a long duration of action, which lasts into the postoperative period [24]. Earlier recommendations of using high dosages (>20–25 mg/70 kg body weight) of droperidol during classical neuroleptanalgesia (NLA) are not being promoted any more. In addition, in 2001 the Food and Drug Administration began requiring that droperidol labeling include a "black box"warning stating that the drug may cause death or life-threatening

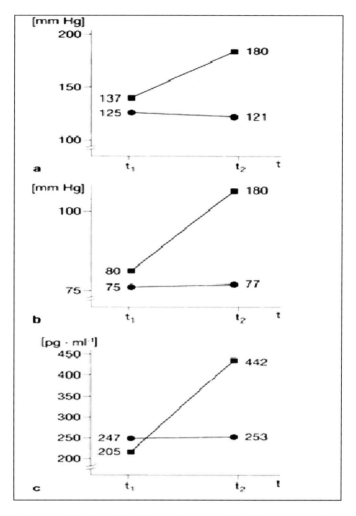

Figure III-10. Mean systolic (**a**) and diastolic blood pressure (**b**), and the corresponding plasma levels of norepinephrine (**c**), with and without the opioid fentanyl (0.2 mg/kg body weight) injected prior to laryngoscopy and intubation (t_1 = time prior to induction; t_2 = 60 seconds following laryngoscopy and intubation) (Adapted from [20])

events resulting from QTc prolongation and *"torsades de pointes"* with possible ventricular fibrillation. The labeling requirement was based on 10 reported cases associated with droperidol use (at doses of 1.25 mg) during its approximately 30 years on the market [25]. Although, no case reports in peer-reviewed journals have linked droperidol with QTc prolongation, cardiac arrhythmias, or death at the doses used for anesthesia or the management of postoperative nausea and vomiting (PONV), the company has stopped all marketing and distribution.

Use of Benzodiazepines

All benzodiazepines (i.e., midazolam, diazepam, chlordiazepoxide, fluni-trazepam, flurazepam, nitrazepam, temazepam lorazepam, medazepam, chlorapzeptate) induce a potentiation of opioid effects [26]. Extrapyramidal symptoms, as sometimes seen after potent butyrophenones, are not observed, and the contractility of the myocardium is not depressed. However, due to their long duration of action, respiratory depression is prolonged. The benzo-diazepine midazolam is the only agent with a relatively short elimination half-life of 1.3–2.3 h [27], and has no pharmacologically active metabolite such as diazepam. Another advantage is the availability of the specific antag-onist flumazenil, which competitively displaces any benzodiazepine from its receptor site resulting in a reversal of effects [28, 29, 30].

Because benzodiazepines not only increase the analgesic depth of a narcotic analgesic [31], the combined use of an opioid with a benzodiazepine is a conceivable technique for their combined use in the intensive care unit (ICU), especially since development of opioid tolerance and dependence liability is inhibited [32]. However, it has been demonstrated in the animal that during their long-term use, an anti-analgesic action becomes apparent [33, 34, 35]. Although this remains to be demonstrated in patients, the proposed mechanism of supraspinal inhibitory effect of midazolam on opioid-induced analgesia purportedly is discussed as a potential mode of action of development of opioid tolerance regularly seen in ICU patients [36].

Use of Volatile Anesthetics

Trying to cover all basic four components of anesthesia (analgesia, uncon-sciousness, autonomic nervous system stabilization and muscle relaxation) with the sole use of a volatile anesthetic is bound to end in a relative overdose. Because volatile anesthetics cannot be considered as analgesics the concen-tration has to be increased to such a degree that toxic levels are reached, which by means of a direct depressive effect on the myocardium results in marked cardiovascular depression. While volatile anesthetics non-specifically inhibit ion flux and the metabolic activity of nerve cells, their depressive effect starts at the neocortex. With increasing concentrations, deeper subcortical brain areas such as the limbic system are affected, resulting in non-responsiveness to stressful nociceptive stimuli. Finally, the respiratory and the cardiovas-cular regulating centers in the brainstem are depressed, which causes a further decline in blood pressure and impairment in respiration. Halothane, enflurane but also the newer volatile agents such as desflurane and sevoflurane all induce such a concentration-dependent depression starting at the highly developed cortical centers in the neocortex, then descending down to the deeper subcor-tical layers. The only volatile agent, which in an inspiratory concentration of up to 50%, does not depress the contractility of the heart, but at the same time potentiates opioid action, is nitrous oxide [37].

Because of the potential negative-inotropic activity of volatile anesthetics, often the dose of the opioid is increased in order to reduce the concentration of the gaseous agent. And while its hypnotic component is used solely as a supplement, the addition of the opioid reduces minimal alveolar concentration (MAC; Figure III-11) of the volatile agents [39, 40]. For instance, during administration of halothane sufentanil can reduce its MAC by up to 90% [41]. The so-called balanced anesthesia technique consists of low concentrations of a volatile agent given in conjunction with a potent opioid such as fentanyl, remifentanil or sufentanil resulting in analgesia, unconsciousness and a stable autonomic nervous system [42, 43, 44, 45]. Muscle relaxation is induced superlatively by a non-depolarizing agent with such a technique it is possible to eliminate the usual side effects of volatile anesthetics such as a drop in blood pressure and/or arrhythmia, while at the same time maintaining a sufficient deep level of unconsciousness avoiding the risk of intraoperative awareness (Figure III-12).

In order to obtain the obvious advantages of a combined or balanced type of anesthesia, the potent opioid should be given in a sufficiently high loading dose before surgery begins (Figure III-13; Table III-2). Such a high dose is able to sufficiently block all nociceptive afferences during the induction procedure, resulting in cardiovascular stability. In addition, postoperative analgesia is already initiated since residual occupation of opioid receptors is still present at the end of surgery. Lastly, there is a reduction in the incidence of postoperative shivering, which is regularly seen after a volatile anesthetic regimen.

Use of α_2-Agonists

Primarily used as an antihypertonic, clonidine in addition to its centrally-induced sympatholytic activity can be added to an opioid since it also has a sedative-analgesic component. Their main sites of action are specific receptor sites in the reticular activating formation of the medulla oblongata, where

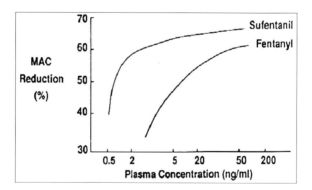

Figure III-11. The effects of increasing concentrations of fentanyl and sufentanil on minimal alveolar concentration (MAC) of enflurane. As depicted, the sufentanil MAC reduction plateaus at plasma concentrations of 2 ng/ml, which corresponds to an infusion rate of 0.045 μg/kg body weight in dogs. Sufentanils slightly greater ability to reduce MAC suggests that it is a more favorable anesthetic than fentanyl (Adapted from [38, 39])

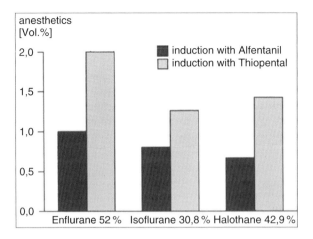

Figure III-12. Combined use of different volatile anesthetics with the opioid alfentanil. There is a significant reduction in MAC. Similar effects can be induced with other narcotic analgesics (Adapted from [46, 47])

pressor-regulating centers control the sympathetic outflow. These centers are connected via the nucleus tracts solitarii with the baroreceptors of the carotid sinus and the aortic arch. Additional afferents link to the nucleus ambiguous and the nucleus dorsalis nervi vagi, resulting in an activation of the cardiac vagal input. Since the activity of the nucleus tractus solitarii is controlled by α_2-adrenoreceptors, there is an activation of the cardiac vagal nerve and an inhibition of the central sympathic outflow, followed by a reduction in blood pressure. The anxiolytic and analgesic activity is mediated

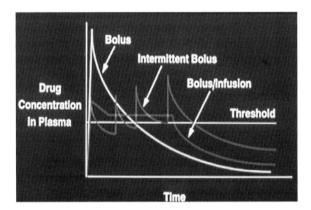

Figure III-13. Contrary to intermittent small doses of an opioid, a high loading dose is recommended at the beginning of anesthesia. At the end of surgery plasma concentrations are below the respiratory depressive threshold

Table III-2. Representative example of a balanced type of anesthesia with a mean duration of 2 h using an opioid as the main anesthetic agent

Premedication	Midazolam 0.2 mg/kg BW 30–60 min before operation
Priming with an opioid – Opioid loading dose	2–4 μg/kg BW fentanyl or 0.2–0.5 μg/kg BW sufentanil or 0.5 mg/kg BW remifentanil
Priming with a muscle relaxant	0.01 mg/kg BW vecuronium or 0.01–0.02 mg/kg BW alcuronium
Induction of anesthesia	0.2–0.3 mg/kg BW etomidate or 2 mg/kg BW propofol followed by full dose of muscle relaxant
Preoxygenation	Mask ventilation with 100% O_2
Maintenance of anesthesia	Ventilatory support $N_2O/O_2 = 2 : 1$ 0.3–0.8 vol% enflurane or 0.7–1.0 vol% sevoflurane
2nd Opioid dose before surgery begins	2–4 μg/kg BW fentanyl or 0.2–0.5 μg/kg BW sufentanil or remifentanil by continuous drip
Reduced analgesia	0.15–0.7 μg/kg BW sufentanil or 1–2 μg/kg BW fentanyl
<45 min to end of operation "on-top" opioid when necessary	7.0–25 μg/kg BW alfentanil or 1–2 μg/kg BW remifentanil
Postoperative pain therapy in the postoperative care unit (PACU)	First peripheral analgesic (i.e. metamizole) followed by titration to effect using morphine or oxymorphone or hydromorphone

via the locus coeruleus since specific binding sites for opioids for serotonin, GABA, substance P, catecholamines, and acetylcholine are found in this area (Figure III-14).

By binding to the α_2-receptors, clonidine as well as dexmedetomidine and mivazerol inhibit the activity at the locus coeruleus resulting in an inhibition of activity at corresponding cortical area, the hypothalamus and the limbic system. On the other hand specific α_2-binding sites have also been identified in the spinal cord, whereby the successful epidural administration of clonidine with morphine for therapy of acute and chronic pain is justified [49, 50, 51].

Combined use of opioid-based anesthesia with an α_2-agonist in general results in a reduction of the hypnotic by 45% and the necessary dose of an opioid by 40%–70% [52, 53, 54, 55]. The recommended dose of clonidine should be between 1.5 and 3.0 μg/kg body weight and for dexmedetomidine 0.25–1.0 μg/kg body weight, resulting in a mean duration of 9 h. The lower dose of dexmedetomidine is explained by its higher receptor specificity. While clonidine demonstrates an affinity for the α_1/α_2 receptor subsites of 200:1, dexmedetomidine has a higher selectivity and affinity of 1600:3 with a much shorter half-life of around 2 h. This higher selectivity and the shorter duration of action result in lesser side effects and a better control. Mivazerol with selectivity for the α_1/α_2 receptor of 119:1 shows higher specificity than clonidine. Due to its selective binding at the imidazole $\alpha_{2/A1}$ receptor subsite with a value of 213 compared to 32 of dexmedetomidine and to 16

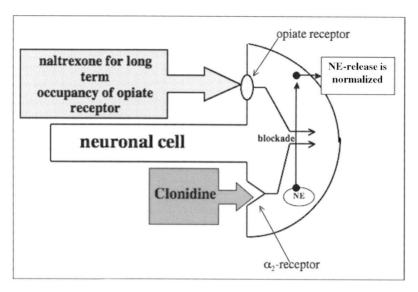

Figure III-14. The mode of action of α_2-agonists within the locus coeruleus, being in close vicinity of opioid binding sites, where they induce a central sympatholytic action, resulting in a reduction of norepinephrine (NE) release (Adapted from [48])

of clonidine [55], a large multicenter trial has documented significant myocardial ischemic-protective activity [56].

Following the administration of an α_2-agonist, the following side-effects can been seen:

1. A short-term hypertonic reaction originating from central α_2-receptors with vasoconstriction.
2. This is followed by a hypotonic action by means of a vasodilatatory effect, which can be reversed by the administration of norepinephrine.
3. The marked, centrally-mediated bradycardia is due to the increased activity of the vagal nerve. Such side effect can be rapidly reversed by the vagolytic agent atropine.

Because of such side effects and due to the site of action, α_2-agonists are contraindicated in the following patient population:

1. sinus bradycardia (sick-sinus syndrome),
2. AV–conduction pathology,
3. hypovolemia and/or low blood pressure,
4. a hypersensitive carotid sinus,
5. aortic valve stenosis (preexistent bradycardia).

In summary, combination of an opioid with an α_2-agoníst results in the following advantages:

1. Sufficient protection of the cardiovascular system from stressful response induced by laryngoscopy and intubation (clonidine $5\,\mu g/kg$ body weight)

2. Clonidine, when used peridurally in dosages of 450 μg, prolongs and potentiates the analgesic action of locally applied anesthetics [57] and morphine [58].
3. It does not prolong the respiratory depressive effects of an opioid.
4. It reduces the dose of the opioid necessary for a sufficient deep level of analgesia by 40%.
5. The α_2-agoníst induces a sedative effect, which adds to the sedative effect of the opioid or the volatile anesthetic [59].
6. It protects the myocardium against a possible ischemic event.
7. It reduces minimal alveolar concentration (MAC) of volaile anesthetics in a dose-related manner by 40%–70% [60].
8. Preclinical data suggest a neuroprotective effect in case of carotid occlusion [61].
9. It has a cardioprotective effect because of its anti-arrhythmic properties [62].
10. Clondine is regularly used in the therapeutic armamentarium during the alcohol abstinence syndrome [63] and for the prevention/reduction of opiate withdrawal symptoms [64, 65].

Because of their favorable actions, in the future α_2-agonists will be of benefit in anesthesia, pain therapy, and sedation in the intensive care unit [66, 67]:

- For premedication since they induce sedation and amnesia.
- In the perioperative period because they reduce the MAC of volatile anesthetics and the amount of the opioid necessary for analgesia.
- Postoperatively, they reduce the dose of peridurally applied local anesthetics and neuraxial opioids for postoperative pain therapy.
- In the intensive care unit they potentiate analgesia, and reduce the dose of the opioid necessary for sufficient sedation (dexmedetomidine 0.2–0.7 μg/kg body weight/hour).
- As an adjunct in the opioid weaning period, they reduce abstinence symptoms following long-term opioid administration.
- Postoperatively they reduce muscle shivering.
- For therapy in chronic pain states, they potentiate all peridurally-applied opioids.
- For anesthesia in rapid opiate detoxification (ROD) they are a necessary adjunct to reduce acute abstinence symptoms.

Pharmacokinetics of Opioids: Significance for Clinical Use in Anesthesia

In order to bind to the specific receptor sites within the CNS, opioids either given intravenously (i.v.), intramuscularly (i.m.), subcutaneously (s.c.) or orally (p.o.), have to penetrate various lipid layers. These barriers present a physiological obstacle, which all centrally active agents need to overcome (Figure III-15).

When a drug is administered, a portion is bound to plasma proteins and a portion remains free in the plasma. The portion of the drug, which is free in the plasma, is then available to cross membranes to reach several destinations of interest. First, it

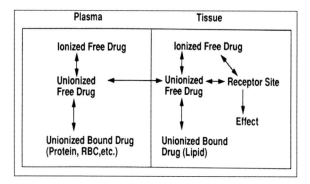

Figure III-15. When a drug is administered, a portion is bound to plasma proteins and a portion remains free in the plasma. This unbound portion is then available to cross membranes while also being delivered to the liver and kidney for metabolism and elimination. At the same time it is delivered to miscellaneous non-target tissues, where it is bound like a plasma reservoir. And finally, it is delivered to the target organ, the CNS, where the desired effect is produced

may be delivered to the liver and kidney for metabolism and elimination. Second, it may be delivered to miscellaneous non-target tissues where it may be bound or produce unwanted effects. Third, it may be delivered to the target organ where the desired effects are produced. The pharmacokinetics of a drug is affected by the uptake, distribution, elimination, and biotransformation of the drug within the biological system. Pharmacokinetic variables determine the drug concentration in plasma and tissue that result from a given dose.

Pharmacodynamics describes the relationship between drug concentration and drug response. It affects the intensity and duration of response produced by the drug at the receptor site. In order to induce an action, the opioid has to pass through the blood-brain barrier (BBB) membrane. The following factors affect the rate of membrane penetration:
- Molecular size
- Lipid solubility
- Plasma protein binding and hence the portion of free drug
- Degree of ionization, since only non-ionized molecules can cross the BBB.

For a drug to produce an effect, it must leave the plasma and pass through membranes to reach its eventual receptor site. The rate and extent to which a drug penetrates membranes is determined by the above listed factors. Thus molecular size, lipid solubility, plasma protein binding, and the degree of ionization ultimately determine the rapidity of onset, time to peak effect, and duration of action of any given drug. A smaller molecule will tend to pass more readily through cell membranes. Greater lipid solubility allows a drug to pass through lipid containing biological membranes including the blood-brain barrier with greater ease. Binding of drugs to plasma proteins and red cell membranes leaves less free drug available to penetrate and reach receptor sites. Similarly, ionization of a drug hinders its ability to cross cell membranes. Charged molecules will either be repelled by like charges on membranes or attracted to unlike charges on membranes, and in either case, be less effective in passing through membranes to reach receptor sites.

There is a dynamic relationship between these four factors. Ideally, if a drug is to have a rapid onset of action (i.e., be able to penetrate membranes rapidly) it would have a very small molecular size, a high degree of lipid solubility, have minimal protein binding and minimal ionization at physiologic pH. Clinically, alfentanil as well as remifentanil have the most rapid onset of action of any of the opioids, primarily because of their minimal ionization at physiologic pH. Fentanyl, on the other hand, in spite of its extraordinary lipid solubility, has a slower onset of action, compared to alfentanil and sufentanil, largely due to a high degree of protein binding and a high degree of ionization at physiologic pH. Sufentanil's onset of action is intermediate between fentanyl and alfentanil because of intermediate lipid solubility and ionization. All of the newer opioids are more lipid soluble than morphine and, as a result, in spite of modest differences in ionization and protein binding, all will be expected to have a more rapid onset of action following intravenous administration.

Lipid solubility also plays a role in affecting the elimination of a drug. A drug with a high degree of lipid solubility will be readily stored in lipid containing tissues and, as a result, will be released from those tissues more slowly into plasma and consequently will be eliminated at a slower rate. In general, drugs with a high degree of lipid solubility will therefore have a longer beta elimination half-life than those drugs with relatively small lipid solubility. The lower lipid solubility of alfentanil contributes to its shorter beta elimination half-life compared to fentanyl. Since alfentanil is significantly less lipid soluble, its volume of distribution is smaller and, as a result, more of the administered drug will be delivered to the liver for metabolism and elimination resulting in a faster decay of concentration and termination of effect.

All the opioids have a relatively small molecular size. Lipid solubility is defined as the octanol/water coefficient at pH 7.4 for each drug. Morphine has poor lipid solubility resulting in slow membrane penetration. Thus, morphine enters the CNS slowly and displays a slow onset of action. Sufentanil, fentanyl, and to a lesser degree alfentanil, have much higher degrees of lipid solubility and on this basis would be expected to have a more rapid onset of action following intravenous administration.

Protein binding at pH 7.4 represents the percentage of drug, which will be either bound to plasma proteins, including albumin and alpha-1 acid glycoprotein, or to red cell membranes. All of the new short-acting opioids have a relatively high degree of protein binding. A pharmacokinetic consequence of high protein binding is that lesser amounts of drug will be available in free form to penetrate membranes to produce a CNS effect. High protein binding also contributes to a smaller volume of distribution. Finally, plasma protein binding limits the amount of free drug available for elimination by the hepatic and renal systems, which would tend to reduce clearance rate. The percent of a drug that is non-ionized at pH 7.4 is tabulated

Table III-3. Difference in lipophilicity of various opioid agonists and antagonists as reflected in the heptane/water and heptane/phosphate buffer distribution

Agonist	Heptane/water distribution-coefficient
Methylmorphine	0.00001
Normorphine	0.00001
Dihydromorphine	0.00001
Morphine	0.00001
Levorphanol	0.0092
Etorphine	1.42
Pethidine	3.4
Fentanyl	19.35
Methadone	44.9
Antagonist	Heptane/phosphate buffer distribution coefficient
Naltrexone	0.008
Naloxone	0.02
Diprenorphine	0.24

Adapted from [68]

in Table III-3. A drug, which is non-ionized at physiologic pH, will more readily cross membranes to reach receptor sites and produce an effect. Fentanyl at a pH of 7.4 is approximately 90% ionized and 10% non-ionized. Alfentanil is just the opposite, i.e., approximately 90% non-ionized and 10% ionized, with sufentanil intermediate. The minimal ionization of alfentanil at physiologic pH contributes to its ease of membrane penetrance and partially explains its rapid onset of action. Since sufentanil's degree of ionization is intermediate, it would be expected to have a more rapid onset of action than fentanyl, although perhaps not as fast as alfentanil. All of these factors must be considered when determining the eventual clinical properties of an administered opioid.

Since the rate of penetration of physiological membranes closely correlates with lipophilicity of agents, the character of the opioid determines the amount of molecules being able to dissolve in a fatty solution. Since the central nervous system mainly consists of fatty-like substances, i.e. the cerebrosides, more of an agent with a high lipophilic character will enter brain tissue, where it mediates its pharmacological activity. For instance, an agent like morphine is a more hydrophilic compound, suggesting that it takes relatively long to enter the brain (Table III-3). Indeed about 45 min will elapse before a maximum effect is seen clinically. An agent like fentanyl is highly lipophilic; it therefore quickly enters the brain initiating a maximal effect within five minutes.

Following intravenous injection, approximately 85% of the drug is bound unspecifically to plasma and tissue proteins. Of the residual 15% only a portion is bound in the plasma in a non-ionized form. As a remainder, approximately only 1% of the originally injected amount will penetrate the blood-brain barrier, where

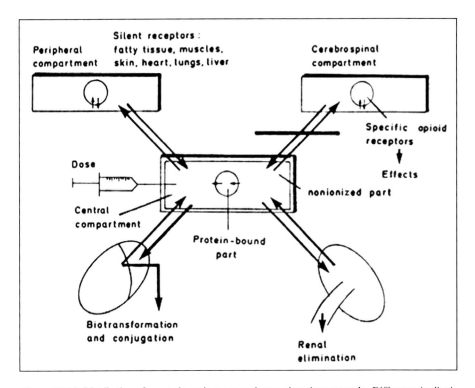

Figure III-16. Distribution of agents in various organ tissues given intravenously. Difference in distribution depends on physicochemical properties such as the degree of binding to protein-rich organs, their lipophilicity, and the degree of ionization. Note, many centrally active agents unspecifically bind to peripheral protein rich organs from where they later re-enter the blood stream, and after crossing the blood-brain barrier are able to induce an effect

the lipophilicity determines the speed of transfer from the plasma into the biophase, i.e. the central compartment in the CNS where the agent binds to the receptor sites. From the different pharmacokinetic properties of the various opioids (Figure III-16) different pharmacodynamics with different time of onset, the time until maximal effect and the duration of effect will evolve.

While lipophilicity is one determinant affecting the speed of onset, (i.e. how fast the molecules cross the blood-brain barrier), the other determinant is the amount of drug being present in a free, non-ionized form (i.e. the amount of molecules being able to penetrate the blood-brain barrier). Therefore, high amounts of non-ionized molecules in the plasma result in a fast onset of action. For instance, alfentanil and remifentanil have > 80% of the drug being present in a non-ionized form (Table III-4). Besides their lipophilicity, it is because of this property that these two agents demonstrate the fastest onset of action, being around 1 min.

Following injection, there are two distinct phases of declining drug concentrations in the plasma (Figure III-17).

Table III-4. Comparative pharmacokinetic data of various opioids

Opioid	Elimination half life (min; $t_{1/2\beta}$)	Clearance (Cl; ml/kg/min)	Volume of distribution (Vd; L/kg)	Protein binding (%)	Distribution coefficient (lipophilicity)
Fentanyl	219	13.0	4.0	84	955
Alfentanil	94	6.4	0.86	92	129
Sufentanil	64	12.7	2.0	92	1727
Morphine	177	14.7	3.2	60	1.0
Remifentanil	5–14	30–40	0.2–0.4	70	18
Pethidine	192	12.0	2.8	?	32
Meptazinol	124	132	4.99	27	65
Methadone	50–4500	?	3–4	60–90	57

Adapted from [70, 71, 72]

The time required for the plasma concentration to decline by 50% is referred to as its "half-life". The alpha half-life (t 1/2 α) represents the rate of distribution, while the terminal elimination or beta half-life (t 1/2 ß) represents the rate of elimination. The half-life for the distribution and elimination phases can be calculated from the straight lines in the Figure III-17 which are extrapolated from the plasma concentration decay curve [69]

Following injection and binding to the receptor site, a pharmacodynamic effect is initiated. The offset of action, however, is determined how fast the drug dissociates from the receptor and how fast it leaves the cerebral compartment returning

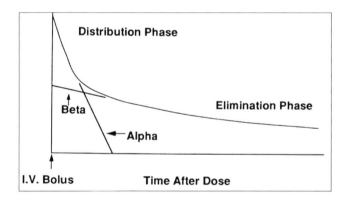

Figure III-17. Depicted is a plot of plasma concentration, using a two-compartment model for distribution, following an intravenous bolus dose of a drug. There are two distinct phases of declining drug concentration in the plasma. The first phase (alpha phase), the distribution phase, represents the rapid movement of drug from the plasma into the tissues. The second phase (beta phase), the elimination phase, represents a less rapid decline in drug plasma concentration due to removal of the drug from the body via metabolism and excretion

into the blood stream from where it is metabolized by the liver which inactivates the agent. For instance, another highly lipophilic agent is buprenorphine. Its offset of action, however, is mainly determined by the rate it dissociates from the receptor. This rate is very slow, resulting in a long duration of action of up to 10 h. Another highly lipophilic opioid is fentanyl, which enters brain tissue relatively fast it, however, also leaves the brain relatively fast. Because most of the drug is being stored in protein-rich organs, which act like reservoirs (Figure III-18), And, because there is always a flow of molecules re-diffusing into the blood, the opioid enters the brain. Because of this redistribution from the storage sites, and in spite of a high clearance, duration of action is long. The longest duration of action, which is due to the high amounts of storage sites, is that of methadone. Exceeding all other opioids (Table III-4) its duration of action is about 24 h. It is because of this long duration, that this opioid needs only to be taken once a day.

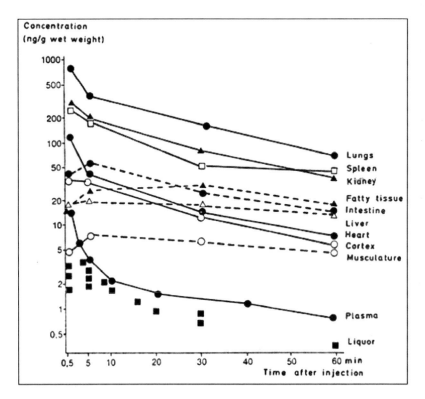

Figure III-18. Following intravenous injection of a highly lipophilic agent like fentanyl most of the drug is bound non-specifically by protein-rich organs. Only the concentration in the cerebrospinal fluid actually reflects the concentration present at the receptor sites, which is lower by the order of several magnitudes than plasma concentration. Data derived from the animal and adapted from [74]

When using fentanyl for anesthesia, it is of major importance to recognize that the speed of recovery is closely linked to recirculation of the opioid from peripheral storage sites into the blood stream. This is because, after initial injection, most of the drug is bound to protein-rich organs with a volume of distribution (Vd) of 4.0 L/kg. These parts of the body do not participate in the mediation of opioid effects. For instance, the lungs act like a filter after initial intravenous injection [73] (Figure III-18).

This volume of distribution is in contrast to alfentanil, which has a value of only 0.89 L/kg. Since most of the drug, which quickly enters the brain, also leaves it very fast, there is a fast onset and a short duration of action. Also, because the drug is accessible for metabolization and does not hide within the storage sites, it is inactivated by the liver. In contrast, fentanyl with its high volume of distribution may induce late effects when residual amounts of fentanyl diffuses from skin, musculature or fatty tissue, inducing a "rebound" of effects. Therefore, the end of action of an opioid is not only determined by receptor concentration. The volume of distribution of the agent is a pharmacokinetic variable, which has the most of impact on the duration of action. It therefore is conceivable that this duration of action is less predictable with fentanyl.

Aside from the volume of distribution, biotransformation within the liver is the important rate-limiting step in the degradation of fentanyl and many other opioids (Figure III-19). After fentanyl prolonged recovery times are possible

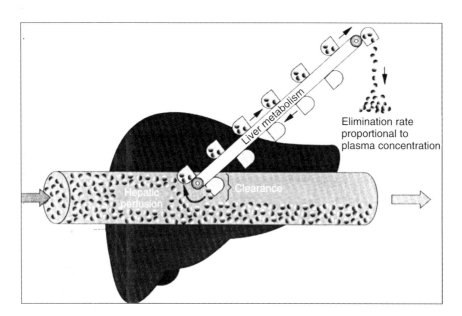

Figure III-19. Schematic representation of biotransformation within the liver, and why elimination of an opioid from the central compartment depends on hepatic flow and why clearance rate depends on the activity of liver enzymes

[75] because only the amount of the drug present in the circulation can effectively be removed from the blood via metabolism. Since the metabolism rate within the liver is greatly affected by local perfusion changes or by a decreased metabolism capacity (e.g. liver insufficiency), this may result in a decrease in the elimination rate (i.e. clearance) with a corresponding increase in the duration of action [76].

There are two opioids where plasma and receptor concentrations lie close to each other, i.e. alfentanil and remifentanil. This is because the volume of distribution for alfentanil is very low (Table III-4) while remifentanil is rapidly metabolized by tissue and plasma esterase. It is because of this close correlation of plasma concentration and pharmacodynamic effects that the onset and the offset of these two agents can be predicted [77].

From such data it can be concluded that the plasma concentration of an opioid does not reflect the actual concentration at the receptor site, the amount that actually induces a pharmacodynamic effect. It was because of this difference that the concept of "effect-site concentration" (the actual biophase) was developed. Whereby the effect-site concentration (Ce) "tries" to equilibrate with plasma concentration (Cp) but only attains a fraction of the original Cp at its peak concentration, afterwards Cp falls below Ce. At this point, no further effect site uptake occurs, and a reverse diffusion out of the effect site may begin. Such pharmacokinetic changes explain the following phenomena:

- A delay in drug effect after a bolus injection.
- Initial drug plasma concentration is far in excess of the biophase required to induce an effect.
- The biophase is only a fraction of plasma concentration, an effect, which is due to redistribution to other compartments.
- Drug effect depends more on other factors than just plasma drug concentration such as partition coefficient, volumes of distribution, etc.

Such difference of concentrations in the various compartments also is seen after bolus injection of fentanyl in human volunteers. There, the distribution of the opioid in the central blood compartment and its accumulation in the peripheral organ compartment underlines the importance of the peripheral compartment site (Table III-5).

Several investigators set out to create a conceptual and mathematical model to depict the data derived from experimental drug plasma concentration decay curves. This resulted in the conceptual three-compartment model (Figure III-20) using the mathematical descriptor

$$C_p(t) = Ae^{-xt} + Be^{-yt} + Ce^{-z}$$

Drug kinetic behavior is described conceptually thru this model (Figure III-20). Right after an intravenous bolus the drug leaves the central compartment (CA_1) via three routes:

1. Exponentially from CA_1 (blood compartment) to CA_2, the vessel-rich compartment consisting of muscle, lungs, gut, kidney, spleen.

Table III-5. Difference of distribution of the opioid fentanyl in the various compartment sites in a volunteer. Note, the high concentration in the peripheral compartment site 60 minutes after application

Time (min.)	Percent of initial dose		
	Central compartment	Peripheral compartment	Elimination
0	100	0	0
0.5	69.8	24.7	5.5
1.0	49.2	41.5	9.3
2.0	25.2	60.8	14.0
3.0	13.9	69.7	16.4
5.0	6.0	75.2	18.8
10	3.7	74.8	21.5
60	2.7	55.5	41.8
120	1.9	38.7	59.4
240	0.9	18.2	80.3

Adapted from [78]

2. Exponentially from CA_1 to CA_3, the vessel poor compartment (i.e. the fatty tissue acting like a reservoir)
3. Exponentially from CA_1 to the environment (i.e. the elimination) also a blood vessel rich compartment consisting of hepatic or renal clearance, enzymatic and/or non-enzymatic degradation.

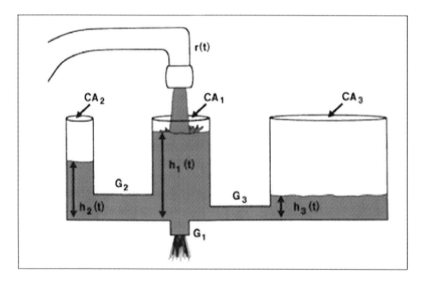

Figure III-20. Schematic illustration of the three-compartment model with the central (blood), the peripheral compartment – a virtual space comprising of internal organs, fatty tissue, musculature and connecting tissue – and the CNS compartment. They are saturated differently with the agent, while there is a rapid exchange of concentration among the different compartments

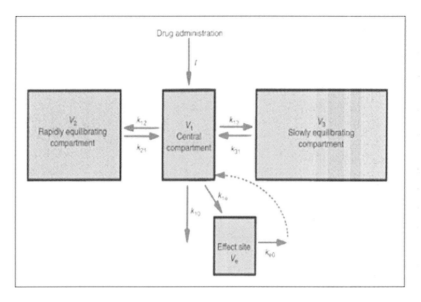

Figure III-21. The different compartments participating in the pharmacokinetics of an opioid, where the effect-site (Ve) is the actual site of action, and after binding, a pharmcodynamic effect is initiated

Only a tiny fraction goes from CA_1 (blood compartment) to Ve (i.e. the brain receptors). It is the conceptual effect site Ve, which as a compartment is very small when compared to V_2, V_3 and elimination (Figure III-21).

SIGNIFICANCE OF PHARMACOKINETIC DATA FOR PRACTICAL USE

While terminal elimination half-life (t 1/2ß) is only a single variable based on the beta slope of only the decay curve of an agent, it does not take into account redistribution and compartment kinetics (Table III-6). Time course of anesthesia related to intravenous bolus use is far less than the time course for terminal half-life. One would expect effects and recovery within seconds and minutes not hours. Anesthesia intravenous bolus time frame is determined by redistribution and mixed kinetics phase. Therefore elimination half-life is irrelevant in discussing effects of i.v. boluses within anesthesia. In the literature, the guidelines doses for i.v. boluses are based on volumes of distribution, overdose limits, peak effect concentrations but not necessarily duration considerations. It is therefore necessary to balance between side effects of overdose and duration of desired effects to choose a bolus dose.

Table III-6. Classical phramacokinetics of different opioid agonists as they are often described in the literature

Opioid	Rapid distribution half-time (min) $t_{1/2\alpha}$	Slow distribution half-time (min)	Elimination half-time (hours) $t_{1/2\beta}$
Morphine	1.2–25	9–13.3	7.2–22
Pethidine (meperidine)	4–17	?	3.2–7.9
Fentanyl	1.0–17	13–28	3.1–7.9
Alfentanil	1.4	17.7	2.7
Sufentanil	0.7–35	8.2–16.8	1.2–1.9

For example, why is alfentanil shorter acting and faster than fentanyl. Looking at traditional elimination half-life, one would explain this phenomenon by stating that this was due to alfentanil's shorter elimination half-life. Not so! Notice alfentanil and fentanyl's decay curves are almost identical until after 90 min. But we are explaining phenomena within the 3–10 min range. The fact is that alfentanil peaks earlier at a higher percentage of the initial plasma concentration Cp. Alfentanil effect is more rapid due to its smaller volume of distribution and rapid uptake into the effect compartment. Therefore, the clinician needs relatively less drug to get the same effect.

Therefore, the clinician underdoses alfentanil relative to fentanyl and sufentanil to get the same effect, and its duration of effect is shorter since less drug needs a shorter time decay to achieve subapnea levels. This shows that elimination half-life is a poor predictor of describing drug disposition in time frames relevant to anesthesia where redistribution and mixed kinetics are more relevant. Alfentanil's rapid onset and shorter duration of effect is due to distribution kinetics and not due to elimination kinetics only. When using a bolus dose of an agent, three different scenarios can be created:

1. Only one huge dose is given in order to cover the projected procedure time. This necessitates a very large initial overdose, creating both a prolonged elimination and recovery time.
2. A single bolus for rapid short-term effect is given, which rapidly redistributes and falls below the therapeutic target window allowing quick recovery.
3. Repeated boluses are given to maintain an effect-site concentration within the therapeutic window frame, however, creating a seesaw effect with repeated boluses with possible subsequent build-up of the drug and a prolongation of effects.

Since the key points of any injection is that the effect-site concentration, and not the plasma concentration, determines drug effect. Since a three-compartment model best describes most intravenous drugs, the terminal elimination half-life is *not* the basis for comparing durations of effect of i.v. boluses, especially since i.v. boluses balance overdose with duration.

Table III-7. Approximate opioid loading doses (bolus) and maintenance infusion rates for total intravenous anesthesia (TIVA)

Drug	Loading dose (μg/kg)	Maintenance dose (μg/kg/min)
Alfentanil	50–150	0.5–1.0
Fentanyl	5–15	0.33–0.1
Sufentanil	1–3	0.01–0.05
Remifentanil	0.5–1.0	0.1–0.4
Ketamine	1500–2500	25–75
Propofol	1000–2000	50–150
Mivacron	50–150	0.25–1.5
Methohexital	1500–2500	50–150

Adapted from [79]

ADVANTAGES OF "MAINTENANCE PHASE" INFUSIONS COMPARED TO INTERMITTENT BOLUS DOSE

During *an infusion*, the effect-site concentration mirrors plasma concentration, except following changes in rates or following supplemental boluses. This is due to the fact that either from a high loading dose or a long infusion time (Table III-7), the different compartments of the three-compartment model have been filled. Therefore, the kinetics are now mostly on the lower end of the decay curve (i.e., beta slope). Indications for the intravenous infusion of an opioid for anesthesia are as follows:
• When duration of effect is the key consideration
• When overdose effects are undesirable
• When rapid onset time is not critical
• For malignant hyperthermia patients, for patients with high risk of post operative nausea and vomiting, or for use in an ICU sedation setting
The advantages of a continuous opioid infusion in anesthesia are as follows:
• Decreased total dose of a drug
• Greater hemodynamic stability
• Decreased side effects (e.g. rigidity with opioids)
• Decreased need for supplementation with other anesthetics
• More predictable recovery of consciousness
• Possible less pain in the post-operative period
• Possible decreased discharge time
For continuous intravenous infusion one therefore needs to know the target infusion rates to achieve a desired plasma concentration by replacing what is lost to elimination. Cp50 is the concentration that prevents reaction to stimulus in 50% of the population (analogous to minimal alveolar concentration or MAC). Infusion rates are calculated based upon elimination kinetics only. The initial part of the infusion will have to overcome redistribution kinetics prior to achieving its desired target concentration. So, initially, one would woefully be in the subtherapeutic range due to redistribution of the infusion rate. And unless a higher rate is used, the target Cp 50 may never be reached since elimination is still occurring at the

Table III-8. The approximative effective drug plasma levels at different situations when combined with 65%-70% nitrous oxide in order to reach sufficient effect site concentrations. Effective plasma concentrations may differ markedly depending on premedictation and intraoperative drug combinations

Drug (ng/ml)	Skin incision	Major surgery	Minor surgery	Recovery	Analgesia-sedation
Alfentanil	200–300	250–450	100–300	–	50–100
Fentanyl	3–6	4–8	2–5	–	1–2
Sufentanil	1–3	2–5	1–3	–	0.02–0.2
Remifentanil	4–8	2–4	2–4	–	1–2
Propofol	2000–6000	2500–7500	2000–6000	800–1800	2000–3000
Methohexital	5000–10.000	5000–15.000	5000–10.000	1000–3000	2000–3000
Thiopental	7.500–12.500	10.000–20.000	10.000–20.000	4000–8000	7.500–15.000
Etomidate	–	500–1000	300–600	200–350	100–300
Midazolam	400–600	50–250 (+opioid)	50–250 (+opioid)	20–70 (+opioid)	40–100
Ketamin	–	–	1000–2000	–	100–1000

Adapted from [79]

same time as redistribution. But loss to compartments is greatest initially, and then decreases with time. Eventually accumulation of drug will occur due to saturated peripheral compartments returning drug to central compartment plus the ongoing fixed rate infusion. So the infusion must adapt or be either ineffective or eventually toxic. When choosing the appropriate infusion rate in order to achieve the proper target Cp 50 (Tables III-7 and III-8) the following considerations have to be taken into account:

1. What kind of agent is being used?
2. What kind of stimulus has to be blocked (i.e., skin incision, intubation, major/minor surgery, etc.)
3. What kind of reaction is one trying to prevent (i.e., movement, tachycardia/hypertension, pain in the postoperative care unit, etc.)
4. What kind of synergy exists with other anesthetics being given (i.e., nitrous oxide, volatile agents, other i.v. agents, premedication, etc.)

> **One cannot simply start an infusion rate and expect the plasma concentration (Cp) to stay at the correct level!**

The initial bolus should establish a therapeutic level. The bolus would rapidly fill compartments to get to the elimination kinetic part of the curve primarily, while the infusion must replace what is lost through:
• Elimination clearance (i.e. liver, kidney, enzymes)
• Transfer to compartment 1 (Fast)

- Transfer to compartment 2 (Slow)

Unfortunately, the last two processes are changing exponentially with time. Fortunately, inter-individual pharmacokinetic variability is large since parameters are derived from population studies. And since pharmacodynamics are also highly variable especially for narcotics (a good Cp for one patient may not be a good Cp for another). Therefore, a large adjustment factor or tolerance margin is available during infusion, and precision is not absolutely required. The therapeutic window for opioids is large (a *little* overdose is o.k.) during anesthesia since patients can be mechanically ventilated. The anesthesiologist therefore must titrate to effect by recognizing signs of inappropriate depth. One can always add a bolus and can always titrate the infusion rate to meet one's clinical targets. However, there is no current direct measurement real time monitor for plasma concentrations. Clinical monitors such as bispectral index or BIS, EEG, and anesthetic MAC titration currently being used, are all indirect measurements of Cp.

One also has to consider that combinations of narcotic infusions and inhalational anesthetics or other hypnotics allow synergistic interactions, which will reduce the required doses of both agents. Lower doses allow faster and more dependable recovery/emergence times. Infusions can be titrated to keep anesthetic MAC low throughout surgery and allow rapid elimination on emergence.

In summary, the following points have to be considered when using an infusion regimen for maintenance of anesthesia:

1. The effect site concentrations closely parallel plasma concentration in intravenous infusions.
2. Steady Cp is not achieved by steady infusion rate. Patients vary in terms of the infusion patterns required for given Cp (pharmacokinetics) and also the required Cp for a given desired drug effect (pharmacodynamics).

Use of Target Controlled Infusion (TCI) Systems in Anesthesia

Computerized pumps are used for infusions containing pharmacokinetic data based on population studies for various drugs. They deliver combinations of boluses and variable infusions to achieve a specified target Cp. The target Cp can be changed to match varying degrees of required depth throughout surgery. They have not been used frequently due to cost and design issues. The computerized pump Diprifusor® for instance requires proprietary propofol ampules/syringe cassettes. What is important is to know the Cp required for surgery and emergence. To awaken the patient one must decrease Cp from the initial surgical Cp to the emergence Cp that results in awakening. Therefore it is necessary to consider:

- If a higher Cp is maintained during the case, then expect a longer recovery.
- If a very low Cp is required for awakening and spontaneous ventilation, then a longer recovery is also expected.

For opioids, one needs a Cp low enough to awaken, but also high enough for postoperative analgesia. The goal is to coincide achievement of target Cp for emergence with intended time of awakening. The rate at which the body eliminates drug is relatively steady so the percent decrease required to awaken will affect greatly recovery time. The percent decrease in opioid concentrations required for emergence may vary from about 50% (balanced anesthesia) to 80% or more (opioid based technique). In this context recovery time depends on a number of things, among which the following are the most important:

- What is the Cp (initial), for maintenance anesthesia,
- what is the Cp (target), for awakening,
- the duration of infusion,
- the different drug pharmacokinetic characteristics
- and lastly the interpatient variability.

Within this framework the greatest drawback is that there is no real-time Cp monitor which may give a clue of what the necessary Cp is, and when to reduce the infusion rate in order to have a recovery at a certain time (Fig. III-22).

For recovery the principle of Context Sensitive Half Time (CSHT) can be used. The context Sensitive Half Time is the time required for a drug to reach to half its plasma concentration following termination of infusion. The "context" is the duration of the infusion and assumes that the infusion was designed to maintain target plasma concentration (e.g., with a computerized pump). Essentially, the longer the infusions, the longer the time needed to take to reduce its plasma concentration by ½. But Context Sensitive Half Time behavior varies between drugs, especially since it cannot be predicted at all by drug's terminal elimination half-life. Even though there is a no relationship between elimination half-life and Context Sensitive Half Time, elimination half-life will always exceed Context Sensitive Half Time, regardless of Context Sensitive Half Time being derived from computer modeling of known pharmacokinetic parameters. It takes into account drug behavior in compartments and redistribution (Figure III-23).

CSHT can be used to support a choice of drug for infusion depending on its projected duration of infusion. Note the propofol, midazolam and thiopental slopes. Propofol's CSHT is under 50 min, even after 9 h infusion. Midazolam has a slower CSHT (60 min) but seems constant after a 6 h infusion. So one can choose the drug with which to infuse for 2 h, 6 h, or 24 h and then allow for expedient awakening.

Fentanyl has a rapid increase in CSHT with infusions even over a short time frame. This causes slow recovery after an infusion due to large reservoirs in fat. However, it still can be used knowing that one must turn off infusions earlier to allow awakening. It would be similar to using halothane or isoflurane vapours. Among opioids, sufentanil may be a good choice for infusions lasting less than 8 h. Alfentanil may be a good choice for infusions over 8 h because its CSHT slope crosses over at around 600 min, while alfentanil's CSHT is fairly flat after 2 h sufentanil's slope continues to rise. Because remifentanil is metabolized by plasma

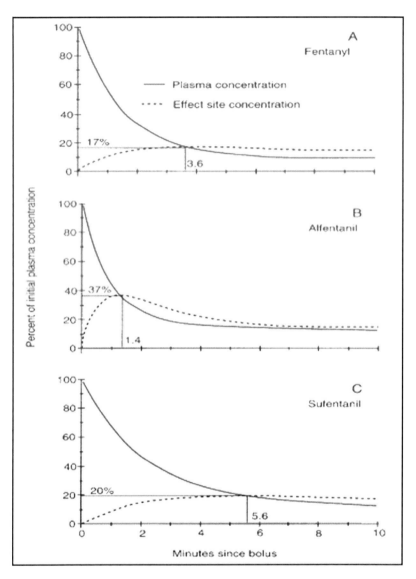

Figure III-22. The different decay curves of opioids after intravenous injection with similar elimination half-lives

esterases it always has a CSHT of only 3–6 min. It rapidly attains target concentration following change in infusion rate and lacks any significant accumulation, i.e. steady infusion rate = steady effect-site concentration. However, it provides no postoperative analgesia. Remifentanil is by far the best opioid for rapid equilibration

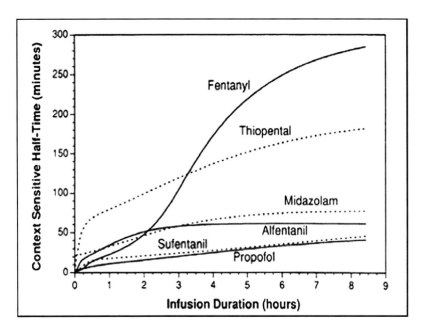

Figure III-23. Context-Sensitive Half Times (CSHT) as a function of infusion duration (the context) derived from pharmacokinetic models of fentanyl, sufentanil, propofol, midazolam, and thiopental (Adapted from [80])

and recovery but one must add a postoperative analgesic such as bolus of fentanyl or morphine.

In summary the following points have to be considered for recovery times when using an opioid infusion:

• It depends on the type of drug being used.
• It depends on the duration of infusion.
• It depends on the effect-site concentration required for surgery.
• It depends on the effect-site concentration required for awakening.

The weak correlation between plasma levels and pharmacodynamic effects can be visualized in the spectral edge frequency of the electroencephalographic recording, where the opioid was administered in volunteers. There, the EEG represents the biophase of pharmacodyamic effects of the opioid, while the plasma concentration reflects the circulating amount of the drug outside the CNS. It can be seen during fentanyl and sufentanil infusion, there is a drop in spectral edge frequency. Being due to a dominance of delta-waves, there is a lag of peak plasma concentration and central changes. And even after rapid decline of plasma levels, there is only a gradual change in pharmacodynamic effect (Figure III-24).

Such lag in effects is in contrast to two other fentanyl analogues, alfentanil and remifentanil. There is a parallel decline of plasma concentration and the

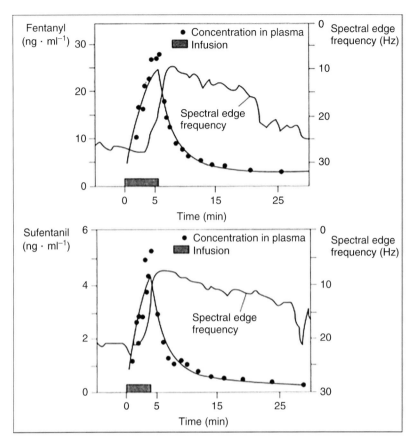

Figure III-24. Opioid plasma concentrations and their corresponding electroencephalographic changes, the spectral edge frequency, following a 5-min infusion of fentanyl (150 μg/min) and sufentanil (15 μg/min) respectively Adapted from [81, 82]

centrally mediated sedative effect, as visualized in a computerized EEG spectral edge frequency (Figure III-25).

"On-Top"-Dose of a Either Alfentanil or Remifentanil in an Opioid-Based Anesthetic Regimen

The demand to ensure a sufficient analgesic level up to the very last minute of an operation, without inducing an overhang of effects, with a delay in recovery, has led to the development of opioid agents, which are characterized by a short duration of action. Due to the pharmacokinetic and physicochemical properties the opioid fentanyl, which is being used most often in neuroleptanalgesia and in an opioid-based anesthetic regimen, often projects into the postoperative period with

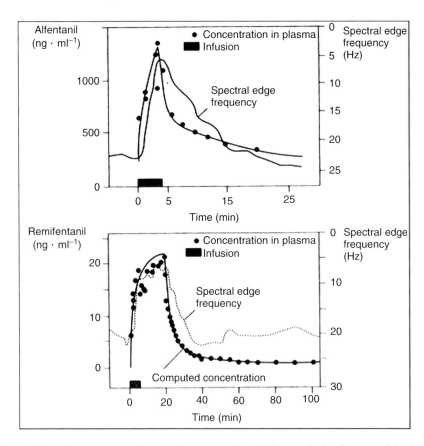

Figure III-25. Plasma concentration and the corresponding EEG-spectral edge frequency following a 5-minute infusion of alfentanil (1500 μg/min) and remifentanil (150 μg/min) respectively (Adapted from [83, 84])

Table III-9. Comparison of pharmacokinetics of different opioids among each other

Opioid	Elimination half life $t_{1/2\beta}$ (min)	Clearance (Cl) (ml/min/kg)	Distribution coefficient Vd (L/kg)	Protein Binding (%)	Non-Ionized (%)
Fentanyl	219	13.0	4.0	84	9
Alfentanil	94	6.4	0.86	92	89
Sufentanil	64	12.7	2.9	92	20
Morphine	77	14.7	3.2	60	24
Pethidine	92	12.0	2.9	?	5
Meptazinol	124	132	4.99	27	10

Adapted from [70, 75]

insufficient recovery of spontaneous ventilation and consciousness. The cause for such overhang is the larger distribution coefficient (Vd) of fentanyl in the peripheral compartment of the body (skin, musculature, and fatty tissue), whereby it hides from the biodegradation resulting in high amounts in the biophase and a long terminal elimination half-life ($t_{1/2\beta}$) with a long duration of action (Table III-9).

To circumvent this disadvantage the anesthesiologist can use the short-acting opioid alfentanil or the ultra-short acting opioid remifentanil. Both of them are fentanyl analogs derived from the group of 4-aniline-piperidines, which are able to blunt the stress response in the very last minute of an operation. Since stress during operation results in a cascade of events, which have been implicated in increasing patient morbidity and/or mortality this results in an improvement of patient care. In comparison to the other potent narcotic analgesics, alfentanil is characterized by a smaller volume of distribution (Vd) and due to the higher clearance rate (Cl), it also results in a shorter elimination half-life ($t_{1/2\beta}$; Figure III-26). Because alfentanil in comparison to the other opioids also has a higher portion of non-ionized molecules, more fractions of the pharmacologically active agent are able to penetrate the blood-brain barrier, reaching the opioid receptor sites within the CNS (Table III-9), thereby inducing an immediate and powerful analgesic effect.

When using the opioid remifentanil, elimination half-life is only 7 min, having an onset of action of about 1 min, which is similar to alfentanil. Independent of liver function, degradation is done by blood and tissue esterase, whereby repetitive doses or an infusion does not result in an overhang of effects.

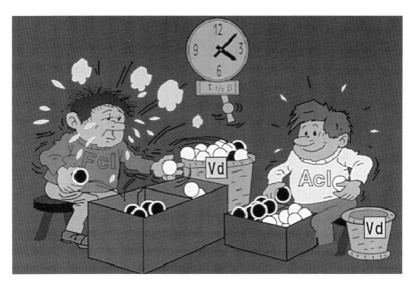

Figure III-26. Low volume of distribution of alfentanil (Vd), when compared to fentanyl, results in more molecules available for degradation, a higher clearance (Cl) via the liver, and a shorter elimination half-life ($t_{1/2\beta}$)

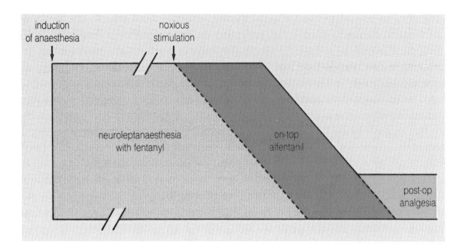

Figure III-27. Principle of the "on-top" administration of alfentanil or remifentanil when given at the end of classical neuroleptanalgesia or an opioid-based anesthetic technique with fentanyl

Due to such a preferable profile, alfentanil or remifentanil can be used to potentiate analgesia when used on-top a preexisting, low analgesic level without inducing an overhang of respiratory depression into the postoperative period (Figure III-27).

The reasons for using either one of these two agents are more obvious than using the potent opioid fentanyl or sufentanil. First, and most of all, the time to maximum effect (onset of action; Figure III-28) is that of circulation time, where after intravenous injection the opioid rapidly enters brain tissue [85] [86]. The opioid can be applied whenever there is a need for an increase in analgesia, directly related to the stage of operation, when there is an increase in nociceptive afferences. Contrary, onset of action of fentanyl starts at 2 min with a maximal analgesic effect clinically seen only after 5 min [77].

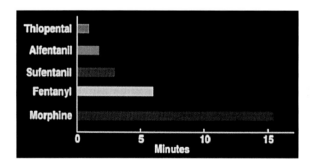

Figure III-28. Comparison of maximal onset times of various opioids compared to a barbiturate. Alfentanil, similar to remifentanil has the shortest onset time till maximal effect, which is comparable to a barbiturate

The obvious advantages of alfentanil as well as remifentanil are also demonstrated in its Context-Sensitive Half Time, reflecting the time at which a drug will induce a biological effect in a patient. Being particularly useful for understanding the impact of a continuous infusion of an opioid and the time until recovery, the "three compartment" phamacological model can be used. Although being derived from data of single dose applications in patients and using a computer stimulation program, it reflects the potential behavior of a drug in patients [87]. There it can be seen that opioids being metabolized by the liver accumulate over time resulting in a longer recovery period. This is especially demonstrated for the opioid fentanyl, which tends to accumulate in the peripheral compartment. Such findings are of clinical significance, as a long infusion time corresponds with a longer duration until the drug decreases by 50% in the CNS (Figure III-29).

A similar beneficial effect is seen with the opioid remifentanil, which does not accumulate in the peripheral compartment since it is an esterase-metabolized opioid (EMO), maintaining a brief period of biological effect without risk of accumulation, regardless of the disease and the time or the duration of infusion [88]. Remifentanil may even be superior to alfentanil since after a similar infusion time, the decay in plasma level of both agents is much faster after remifentanil than after alfentanil. Therefore, regardless of the metabolic status of the patient, a fast decrease in plasma levels can be anticipated with this non-specific esterase metabolized opioid (Figure III-30).

While remifentanil's short duration of action is explained by its rapid degradation via non-pseudocholinesterases, the time that limits the effects of alfentanil is the metabolization by the liver. Due to its high lipophilicity and the higher portion of non-ionized molecules (Table III-9) the blood-brain barrier is rapidly penetrated resulting in immediate binding to the receptor site and the initiation of effects. However, the speed by which alfentanil enters the brain is also in the reverse direction. Alfentanil rapidly leaves the CNS back to the central compartment of the blood, from where the liver eliminates the agent by metabolism [75]. Although being redistributed to protein-rich organ sites (i.e. musculature, liver, kidney, lungs) as other opioids like fentanyl, the amount of this redistribution is much less. Therefore alfentanil cannot hide from metabolism as fentanyl does, resulting in a faster elimination with a loss of effects. Its short duration on respiratory drive is demonstrated in mean end-expiratory CO_2-concentrations in volunteers following different dosages of alfentanil, while using the rebreathing technique as originally described by Read [89]. There it can be seen that a dose of $10\,\mu g/kg$ body weight of alfentanil, the respiratory depressive effect is of short duration and of lesser magnitude as an equianalgesic dose of fentanyl ($2\,\mu g/kg$ body weight). The respiratory depressive effect of fentanyl was 13fold more intense and of longer duration (Figure III-31).

Since theoretically "on-top" administration of alfentanil on a fentanyl-based anesthesia results in an interaction of both opioids on receptor sites, this may provoke a prolongation in an impaired respiratory drive and a long-lasting impairment of vigilance. In a clinical study alfentanil ($10\,\mu g/kg$ body weight) or fentanyl ($1.5\,\mu g/kg$ body weight) was given to patients during classical neuroleptanalgesia

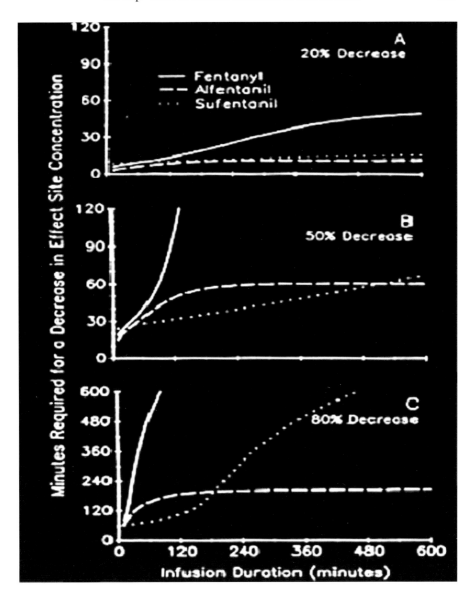

Figure III-29. Difference in time required for a 20%, a 50% or an 80% decrease in the biophase, when using different opioids at different infusion times (Data adapted from [87])

with fentanyl within the last 50 min of the procedure [91]. Postoperatively the electroencephalogram was used to determine any difference in vigilance, while plasma levels were determined to evaluate difference in the metabolic rate of the liver.

Alfentanil as well as fentanyl initially induce a characteristically slowing in EEG activity with dominance of delta-waves (0.5–3 Hz) as described by others

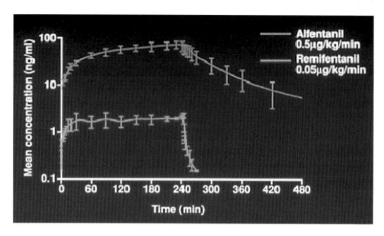

Figure III-30. Decay in plasma concentration following similar infusion times of alfentanil (0.5 µg/kg/min) and remifentanil (0.05 µg/kg/min) (Adapted from [84])

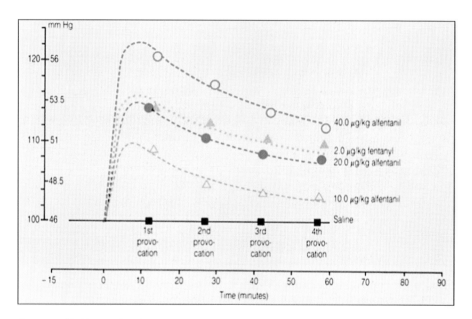

Figure III-31. Mean end-expiratory CO_2-concentrations in volunteers receiving either fentanyl or alfentanil, while the responsiveness of the respiratory center was evaluated using an inspiratory concentration of 4% CO_2 at four different time intervals. Sensitivity of the respiratory center was only reduced 10 and 20 min after alfentanil. After an equianalgesic dose of fentanyl respiratory impairment lasted significantly longer (Adapted from [90])

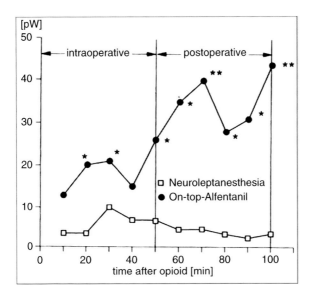

Figure III-32. Comparative power (picoWatt) in EEG activity in the fast beta-band (13–30 Hz) in two groups of patients having received either on-top alfentanil or fentanyl respectively. Note the significant (*p < 0.05; **p < 0.01) higher activity after the additional dose of alfentanil (Adapted from [91])

[17, 81]. However, contrary to "on-top" fentanyl, alfentanil "on-top" resulted in a faster recovery. This was reflected in the fast beta-domain (13–30 Hz) of the EEG, reflecting a higher state of vigilance in the postoperative period (Figure III-32).

Following "on-top" alfentanil and similar to the faster recovery in vigilance, patients also had a faster recovery of spontaneous respiratory drive (Table III-10). Although the dose of alfentanil necessary to induce a sufficient analgesia in a non-premeditated patients is $40 \pm 20\mu g/kg$ body weight [85, 92], a low dose of $10 \mu g/kg$ body weight is sufficient to potentiate analgesia in patients with receptor sites already preoccupied by fentanyl.

While the electroencephalogram reflects the state of vigilance in a patient, the sensory-evoked potential mirrors the depth of analgesia and the degree of blockade

Table III-10. Postoperative spontaneous respiration (L/min) in patients, following "on-top" alfentanil versus "on-top" fentanyl

Postoperative time (min)	"On-top" alfentanil (L/min)	"On-top" fentanyl (L/min)
10	5.1 ± 0.5	5.4 ± 0.8
20	6.4 ± 0.6	6.3 ± 0.8
30	5.9 ± 0.5	5.5 ± 1.1
40	4.4 ± 0.5	4.6 ± 1.5
50	5.9 ± 0.6	5.0 ± 1.5

Adapted from [91]

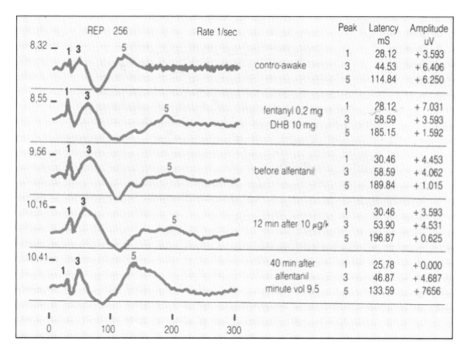

				Peak	Latency mS	Amplitude uV
REP 256		Rate 1/sec				
8,32 – 1 3	5		contro-awake	1	28.12	+ 3.593
				3	44.53	+ 6.406
				5	114.84	+ 6.250
8.55 – 1 3	5		fentanyl 0.2 mg DHB 10 mg	1	28.12	+ 7.031
				3	58.59	+ 3.593
				5	185.15	+ 1.592
9.56 – 1 3	5		before alfentanil	1	30.46	+ 4.453
				3	58.59	+ 4.062
				5	189.84	+ 1.015
10,16 – 3 1	5		12 min after 10 μg/ʰ	1	30.46	+ 3.593
				3	53.90	+ 4.531
				5	196.87	+ 0.625
10,41 – 3 1	5		40 min after alfentanil minute vol 9.5	1	25.78	+ 0.000
				3	46.87	+ 4.687
				5	133.59	+ 7656

Figure III-33. Different peaks of the somatosensory-evoked potential in patients undergoing classical neuroleptanesthesia with fentanyl and a concomitant intraoperative "on-top" administration of alfentanil. Note, the short-term depression of the late peak 5 (> 100m) and its recovery 40 min after administration (DHB = dehydrobenzperidol) (Adapted from [97])

of the electrically-induced stimulus at the median nerve on its way to the cerebral cortex by opioid receptor occupancy [93, 94, 95, 96]. A representative example shows the changes in amplitude height of the late (> 100 ms) evoked peak during neuroleptanesthesia, before and after alfentanil (Figure III-32). From such data it can be concluded, that alfentanil when given "on-top" an opioid based anesthetic regimen, is a safe agent because it induces a short-time increase of analgesia within the last period of an operation, without, however, resulting in an overhang with a depressed vigilance or a prolongation in recovery of spontaneous respiratory drive. With an analgesic potency 40–70fold that of morphine, alfentanil is an agent for short-term potentiation of analgesia given within the last 30 min of operation, while opioids like fentanyl and/or sufentanil should only be given during the anesthetic course, when the duration of operation is expected to last one hour and longer.

Both opioids, alfentanil and remifentanil can safely be given "on-top" an opioid-based anesthesia whenever a reduction in analgesia becomes apparent:
1. Any increase in systolic blood pressure > 15% above the preoperative level before premedication.

2. An increase in heart rate above 90 beats/min, presumed that the patient does not experience hypovolemia.
3. All other vegetative signs of an insufficient depth of analgesia such as lacrimation, transpiration or involuntary movement of extremities.

RECOMMENDATIONS FOR THE USE OF REMIFENTANIL

The ultra-short acting opioid remifentanil can either be given as bolus or by continuous infusion. When giving the opioid as a bolus, a dose of $1\,\mu g/kg$ body weight should be chosen, injecting the drug over a time period of 30 s. This is because a higher speed of injection will result in muscular rigidity. When using the opioid for induction together with a hypnotic (etomidate or propofol) its infusion ($0.5\,\mu g/kg/min$) has the advantage of a sufficient blockade of irritating reflexes induced by laryngoscopy and intubation with lesser stress-related cardiovascular activation. Following induction, anesthesia can be maintained with remifentanil in a dose of $0.25\,\mu g/kg/min$ together with propofol in a dose of 4–$6\,mg/kg/min$, together with artificial ventilation using a mixture of air and oxygen (FiO_2 0.5), or adding a volatile agent such as isoflurane in low concentrations between 0.4 and 0.6 vol% (Table III-11).

Remifentanil is being hydrolyzed by the ever-present blood and tissue esterases, resulting in rapid metabolism. Because of this rapid degradation (Figure III-34) remifentanil should be given as an infusion in order to maintain a stable plasma concentration and a constant occupation of the receptor site.

Table III-11. Suggested dosing of remifentanil for start, maintenance of anesthesia and for postoperative pain therapy in the elderly patient population (> 65 anno) for induction of anesthesia, a reduction of the usual dose by about half is suggested, while for maintenance of anesthesia the dose is adapted to need [98]. In a preexisting renal- and/or liver insufficiency, contrary to alfentanil, no dose-adjustment is necessary, since this opioid is being metabolized by blood- and tissue esterases. In obese patients ($> 30\%$ above lean body weight) and similar as with alfentanil, the ideal weight is used for calculation of the appropriate dose, since it correlates more closely with effects

Balanced anesthesia with remifentanil (TIVA)	Dose for start of anesthesia ($\mu g/kg/min$)	Dose for maintenance of anesthesia ($\mu g/kg/min$)
Induction	1.0 slowly over 30 s	
Maintenance		
With 66% N_2O	0.5–1.0	0.1–2.0
With isoflurane 0.5 MAC	0.5–1.0	0.05–2.0
With propofol $100\,\mu g/kg/min$	0.5–1.0	0.05–2.0
Postoperative Analgesia		
	local analgesic plus 1 g paracetamol or metamizole	Morphine 10 mg before (!) end of anesthesia
Regional or local anesthesia as adjuvans	0.04–0.07	

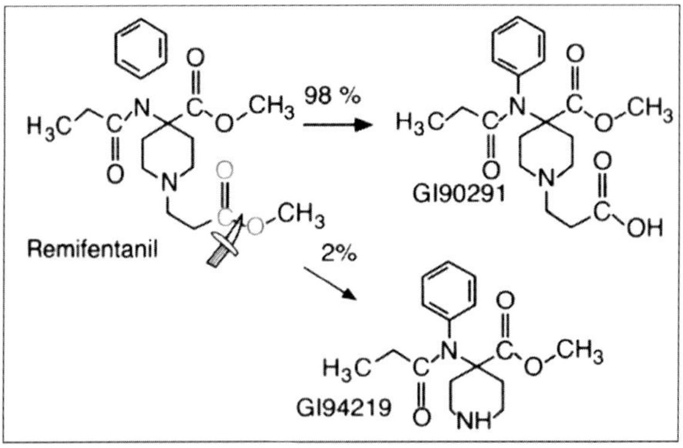

Figure III-34. Pathway of metabolism of remifentanil to two pharmacologically inactive compounds
Adapted from [88]

In general, however, the dose should always be adjusted to the course of operation, and once there is an increased flow of nociceptive afferents, this can be blocked immediately by increasing the infusion rate. Such practice will result in alleviation of any stress-related consequences with blood pressure increase and/or tachycardia. According to need, a volatile anesthetic, a benzodiazepine, or a hypnotic like propofol can be added; however, always keep in mind that analgesia is the primary goal in the course of anesthesia. The rapid onset of action (about 1 min) of remifentanil is due to the high portion of non-ionized molecules, which are able to cross the blood-brain barrier in sufficient amounts occupying the specific receptor sites.

In Summary, remifentanil has obvious advantages; however, there are also certain disadvantages that have to be observed:

Advantages
- Intraoperative judgment of dose versus effect
- rapid adaptation to change of nociceptive flow
- no postoperative overhang
- pharmacokinetics not effected by renal- and/or liver insufficiency

Disadvantages
- In case of unattended stop of infusion, rapid loss of analgesia and increase in awareness
- Postoperative analgesia has to be started already at the last quarter of anesthetic course.
- Preoperative preparation of an infusion system
- Muscle rigidity when administered rapidly as a bolus
- For sufficient postoperative analgesia, surveillance in the postoperative care unit (PACU) is mandatory in order to rapidly adapt the analgesic need of the patient.

Because of its unique short half-life, handling of remifentanil is different than using other fentanyl analogues. With the loss of receptor occupancy there is a sudden loss in postoperative analgesia, sometimes accompanied by abstinence symptoms. Also, use of remifentanil reportedly is accompanied by rapid development of tachyphylaxis [99, 100]. But most of all, postoperative analgesia has to be planned ahead of time. In order to guarantee a smooth pain free state lasting into the postoperative period, the following courses of action are suggested [101]:

1. Towards the end of anesthesia, reduction of the hypnotic with remifentanil given until skin closure.
2. Administration of a long-lasting opioid 10–20 min before end of operation (e.g. morphine 2 mg/kg body weight, buprenorphine 2 μg/kg body weight).
3. Use of a peridural catheter for postoperative pain control with 4 mg morphine plus 10 ml of the local anesthetic bupivacaine 0.25%.
4. Intraoperatively, 30 min prior to the end of anesthesia administration of a NSAID (e.g. metamizole 1.0–2.5 g/70 kg body weight).
5. Use of a patient-controlled analgesia (PCA) system with morphine.
6. In children use of suppositories (1000 mg paracetamol), the opioid tramadol, the partial opioid agonist meptazinol or the agonist/antagonist nalbuphine (0.1 mg/kg body weight).

The clinical utility of most analgesic drugs, and especially that of remifentanil, is altered in the presence of patients with impaired renal or hepatic function not simply because of altered clearance of the parent drug, but mostly through an interaction and the production and accumulation of toxic or therapeutically active metabolites. Some analgesic agents may also aggravate pre-existing renal and hepatic disease. A search was performed, taking in published articles and pharmaceutical data to determine available evidence for managing acute pain effectively and safely in these two patient groups. The resulting information consisted mainly of small group pharmacokinetic studies or case reports, which included a large variation in degree of organ dysfunction. In the presence of renal impairment, those drugs, which exhibit the safest pharmacological profile, are alfentanil, buprenorphine, fentanyl, ketamine, paracetamol (except with compound analgesics), remifentanil and sufentanil. None of these deliver a highly active metabolite load, or suffer from significantly prolonged clearance. Amitriptyline, bupivacaine, clonidine, gabapentin, hydromorphone, levobupivacaine, lignocaine, methadone, mexiletine, morphine, oxycodone and tramadol have been used in the presence of renal failure, but do require specific precautions, usually dose reduction. Aspirin, dextropropoxyphene, non-steroidal anti-inflammatory drugs and pethidine, should not be used in the presence of chronic renal failure due to the risk of significant toxicity. In the presence of hepatic impairment, most drugs are subject to significantly impaired clearance and increased oral bioavailability, but are poorly studied in the clinical setting. The agent least subject to alteration in this context is remifentanil; however the drugs' potency has other inherent dangers. Other agents must only be used with caution and close patient monitoring. Amitriptyline, carbamazepine and valproate should be avoided as the risk of fulminant hepatic failure is higher in this population, and methadone is contraindicated in the presence of severe liver disease.

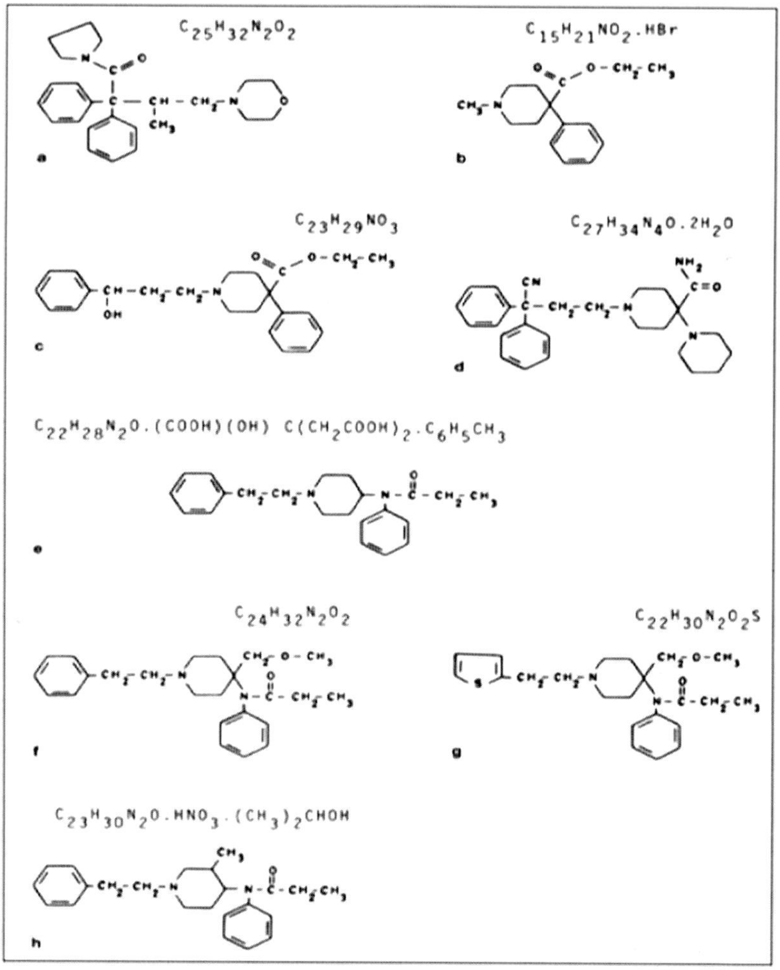

Figure III-35. The basic molecular structure of pethidine, where different substitutions at side-chains result in fully synthetic opioids of the piperidine series with different potency (a = dextromoramide; b = pethidine (meperidine, USP); C = phenoperidine; d = piritramide; e = fentanyl; f = lofentanil; g = sufentanil; h = carfentanil) (Adapted from [106])

The Pharmacology of Sufentanil

Contrary to the short acting opioids alfentanil and remifentanil, the relative long acting and the most potent opioid sufentanil should be used as the basic analgesic agent in all major surgical procedures, which are likely to result in intense nociceptive activity. Due to its high stereospecificity to the receptor site (Figure III-35) it is characterized by the widest therapeutic margin of safety (fentanyl 277, alfentanil 10, 80, sufentanil 26, 716) [13, 102, 103, 104, 105].

Table III-12. Difference in affinity of various opioids to the three main opioid receptior sites μ, κ, and δ as reflected in receptor binding and displacement studies in guinea pig brain homogenates (Ki in nmol/L). The lower the dose, which is necessary to displace 50% of a radioactive labeled ligand from the binding site, the better the affinity. Note, low Ki of sufentanil to the μ-site reflects high affinity

Opioid	Displacement of ^{3}H-D-Ala-Me-Phe-Gly-ol^2-enkephalin at μ-site	Displacement of ^{3}H-D-Ala-D-Leu-enkephalin at δ-site	Displacement of ^{3}H-Ethyl-ketocyclazocine at κ-site
Morphine	1.8 ± 0.26	90 ± 16	317 ± 68
Pethidine	185 ± 51	4345 ± 1183	5140 ± 789
Pentazocine	7.0 ± 1.6	106 ± 10	22.2 ± 4.1
Fentanyl	7.0 ± 0.81	151 ± 21	470 ± 68
Sufentanil	1.58 ± 0.38	23.4 ± 7.2	124 ± 11

Adapted from [107]

At the same time it is a drug with a relative high affinity to and an intense intrinsic activity of the μ-opioid receptor (Table III-12). This accounts for a 800fold higher potency than morphine, and a 5–7fold higher analgesic effectiveness than fentanyl.

Due to its high receptor specificity, which goes in hand with a wide therapeutic margin of safety, clinically this is manifested in practically no cardiovascular depression. In addition, the high intrinsic activity, which parallels with a high analgesic potency, only low amounts of the agent have to be administered in order to achieve a desired effect. This is of advantage as there is a lower load for liver enzymes for degradation. Even in the case of an accidental overdose, no side effects have to be expected from the cardiovascular system.

Being a derivative of the fentanyl series, it has a similar antitussive, respiratory depressive and bradycardiac effect. Also, as demonstrated in the octanol/water partition coefficient (Table III-13), it has a high lipophilicity, suggesting that there is a rapid transfer through the blood-brain barrier, which partly accounts for its fast onset of action within 2 min.

In addition, the higher portion of non-ionized molecules of sufentanil, which accounts for 20%, suggests a faster onset of action than fentanyl where only 8.5% are present in the plasma as non-ionized molecules, which are able to pass through the blood-brain barrier. Therefore, time until max effect is 3–4 min for sufentanil, which however is 5–8 min for fentanyl. Contrary, the hydrophilic compound morphine has an even much longer duration until max. effect being around 15 min, while after remifentanil and after alfentanil time until max. effect is around 1 min.

Aside from the short onset of action, the volume of distribution (Table III-13) also differs among the different fentanyl analogues. With 4.0 L/kg for fentanyl there is a Vd of 2.9 L/kg for sufentanil, suggesting that there is a lesser likelihood of a re-diffusion phenomenon with late opioid-related overhang. This is also reflected in the faster plasma clearance and a shorter terminal elimination half-life ($t_{1/2\beta}$), which is 164 min after sufentanil and 219 min after fentanyl respectively. The lowest volume of distribution is seen with alfentanil (0.86 L/kg) implying little redistribution of the agent from peripheral tissue. Although remifentanil has a relatively large volume of distribution, there is no rediffusion of the agent back into the central blood compartment. This is because the fentanyl analogue is metabolized by blood and tissues esterase resulting in the shortest duration of action being around 7 min [86].

Due to the higher analgesic potency of sufentanil there is a better depression of nociceptive induced stress reactions as mirrored in a more stable blood pressure, pulmonary artery pressure and heart rate [18, 108]. Especially the stress-related hormonal changes such as the usual increase in epinephrine, norepinephrine, corticoids, ADH, vasopressine, and mineralcorticoids are not increased during most intense nociceptive stimulation [109, 110].

It also has been noted that in comparison to fentanyl, sufentanil when given in equianalgesic dosages, results in a longer duration of analgesia, which, however, is accompanied by a lesser respiratory depressive effect (Figure III-36). Such difference is accounted to an uncoupling of analgesia and respiratory depression in the lower dose-range of sufentanil, making this agent a more favorable analgesic in the postoperative period [111, 112].

RESPIRATORY DEPRESSION AFTER SUFENTANIL

Similar to all potent narcotic analgesics, sufentanil dose-proportionally depresses respiratory drive and the responsiveness of the respiratory center to an elevated paCO2-level. In addition it inhibits centers in the pons and the medulla, which regulate respiratory rate and tidal volume. Besides its direct effect on the respiratory center, indirectly sufentanil also affects ventilation via an increase in muscular rigidity, which reduces the compliance of the thoracic cage, resulting in

Table III-13. Comparative pharmacokinetic data of various opioids [70, 72, 88]

Pharmacokinetics	Sufentanil	Fentanyl	Alfentanil	Morphine	Remifentanil
Non-ionized portion (%)	20	8.5	89	23	> 50
Octanol/water- partition coeff.	1727	816	129	1.4	17.9
Protein bound (%)	92.5	84.4	92.1	60	70
Distribution volume (L/kg)	2.9	4.0	0.86	3.2	32.8
Elimination half-time ($t_{1/2\beta}$; min)	164	219	94	177	9.1
Plasma clearance (ml/kg/min)	12.7	13.0	6.4	114.7	2800

an obstruction to gas exchange. In contrast to fentanyl, however, the respiratory depressive effect is less and of shorter duration, while analgesia is still maintained [108, 112]. Such dissimilarity may be due to a selective affinity to alternative opioid sub-receptor sites termed $\mu 1$ and $\mu 2$ respectively [113].

Following the injection of sufentanil the following sequence of effects on spontaneous respiration can be observed:

1. First there is a reduction respiratory rate (bradypnea) with a compensatory increase in tidal volume.
2. This is followed by a phase where only intense stimuli (nociceptive, acoustic) are able to induce a spontaneous respiratory drive.
3. Thereafter the patient "forgets" to breathe, and he will only take deep breaths on command.
4. At the end there is total apnea where the patient has to be ventilated artificially.

Any co-administration of sufentanil with a volatile anesthetic, a barbiturate, a benzodiazepine, a neuroleptic, a hypnotic, an antidepressive agent (MAO-inhibitors), the administration of lithium, or the concomitant use of a cytostatic will result in a potentiation of respiratory depression. Patients with a low protein level, patients with a pre-existing pulmonary disease, or patients who present an alkalosis, a prolongation of sufentanil-related respiratory depression has to be anticipated [114]. Similarly as with any other opioid, respiratory impairment can successfully be reversed with a selective antagonist (naloxone, nalmefene) or a mixed narcotic analgesic such as

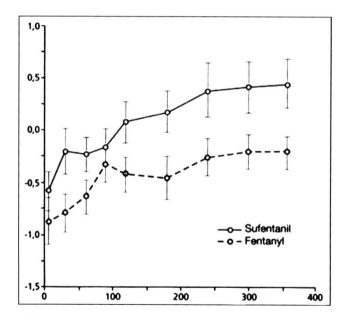

Figure III-36. Difference in steepness of slope of tidal volume to increasing inspiratory concentrations of CO_2 following equianalgesic doses of fentanyl and sufentanil respectively. Note, the faster recovery of the respiratory center response to CO_2 after sufentanil (Adapted from [111])

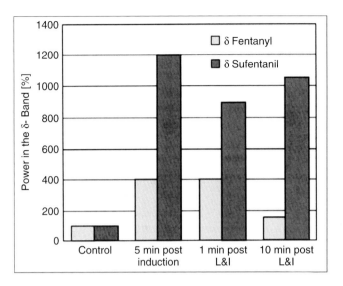

Figure III-37. Relative changes of power in the delta-band of the EEG to control, reflecting a more pronounced hypnosedative effect of sufentanil when compared to fentanyl in patients undergoing open-heart surgery, where the opioid was used for induction of anesthesia (Adapted from [119])

nalbuphine. However, it has to be recognized that the duration of action of sufentanil tends to be longer than the antagonist. This is why, after initial recovery of respiration, there is a rebound of a depressed spontaneous respiration. Therefore, after an initial return of normal ventilation the patient still has to be supervised in order to detect any deterioration of respiratory drive.

THE HYPNOSEDATIVE EFFECT OF SUFENTANIL

The sedative effect of sufentanil is much more pronounced than after fentanyl (Figure III-36). This can be visualized in the EEG where the power spectra within the low delta-band (0.5–3 Hz) are significantly higher when administering equianalgesic dosages of both agents [115, 116]. The more favorable hypnosedative effect of sufentanil clinically can be used for anesthesia and for sedation in the ICU setting, resulting in a lesser need for co-administration of a hypnotic/sedative. This is in contrast to fentanyl where intraoperative awareness and recall has been reported repetitively when using high-dose fentanyl as a sole anesthetic [117, 118].

SUFENTANIL AND MUSCULAR RIGIDITY

Similar as all other potent opioid agents (fentanyl, alfentanil, remifentanil) sufentanil can induce muscular rigidity when administered intravenously as a bolus injection. This rigidity mostly affects striatal muscles of the trunk [120] resulting in difficulty of expanding the thoracic aperture and inflation of the lungs [121]. The incidence of rigidity depends upon:

1. The speed of injection. Bolus injection is more likely to induce this phenomenon.
2. The dose of the administered opioid. High doses will induce muscular rigidity.
3. The age of the patient, since rigidity is seldom seen in the younger patient population; it is, however, regularly seen in patients > 65 years of age.

Muscular rigidity is not due to an epileptogenic action of sufentanil, because in the EEG no spike-and-wave activity is present [122, 123].

The following procedures are proposed in order to prevent/terminate the phenomenon of muscular rigidity:

1. Slow injection of the potent opioid over a period of 2 min.
2. A low dose of a competitive muscle relaxant, before opioid administration, as this partially blocks the increase of neuromuscular transmission.
3. The simultaneous administration of sufentanil and a muscle relaxant.
4. Once muscular rigidity has been established it quickly can be reversed by the intravenous administration of a small dose (20–40 mg/70 kg body weight) of succinylcholine [121].

SUFENTANIL IN SELECTIVE OPERATIONS

Neurosurgery

Sufentanil is a favorable opioid for use in neurosurgical procedures. This is because increasing dosages of the opioid (5–10–20–40 and 80 μg/kg body weight) similar to other fentanyl analogues, induce a dose-dependent significant drop in cerebral perfusion (CBF) and cerebral oxygen consumption ($CMRO_2$; Figure III-38). This close correlation between the reduction in cerebral oxygen consumption and cerebral perfusion is similar to isoflurane in patients undergoing carotid endarterectomy [124]. The beneficial effect of sufentanil on cerebral tissue is especially demonstrated by a reduction of white matter turgor in craniotomized patients under basic isoflurane N_2O/O_2-relaxant anesthesia. Also, sufentanil given as a bolus (0.3 μg/kg body weight) and followed by an infusion (0.3 μg/kg/h) with a stable arterial pCO2 of 28 mmHg, in comparison to a saline infusion, resulted in a lesser protrusion of cortical tissue, a lesser turgor of cortical cells and a lesser perfusion of cerebral vessels. Naloxone as an antagonist is absolutely contraindicated in neurosurgical patients anesthetized with sufentanil. This is because naloxone induces cerebral perfusion, and a significant raise in cerebral metabolic rate with an increase in cerebral oxygen consumption. Also, any opioid-related side effects such as nausea and emesis induce an increase in intracranial pressure, which is of disadvantage for viable neuronal cells.

Although sufentanil reduces cerebral oxygen consumption, perfusion pressure and intracranial pressure in the animal [126, 127], such preferential effects may not be transferred to the poly-traumatized patients with head injury, where the intracranial compliance is reduced and autoregulation of cerebral vessels on different

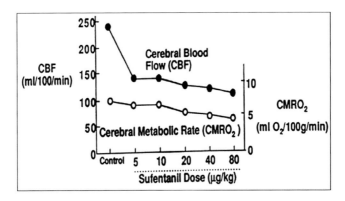

Figure III-38. Sufentanil on cerebral metabolism and perfusion (Adapted from [125])

$paCO_2$ pressure is further reduced by the anesthetic. It therefore is of importance to choose the appropriate anesthetic agent in neurosurgical procedures. Weinstabl and coworker were able to demonstrate conclusively in neurosurgical patients with an increased intracranial pressure (> 20 mmHg) a reduction in perfusion pressure (Figure III-39), which went in hand with a reduction in mean arterial pressure, not affecting intracranial pressure [128].

Such results are in contrast to data of other researchers [129], who after $0.6 \mu g/kg$ body weight of sufentanil observed a short-term increase of intracranial pressure in neurosurgical patients from a mean of 7.1 mmHg to a mean of 13.2 mmHg. Simultaneously with this increase in intracranial pressure mean arterial pressure dropped from a mean of 92 mmHg to a mean of 83 mmHg. Such divergent results very likely are due to a difference in resting intracranial pressure. It seems likely that in certain cases with only a small increase in intracranial pressure there is still a residual compliance in intracranial volume, being able to balance the increase in intracranial volume and pressure. From such data it can be concluded that in patients with an increased intracranial pressure sufentanil does not result in an additional peril of neuronal tissue. The data, however, also demonstrate that cerebral perfusion pressure closely correlates with mean arterial pressure. This fact has to be considered when patients with head trauma have to be anesthetized for operation, using sufentanil as the basic opioid. The opioid, therefore, should be administered in fractional doses in order to prevent a reduction in mean arterial pressure with a borderline perfusion pressure of the cranium.

Also, neurosurgical patients demonstrate a change in reactivity of intracranial vessels on different partial CO_2 pressures in the blood. This may be of utmost importance if forced hyperventilation is needed in order to reduce intracranial volume and intracranial pressure. In this respect sufentanil $10 \mu g/kg$ body weight followed by an infusion rate of $0.35 \mu g/kg/min$ did not reduce the response to different arterial pCO_2 pressures (Figure III-40), results that were similar with alfentanil and/or fentanyl.

Sufentanil in Open-Heart Surgery

In patients undergoing open-heart surgery, the stage of laryngoscopy and intubation as well as sternotomy is characterized by intense vegetative and nociceptive reflex activation. Such effects may be detrimental as they go in hand with hypertension, tachycardia, an increase in pulmonary artery pressure and an increase in peripheral vascular resistance, all resulting in an increase in myocardial oxygen demand (MVO2). As this may further jeopardize the fragile cardiovascular system, every-thing has to be done in order to prevent such a scenario. Therefore an anesthetic agent with no negative-ionotropic action, with a sufficient analgesic potency and a wide therapeutic margin of safety, is a prerequisite for patients with a cardiovascular disease.

Due to its preferable profile, sufentanil seems the most suitable anesthetic because it results in a stable cardiovascular reaction at different nociceptive surgical inter-ventions. This has been demonstrated conclusively in patients with cardiovascular disease, where contrarily to fentanyl (25 μg/kg body weight) given in combi-nation with the muscle relaxant pancuroniumbromide (0.1 mg/kg body weight), sufentanil (5 μg/kg body weight) showed no detrimental effects on the vascular system. A second dose of the opioid (2.5 μg/kg body weight) given prior to an intense nociceptive stimulus such as skin incision and/or sternotomy was able to totally prevent the usual increase in mean arterial blood pressure (MAP) and left

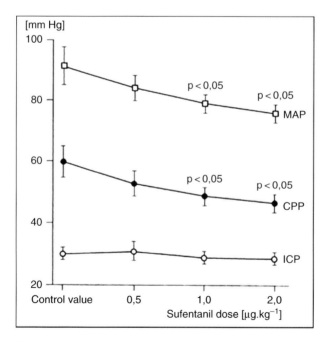

Figure III-39. Effect of increasing doses of sufentanil in patients with increased intracranial pressure (ICP), mean perfusion pressure (MPP), and mean arterial pressure (MAP)

ventricular stroke volume index (LVSWI). Contrarily, after fentanyl ($12.5\,\mu g$/kg body weight) there was a significant increase in vascular variables suggesting insufficient blockade of nociceptive afferences (Figure III-41).

In another study, induction of anesthesia was done in premedicated patients with sufentanil ($1\,\mu g$/kg body weight). Contrarily to fentanyl ($5\,\mu g$/kg body weight) laryngoscopy and intubation induced a significant lesser increase in reflex mean arterial pressure (mmHg) and heart rate (beats/min) (Figure III-42).

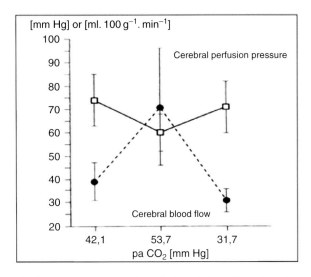

Figure III-40. Cerebral perfusion pressure and cerebral perfusion volume in patients with hypo- and hypercapnia respectively. There is no diminution of autoregulation of intracranial vessels (Adapted from [130])

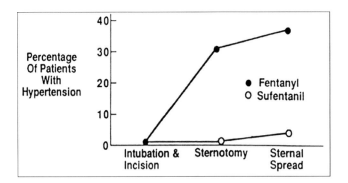

Figure III-41. Incidence of a hypertensive episode (increase in systolic blood pressure > 20% over preanesthetic values) following sternotomy and sternal spread in patients undergoing aortic valve replacement with either fentanyl and equipotent sufentanil respectively (Adapted from [19])

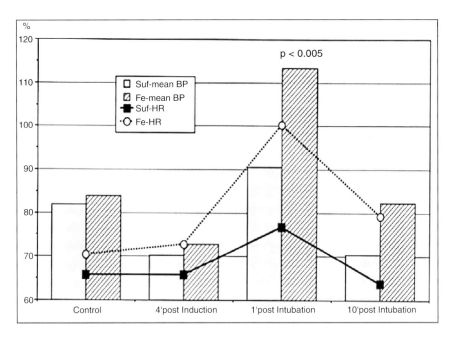

Figure III-42. Relative power in the fast beta-domain (13–30 Hz) of the EEG, following endotracheal laryngoscopy and intubation in patients undergoing open-heart surgery with sufentanil compared to fentanyl, BP = blood pressure, HR = heart rate (Adapted from [131])

Such beneficial effects in blockade of nociceptive afferents are also mirrored in the event-related somatosensory potenial (SSEP) in patients undergoing open-heart surgery with either sufentanil or fentanyl for induction of anesthesia. Patients with sufentanil demonstrated a better blockade of the intubation-related increase in sensory nervous afferent volleys resulting in a lesser increase in amplitude height of the SSEP (Figure III-43).

INTERACTION OF SUFENTANIL

Volatile Aspects

Combining the opioid sufentanil with a volatile agent such as desflurane or sevoflurane, minimal alveolar concentration (MAC) dose-proportionally is reduced, whereby a high dose of sufentanil reduced requirements of the volatile agent by 60–70% (Figure III-44). When compared to fentanyl this MAC reduction is much more pronounced [41] which is why in a balanced type of anesthesia the usually administered concentration of the volatile anesthetic can be reduced by at least 50%.

Muscle Relaxants

The simultaneous application of sufentanil and a muscle relaxant such as pancuro-niumbromide results in blunting the usual bradycardic and hypotonic action of the

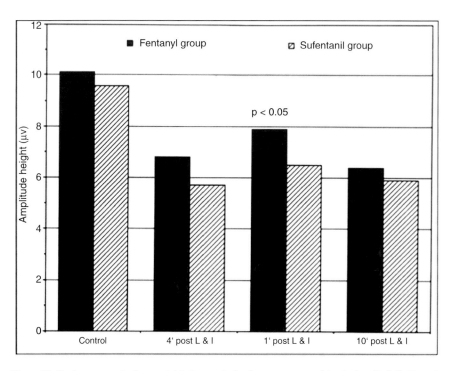

Figure III-43. Sensory-evoked potential before and after laryngoscopy and intubation (L & I). Note the significant higher increase in late amplitude height in patients with fentanyl, suggesting a higher sensory impulse flow of nociceptive activity to the CNS (Adapted from [119])

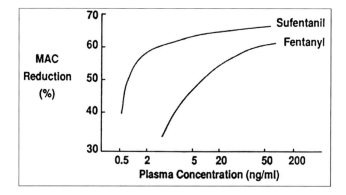

Figure III-44. Dose-related comparable reduction of enflurane following increasing doses of sufentanil or fentanyl (Adapted from [132])

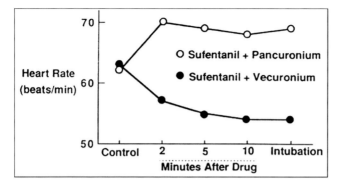

Figure III-45. Heart rate changes following the combined application of sufentanil with pancuronium-bromide and vecuronium respectively (Adapted from [134])

opioid (Figure III-45). While such compensatory effect is due to the vagolytic and sympathomimetic action it is not seen when the muscle relaxant vecuronium is co-administered with the opioid. This lack in effect is related to negligible autonomic reactions of this muscle relaxant. Because pancuroniumbromide is able to counteract the vagomimetic effects of sufentanil, such a combination is preferred in patients, where a pronounced decline in blood pressure has to be anticipated. Therefore, the combination of sufentanil with vecuronium or atracurium sometimes can result in a major drop in mean artrial pressure with bradycardia than the combination with pancuroniumbromide (Figure III-45).

In summary, it has to be clarified that in spite of the decline in blood pressure after sufentanil, this can not be taken as an indicative sign of myocardial ischemia [133].

The simultaneous and rapid injection of sufentanil with the polarizing muscle relaxant succinylcholine, due to the bradycardic effect of the latter, results in pronounced bradycardia than seen after sole injection of the opioid. Also, when given together with sufentanil, due to the succinyl-induced rise of potassium and histamine, which by itself already induces a decline in mean arterial pressure, there is a potentiation of the hypotensive effect. The hypotensive effect of sufentanil can be diminished by the slow injection over a period of 2 min or by titration of the opioid to the desired amount.

Barbiturates

Because a barbiturate like thiopental, when administered together with a muscle relaxant for the induction of anesthesia results in a significant increase in heart rate and systolic pressure, the product of both (the rate-pressure product) can be considered as an index of myocardial oxygen demand (MVO2) exceeding significantly the awake-control situation (Figure III-46). This increase can significantly be reduced or even totally attenuated when a small dose of sufentanil of 0.5–1.0 µg/kg body weight is given prior to both induction agents (Figure III-46).

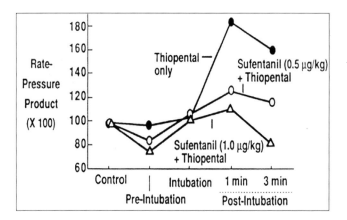

Figure III-46. Hemodynamic consequences during the induction of anesthesia with thiopental in combination with different doses of sufentanil (Adapted from [135])

Due to the attenuation of the hemodynamic responses following laryngoscopy and intubation, sufentanil is able to preferably block the nociceptive reflex mechanism, which is usually observed during the induction period. However, when using a combination of a barbiturate and sufentanil, one should realize that the dose of the hypnotic should be reduced accordingly. For the induction of unconsciousness, usually a sole dose of thiopental of 4.08 mg/kg is necessary. Adding sufentanil (0.5–1.0 μg/kg body weight) to the induction agent there is a significant reduction of the dose of the barbiturate to 1.99–1.32 mg/kg body weight [135].

Anesthesia, however, can also be induced by the sole use of sufentanil. When using 2–8 μg/kg body weight of sufentanil this especially is of advantage in cardiac patients, because coronary sinus blood flow (CSBF), an index of coronary perfusion, mean arterial pressure and heart rate are not affected because of intubation, and following sternotomy [136]. Since the decline in mean arterial pressure correlates with a decline in myocardial oxygen demand (MVO_2) it can be concluded that sufentanil is a preferable agent for the induction of anesthesia in patients undergoing coronary artery by-pass graft operation (Figure III-47).

In summary, drug-drug interactions with sufentanil differ significantly resulting in either a decrease or an increase of hemodynamics. Most of all it is important to know, which of the additionally used agents result in a prolongation of effects, so that there is no overhang and the patient needs additional time on the ventilator, supervision, or there is retarded awakening (Table III-14).

PRACTICAL CONSIDERATIONS FOR THE USE OF SUFENTANIL

The following recommendations for the use of sufentanil in anesthesia, depending on the type and the duration of surgery are given in the next table. If sufentanil is

Table III-14. Summary of interaction of sufentanil with other agents affecting the cardiovascular system and the possible potentiation and duration of action. None (0), small (+), medium (++), pronounced (+++) potentiation and/or duration of action

Agent	Blood pressure	Heart rate	Potentiation of action	Duration of action
Succinylcholine	Increase	Increase	0	0
Vecuronium	0	0	0	0
Curare	decrease	decrease	0	0
Atracurium	decrease	decrease	0	0
Pancuronium	increase	increase	0	0
Barbiturates	decrease	decrease	++	++
Droperidol(> 5mg)	0	0	(+)	0
Benzodiazepines	decrease	decrease	++	+++
Propofol	(decrease)	(decrease)	++	++
Volatile agents	0	0		+++
N₂O	0	0	++	(+)
ß-Blocker	decrease	decrease	++	++
Ca⁺⁺-Antagonist	decrease	decrease	++	++
α₂-Agonist	(decrease)	(decrease)	+++	(+)
MAO-Inhibitors	0	0	+	+++

Modified from [138, 139, 140, 141]

given in combination with a muscle relaxant, however, without nitrous oxide and the patient is ventilated with pure oxygen, induction of anesthesia is started with a loading dose of 0.8–1.0 µg/kg body weight. For maintenance of anesthesia in case of a reduction of analgesia, a repetitive dose of 0.35–0.7 µg/kg body weight is suggested. When sufentanil is being used in total intravenous anesthesia (TIVA),

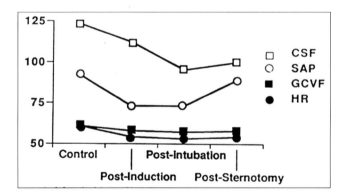

Figure III-47. Hemodynamic measurements in patients undergoing coronary artery by-pass grafting before, and after receiving sufentanil (2 µg/kg). Measurements were done before and after the total dose of sufentanil, after endotracheal intubation, and 5 min after sternotomy. HR = heart rate (beats/min); SAP = systemic atrial pressure (mmHg); CSF = coronary sinus flow (ml/min), GCVF = great coronary vein flow (ml/min). CSF is used as an indicator of global myocardial perfusion, and GCSF denotes left ventricular perfusion (Adapted from [137])

where it is combined with a hypnotic like propofol and the patient is ventilated
with 100% oxygen, a loading dose of 1 μg/kg body weight is advocated. This is
followed by a continuous infusion via a motor-driven pump administering a dose
of 0.1–0.15 μg/kg/min. When using this type of anesthesia, it is apparent that the
usual dose of the hypnotic can be reduced significantly, because sufentanil by itself
already has a pronounced sedative effect. In case of a balanced type of anesthetic
technique, where the agent is being used in combination with a volatile anesthetic,
initially sufentanil should be administered in a dose of 0.5–0.7 μg/kg body weight,
the first half for intubation and the second half just prior to skin incision. With a
maintenance dose of sufentanil of 0.26 μg/kg, intraoperatively the concentration of
the volatile anesthetic can significantly be reduced (i.e., isoflurane 0.3 vol%), in
order not to encounter an overhang at the end of the procedure.

It has to be pointed out that with the start of anesthesia, sufentanil should be
given in a high enough loading dose. This has several advantages:

• A sufficient high loading dose, given at the start of anesthesia, results in the
occupation of all receptor sites, causing a deep level of analgesia with lesser need
for additional doses of the opioid.
• Laryngoscopy and intubation by themselves already present a very intense
nociceptive stimulus, which can only be blocked sufficiently by a high dose of
the opioid.
• The secretion of excitatory transmitters and the subsequent potentiation of
nociceptive afferences through "wind-up" can be inhibited before the first burst
of nociceptive impulses is being generated.
• Forty five minutes before the end of operation, the patient is in no further need
of an additional dose of the opioid. At the end of anesthesia an antagonist will
not be necessary and the patient will breathe on his own, showing a sufficient
level of wakefulness.

Table III-15. Recommendations of the appropriate dose of sufentanil for different types of operations
using a N_2O/O_2 based anesthetic regimen. 50%–70% of the titrated dose of sufentanil should be given
for induction, the second half just prior to skin incision

Duration operation (h)	Type of operation	Induction dose (μg/kg)	Maintenance dose (μg/70 kg)
1–2	Hysterectomy, cholecyctectomy, osteosynthesis	0.55–1.0	Clinical signs 10–25
2–8	Endarterectomy, colectomy, nephrectomy, gastrectomy	1.0–5.0	Clinical signs 10–25
4–8	AC by-pass, valvular replacement, thoraco-abdominal aneurysm repair (TAA)	4.0–10.0	Before sternotomy 5–10 μg/kg; clinical signs 10–25

Adapted from [108, 19, 130, 133, 142, 143]

- Already during the course of anesthesia the opioid is being metabolized and inactivated. Those amounts of the opioid, which have accumulated in the peripheral compartment, intraoperatively diffuse into the central blood compartment where they do not hide from metabolism via the liver.
- The usual dose of the hypnotic, being necessary for the induction of anesthesia, can be reduced by at least 50%.
- In balanced anesthesia the concentration of the volatile agent can be reduced by 59% because sufentanil has a hypnotic action of its own.
- Sufficient analgesia is maintained throughout the whole procedure and there is no need for re-administration of the opioid in order to sustain a sufficient level of analgesia.
- There is no need for re-administration of the opioid, which otherwise would results in an additional accumulation of the drug in the peripheral compartment, acting like a reservoir (muscles, connecting tissue, fat tissue). From there the drug will flow back into the blood compartment, which may result in a rebound of effects with late respiratory impairment.

In summary it is important to consider the following points when using sufentanil for anesthesia:

1. High loading dose lessens repetitive reinjection, which should be avoided.
2. In TIVA with propofol reduce the amount of the hypnotic
3. In patients with a shock-like state, reduce the usual dose by at least 50% or titrate according to need.
4. In patients with hypovolemia titrate according to need.
5. In patients with marginal myocardial function give a lower dose of the opioid than usual.
6. Combining the opioid with a volatile agent the MAC can be reduced by 50%–60%.
7. In high doses the opioid mediates an antiarrythmic action.

EXAMPLES FOR THE USE OF SUFENTANIL IN ANESTHESIA

Balanced Anesthesia for an Abdominal Operation

Medication (mg/70 kg)	Induction dose	Maintenance dose	Post-operative In PACU
Sufentanil	0.03–0.5	0.01–0.03	
Thiopental	70	when necessary	5–10–15 mg iv until VAS < 3.0
Vecuronium	4–8	0.2–0.4 vol% or N$_2$O/O$_2$ = 50/50	
Isoflurane (vol%)	100% O$_2$		
Morphine			

Total intravenous anesthesia (TIVA) for open-heart surgery

Medication (mg/70 kg)	Induction dose	Sternotomy phase	Maintenance Dose	Post-op analgesia
Sufentanil	0.1	0.1	0.1 mg/h	0.05 mg/h
Midazolam	5–10	$->5-10$	if necessary $->5\,mg/h$	FiO2 according to gases
Pancuronium	2			
Propofol	$->15$			
Ventilation	100% O2			

Opioids for Use in Postoperative Pain Management

Postoperative pain is a good example of acute nociceptive pain, which demands immediate therapy. Aside from peripheral nociceptor activation of the skin and the muscles, by means of traction at the peritoneum and muscles during the operation, also visceral and spastic painful afferences are triggered. Therefore, any sufficient postoperative pain strategy should consider all these origins of nociception. The most simple and effective way to reduce postoperative pain is the installation of local anesthetics at the site of incision [144]. Although not being confirmed in a controlled study, such intervention has been claimed to result in a delay of healing process [145]. In general, however, the expected pain in the postoperative period depends on:
1. The site of the incision,
2. The type of anesthetic being used during operation.
About 74% of all patients following a thoracotomy are in need of an analgesic. After upper abdominal operations 63% and after lower abdominal operations 51% ask for some kind of pain relief. The figure even drops further to 27% when an operation is done on the upper or lower extremities, and following an urological or general surgical intervention up to 36% and 49% respectively will need no analgesic at all [146]. According to Ferrari and coworkers, aside from the site and the size of operation, the type of anesthesia has a major impact on the incidence of postoperative pain. Following anesthesia with the volatile anesthetic methoxyflurane 90% and after halothane, 85% need some kind of postoperative pain management. However, after neuroleptanesthesia, when using the opioid fentanyl, only 50% were in need of an additional analgesic within the first 8 postoperative hours [147]. Especially when using the more potent opioid sufentanil as the main anesthetic intraoperatively, in contrast to fentanyl, the duration of postoperative pain relief is significantly prolonged [148].

In spite of the vast number of potent opioid analgesics available for postoperative pain therapy, over the past decade there has been little improvement in reducing the incidence of postoperative pain. Similar as in 1980 where Cohen and coworkers described an unsatisfactory pain relief in about 75% of all patients having undergone a surgical procedure [145], there has been little improvement in its management over the past years. This is underlined by data from the year 1983 where in spite of all the knowledge on pain transmission and upload receptors being involved in its alleviation, still 41% of all patients complained of insufficient postoperative pain relief [149]. Even in 1990 no improvement in overall pain therapy in the PACU was noted and even today, in 2008 it is suggested that around 40% of all patients unnecessarily still have to undergo pain in the immediate postoperative period [150]. This is supported by data in the literature, which demonstrate insufficient pain relief and its therapy in up to 21%–43% of all patients [151, 152, 153]. Such data should not lead to the conclusion of non-existing potent analgesics for postoperative pain management; it rather implies that other aspects have an effect on the quality of pain management (Figure III-48):

- First and most of all there is insufficient knowledge of the medical personnel in handling potent opioid analgesics.
- There is a non-justified fear of potential side effects from potent opioid analgesics, especially the development of addiction and respiratory depression.
- In addition, there is insufficient knowledge on the duration of action of the different analgesics.
- Lack of use of a non-rating scale (NRS) for determining individual pain intensity results in insufficient monitoring the efficacy of pain strategy.
- No additional alternative therapeutic strategies such as epidural analgesia, regional blocks etc. are integrated in pain management.
- Lack in co-administration of peripheral non-opioid analgesics (e.g. cyclooxygenase inhibitors) would result in an opioid-sparing effect.

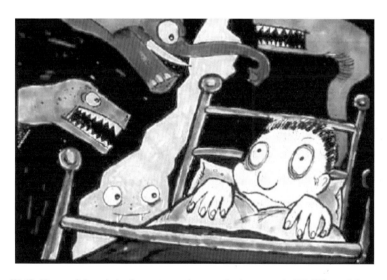

Figure III-48. Hours of despair in the postoperative anesthesia care unit (PACU), a nightmare if not given the proper pain treatment

Although the anesthesiologist, due to his knowledge on the pharmacology of potent analgesics, the type of drugs being used intraoperatively, the patients individual reaction to a specific agent, very likely is the most experienced person to deal with postoperative pain, he no longer is responsible for postoperative pain therapy on the ward (Figure III-49). It is therefore that often in a patient's file recommendations for postoperative pain therapy simply consists of an analgesic given "pro re nata (PRN)". Finally, it is the nurse on the ward who, according to her knowledge and her past experiences, decides when and which analgesic should be given. Common thinking like

- the potential of addiction liability by an opioid analgesic
- the potential of side effects such as
  - respiratory depression
  - urinary retention
  - extreme sedation
- constipation

often results in underdosing the opioid rather than resulting in sufficient pain relief [154, 155].

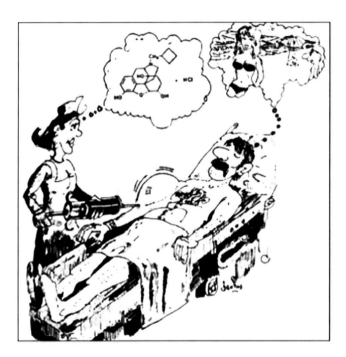

Figure III-49. The way it should be in the PACU – a care-taker educated in opioid use results in a satisfied patient with no pain

ADDICTION LIABILITY BY USE OF OPIOIDS FOR POSTOPERATIVE PAIN

In a large multicenter trial it has been demonstrated conclusively that patients, who received an opioid for postoperative pain management unlikely developed an addictive behavior [155]. The incidence for the development of addiction was below 0.03%. The reason for such low percentage is the fact that potent opioids are only taken during the acute phase of intense pain, when the organism is in need of an additional analgesic, a time when his own endogenous opioid system is not able to sufficiently cope with the nociceptive bombardment. And only 4 out of 1200 patients showed signs of abuse, while only one individual developed true dependency [156]. Especially insufficient dosing of opioids in non-malignant pain is considered the main cause in the development of psychic habit forming while often a non-opioid is involved in such pathology [157, 158].

TIME-CONTINGENT DOSING OF OPIOIDS FOR POSTOPERATIVE PAIN

Administering an opioid only on demand ("pro re nata") is considered a sufficient rationale to treat individual pain. This is because the patient by himself is the best monitor to judge pain intensity in the postoperative period, and he is more likely to determine when pain becomes unbearable and chooses the time when to administer the opioid. Being the only person to judge when its is necessary to treat pain, it is only after expressing his desire that the medical personal with some time delay will respond to his aspiration. It is because of these administrative delays, that patients will experience a period of insufficient pain relief, where increasing pain intensity is experienced between times of therapy (Figure III-50).

The goal of every postoperative pain management therefore should be to administer the agent before the patient perceives pain (principle of time-contingent

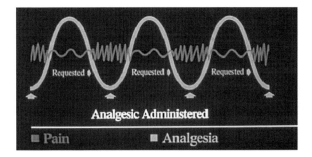

Figure III-50. Schematic presentation of postoperative pain cycles with periods of sufficient relief, which, however, is followed by a breakthrough with increased pain sensations. There is a lag between the need and the time of application using the pro re nata (PRN) schedule

dosing). Time-contingent dosing is based on an overlap of the declining plasma concentration of the opioid, resulting in a constant and steady occupation of receptor sites, and a long-term blockade of all incoming nociceptive afferents. Such practice guarantees:

1. A constant and stable plasma concentration,
2. A reduction in stress-related disorders and complications in wound healing.
3. A reduction in the amount of the opioid necessary to maintain analgesia. There is no need to pursue the pain as this regularly leads to higher doses than usually necessary.
4. No development of a so-called "wind-up" phenomenon, which usually results in a potentiation of nociceptive afferents [159].
5. No development of a chronic pain behavior pattern in the patient, and lastly,
6. A contented patient.

For the patient it is more satisfying to receive an opioid analgesic in sufficient amounts at a time when there is no breakthrough of painful afferences which otherwise would result in an increase of discomfort (Figure III-51).

SELECTION OF THE APPROPRIATE AGENT IN POSTOPERATIVE PAIN MANAGEMENT

In order to answer the intriguing question, which might be the best analgesic for use in postoperative pain therapy, first it is necessary to point out that an opioid still is the optimal agent for the alleviation of pain in the PACU. When using an opioid, it is not the potency of the drug, which is of utmost importance. More importantly, questions like the duration of action, the incidence of side effects and the likelihood of a respiratory depression are queries, which have to be put in perspective. For

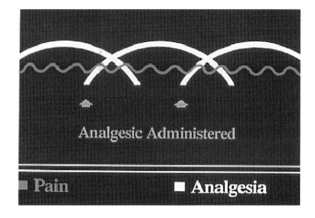

Figure III-51. Postoperative pain therapy and the corresponding plasma levels, using time-contingent dosing. The goal is an overlap of a descending opioid plasma level resulting in sufficient receptor occupation

instance an opioid like sufentanil, although being the most powerful agent available, it however results in severe respiratory depression. Other opioids such as fentanyl or alfentanil have a too short half-life of only 20–30 min and 5–10 min respectively. Pethidine, although having a much longer duration of action and shows a lesser incidence of respiratory depression, has a mean duration of action between 2 and 3 h. However, because of its cardio-depressive effects and especially its tachyarrhythmic potency this is accompanied by an increase in myocardial oxygen consumption (MVO_2). It, therefore, is not considered the optimal agent for postoperative pain management. Although not having the most advantageous profile, some of the standard opioids in this regard, i.e. morphine and/or hydromorphone do have a number of advantages when being used in the postoperative period. First of all the duration of action is between 3 and 5 h and when being used in the lower dose range, they do not induce a clinically relevant impairment of respiration. Due to the histamine liberating effect of morphine, sometimes a relevant drop in blood pressure is encountered, especially in patients, who due to an excessive intraoperative blood loss already have a compromised circulation. While codeine has a similar duration as pethidine, it may be a favorable agent postoperatively in infants and young children [160, 161]. In this respect, also tramadol, because of its negligible respiratory depression and not being a scheduled type opioid, is an analgesic for use in pediatrics but also after minor surgical procedures [162]. The opioid with the longest duration of action of up to 10 h is buprenorphine [163, 164], which has a sufficient potency (40 times morphine) to combat severe postoperative pain after large surgical interventions (Figure III-52).

When using buprenorphine one has to realize that its onset of action is fast within 2–5 min, however its full effect will be seen after a period of 45 min. This is because the agent has a very slow association characteristic before it is fully bound to the opioid receptor [165]. It is therefore mandatory not to administer a

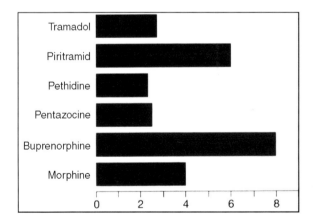

Figure III-52. Mean duration of action (hours) of various opioids for use in the postoperative time period

second injection or give another buccal tablet within this time frame in order not to induce an overdose with all the sequelae of any excessive opioid intake (i.e., respiratory impairment). This especially has to be recognized in the elderly patient because he is more sensitive to develop an insufficient respiratory drive. Although a selective antagonist such as naloxone can easily antagonize such event, one has to realize that higher dosages (1–2 mg/70 kg body weight) than normal may become necessary in order to displace buprenorphine from its receptor. If an antagonist is not available, also a non-specific analeptic such as doxapram (Dopram®) can be used because it stimulates respiratory drive via activation of chemoreceptors at the glomus caroticus, which in turn activates the respiratory center. At the same time it also affects blood pressure via pressor receptors in the aortic arch (Figure III-53). In addition almitrine (Vectarion®), another non-specifc analeptic can be used, which has similar properties as doxapram. Aminophenazole (Pamadine®) directly stimulates the medullary respiratory center and the agent physostigmine induces

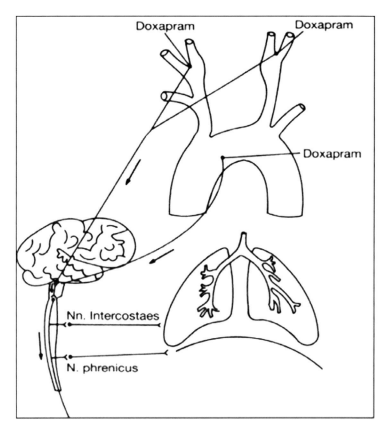

Figure III-53. Mode of action of the analeptic agent doxapram resulting in a nonspecific activation of respiratory drive

an overall decrease in acetylcholine (ACh) turnover, specifically in the medulla, counteracting opioid-induced reduction of ACh-release.

Especially after ambulatory surgery the patient needs some back-up agent, which is sufficiently potent for pain alleviation, however, at the same time does not compromise the cardiovascular or the respiratory system. Since those patients usually have undergone minor surgical procedures, often a peripheral NSAID is sufficient for pain therapy especially if the patient uses the analgesic as a self-medication. However, sometimes an opioid becomes as necessary as the pain becomes intense. Preliminary results with a time-controlled release formulation of dihydrocodeine seem to be promising. This agent not only results in a time-contingent long duration of action after minor surgical procedures such as endoscopic cholecystectomy and/or arthroscopy [166, 167]. When given together with a peripheral NSAID it results in good to optimal pain relief. While its time to max efficacy is between 2 and 3 h, its duration is between 8 and 12 h; it therefore can be used for acute treatment of exacerbating pain without the potential risk of respiratory depression.

In combating postoperative pain, a three-step ladder is proposed, where according to the intensity of individual pain, the proper analgesic can be chosen (Figure III-54).

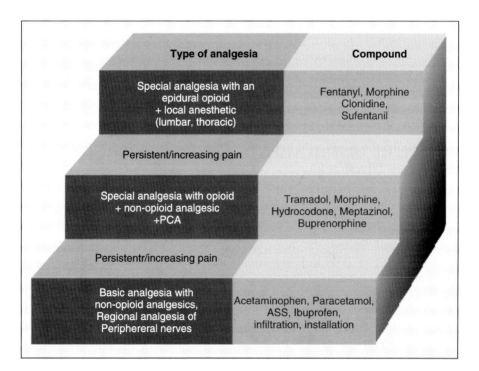

Figure III-54. A three-step ladder in modern postoperative pain management using a multimodal approach

In summary, the following management options are available for post-operative pain management (Table III-16).

Pharmacologic management of mild to moderate postoperative pain should begin, unless there is a contraindication, with an NSAID. However, moderately severe to severe pain should normally be treated initially with an opioid analgesic, with or without an NSAID.

Even when insufficient alone to control pain, NSAIDs, including acetaminophen, have significant opioid dose-sparing effects on postoperative pain and hence can be useful in reducing opioid side effects. If the patient cannot tolerate oral medication, alternative routes such as rectal administration can be used. At present, one NSAID (ketorolac) is approved by the Food and Drug Administration for parenteral use. NSAIDs must be used with care in patients with thrombocytopenia or coagulopathies and in patients who are at risk for bleeding or gastric ulceration. However, acetaminophen does not affect platelet function, and some evidence exists that two salicylates (salsalate and choline magnesium trisalicylate) do not profoundly affect platelet aggregation.

Opioid analgesics are the cornerstone for management of moderate to severe acute pain. Effective use of these agents facilitates postoperative activities such as coughing, deep breathing exercises, ambulation, and physical therapy. When pain cannot be adequately controlled despite increasing the opioid dose, a prompt search for residual operative pathology is indicated, and other diagnoses such as neuropathic pain should be considered. Opioid tolerance and physiologic dependence are unusual in short-term postoperative use in opioid naive patients. Likewise, psychologic dependence and addiction are extremely unlikely to develop after the use of opioids for acute pain.

CHOICE OF OPIOID AGENTS FOR POST-OPERATIVE PAIN TREATMENT

Morphine is the standard agent for opioid therapy. However, it has to be taken into account that this drug needs a long period to pass through the blood-brain barrier in order to bind with the receptor and establish an effect. Therefore one should not readminister small doses at short intervals [168]. If morphine cannot be used because of an unusual reaction or allergy, another opioid such as hydromorphone can be substituted. Pethidine (meperidine, USP) should be reserved for very brief courses in patients who have demonstrated allergy or intolerance to other opioids such as morphine and hydromorphone. Pethidine is contraindicated in patients with impaired renal function or those receiving antidepressants that are monoamine oxidase (MAO) inhibitors. Normeperidine is a toxic metabolite of meperidine, and is excreted through the kidney. Normeperidine is a cerebral irritant, and accumulation can cause effects ranging from dysphoria and irritable mood to seizures.

Table III-16. Scientific evidence and considerations for different interventions to manage pain in the post operative period in adults

Agents		Type of evidence	Considerations
NSAIDs	Oral (alone)	Ib, IV	Effective for mild to moderate pain. Begin preoperatively. Relatively contraindicated in patients with renal disease and risk of or actual coagulopathy. May mask fever.
	Oral as adjunct to opioid	Ia, IV	Potentiating effect resulting in opioid sparing. Begin preop. Cautions as above.
	Parenteral (e.g ketorolac)	Ib, IV	Effective for moderate to severe pain. Expensive. Useful where opioids contraindicated, especially to avoid respiratory depression and sedation. Advance to opioid.
Opioids	Oral	IV	As effective as parenteral in appropriate doses. Use as soon as oral medication is tolerated. Route of choice.
	Intramuscular	Ib, IV	Has been the standard parenteral route, but injections painful and absorption unreliable. Hence, avoid this route when possible.
	Subcutaneous	Ib, IV	Preferable to intramuscular for low-volume continuous infusion. Injections painful and absorption unreliable. Avoid this route for long-term repetitive dosing. Parenteral route of choice after major surgery.
	Intravenous	Ib, IV	Suitable for titrated bolus or continuous administration (including PCA), but requires monitoring. Significant risk of respiratory depression with inappropriate dosing.
	PCA (systemic)	Ia, IV	Intravenous or subcut. routes recommended.
	Epidural, intrathecal	Ia, IV	Good, steady level of analgesia. Popular with patients but requires special infusion pumps and staff education. See cautions about opioids above. When suitable, provides good analgesia. Significant risk of respiratory depression, sometimes delayed in onset. Requires careful monitoring. Use of infusion pumps requires additional equipment and staff education.

Table III-16. (continued)

Agents		Type of evidence	Considerations
	Epidural, intrathecal	Ia, IV	Limited indications. Expensive if infusion pumps employed. Effective regional analgesia. Opioid sparing. Addition of opioid to local anesthetic may improve analgesia. Risks of hypotension, weakness, numbness. Use of infusion pump requires additional equipment and staff.
Local anesthetics	Peripheral nerve block	Ia, IV	Limited indications and duration of nerve block action. Effective regional analgesia. Opioid sparing

Key for type of evidence:
Ia = Evidence obtained from meta-analysis of randomized controlled trials
Ib = Evidence obtained from at least one randomized controlled trial
IV = Evidence obtained from expert committee reports or opinions and/or clinical experiences of respected authorities

Also one should consider the option of self-medication with intravenous opioids that may include oral or other routes of administration. In this regard patient controlled analgesia (PCA) offers patients a sense of control over their pain and is preferred by most patients to intermittent injections.

> **Morphine needs about 45 min until max effect. In postoperative pain treatment repetitive small doses given at short intervals may accumulate resulting in respiratory depression**

DOSAGE OF OPIOID ANALGESICS IN POST-OPERATIVE PAIN TREATMENT

Patients vary greatly in their analgesic dose requirements and responses to opioid analgesics. The recommended starting doses may be inadequate. Subsequent opioid doses must be titrated to increase the amount of analgesia and reduce side effects. Relative potency estimates provide a rational basis for selecting the appropriate starting dose, for changing the route of administration (e.g. from parenteral to oral), or for changing from one opioid to another. Patients who have been receiving opioid analgesics before surgery may require higher starting and maintenance doses postoperatively.

Lastly, there is evidence that opioid receptor polymorphism also influences analgesia need in the postoperative period. Therefore, genetic variation in the μ-opioid receptor may contribute to the differences seen in post-operative morphine consumption for pain management among individuals, researchers report [169]. This connotation is underlined by previous studies, which suggested that cancer patients homozygous for the 118G allele, caused by the single nucleotide polymorphism at nucleotide position 118 in the μ-opioid receptor gene, require higher doses of morphine to relieve pain. The contribution of this allele to morphine efficacy in 80 women scheduled to undergo general anesthesia for elective total hysterectomy surgery. All, 43 of the women were homozygous for A118 (AA), 19 were heterozygous (AG), and 18 were homozygous for G118 (GG). The overall G allelic frequency was 34.4%. Women homozygous for G118 needed more doses of morphine to achieve adequate pain relief in the first 24 h than those homozygous for A118, at 33 mg versus 27 mg, respectively. At 48 h, however, there was no statistical difference in morphine consumption between the two groups of women. Although other potential contributing factors such as mood and anxiety may also alter patients' opioid requirements, the genetic variation of the μ-opioid receptor was associated with the different response to intravenous patient-controlled analgesia morphine therapy for surgical pain.

The following points have to be considered when using an opioid for postoperative pain therapy:

Dosage Schedule in Post-operative Pain Treatment

Opioid administration relying on patients' or families' demands for analgesic pro re nata, or "as needed," produces delays in administration and intervals of inadequate pain control. Analgesics should be administered initially on a regular time schedule. For example, if the patient is likely to have pain requiring opioid analgesics for 48 h after surgery, morphine might be ordered every 4 h around-the-clock (not prn) for 36 h. Opioid administration is contraindicated when respiratory depression is present (less than 10 breaths per minute). Once the duration of analgesic action is determined, the dosage frequency should be adjusted to prevent pain from recurring. Orders may be written so that a patient may refuse an analgesic if not in pain or forget it if asleep. However, since a steady-state blood level is required for the drug to be continuously effective, interruption of an around-the-clock dosage schedule (e.g., during sleep) may cause a resurgence of pain as blood levels of the analgesic decline. Late in the postoperative course, it may be acceptable to give opioid analgesics pro re nata (prn). Switching to PRN dosing later in the postoperative course provides pain relief while reducing the risk of adverse effects as the patient's analgesic dose requirement diminishes. Clinicians should assess patients at regular intervals to determine the efficacy of the intervention, the presence of side effects, the need for adjustments of dosage and/or interval, or the need for supplemental doses for breakthrough pain.

Route of Opioid Administration in Post-operative Pain Treatment

Intravenous administration is the parenteral route of choice after major surgery. This route is suitable for bolus administration and continuous infusion (including PCA). Repeated intramuscular injections by itself can cause pain and trauma and may deter patients from requesting pain medication. Rectal and sublingual administrations are alternatives to intramuscular or subcutaneous routes when intravenous access is problematic. All routes other than intravenous require a lag time for absorption into the circulation. Oral administration is convenient and inexpensive. It is appropriate as soon as the patient can tolerate oral intake and is the mainstay of pain management in the ambulatory surgical population.

Non-pharmacologic Management in Post-operative Pain Treatment

Patient teaching should include procedural and sensory information, instruction to decrease treatment and activity-related pain (e.g., pain caused by deep breathing, coughing) and information about the use of relaxation. Cognitive-behavioral (e.g., relaxation, distraction, imagery) and physical interventions (e.g., heat, cold, massage) are intended to supplement, not replace, pharmacologic interventions. Cognitive/behavioral interventions include a variety of methods that help patients understand more about their pain and take an active role in pain assessment and management. Simple relaxation strategies can be effective in helping to manage pain. Patients benefit from periodic reinforcement and coaching in the use of relaxation techniques. Commonly used physical agents include applications of heat and cold, massage, movement, and rest or immobilization. Applications of heat and cold alter the pain threshold, reduce muscle spasm, and decrease local swelling. Transcutaneous electrical nerve stimulation (TENS) may be effective in reducing pain and improving physical function.

Considerations for Elderly Patients in Post-operative Pain Treatment

Elderly people often suffer multiple chronic, painful illnesses and take multiple medications. They are at greater risk for drug-drug and drug-disease interactions. Pain assessment presents unique problems in the elderly, as these patients may exhibit physiologic, psychologic, and cultural changes associated with aging. Misunderstanding of the relationship between aging and pain is common in the management of elderly patients. Many health care providers and patients alike mistakenly consider pain to be a normal part of aging. Elderly patients sometimes believe that pain cannot be relieved and are stoic in reporting their pain. The frail and oldest-old (> 85 years) are at particular risk for undertreatment of pain. Aging need not alter pain thresholds or tolerance. The similarities of pain experience between elderly and younger patients are far more common than are the differences. Cognitive impairment, delirium, and dementia are serious barriers to assessing pain in the elderly. Sensory problems such as visual and hearing changes may also interfere with the use of some pain assessment scales. However, as with other patients, the clinician should be able to obtain an accurate self-report of pain from most patients. When verbal report is not possible, clinicians should observe for behavioral cues to pain such as restlessness or agitation. The absence of pain behaviors does not negate the presence of pain. NSAIDs can be used safely in elderly persons, but their use requires vigilance for side effects, especially gastric and renal toxicity. Opioids are safe and effective when used appropriately in elderly patients. Elderly people are more sensitive to analgesic effects of opiate drugs. They experience higher peak effect and longer duration of pain relief.

As outlined, modern postoperative pain therapy now consists of several steps using different types of analgesics, all of which play an important role in reducing nociceptive afference. While the basic strategy is to always start with an NSAID as its affects the site of incision, the next step is the addition of an opioid with medium potency (tramadol, morphine, hydrocodone). It is only when this strategy is insufficient to alleviate postoperative pain, that other agents such as ketamine (a non-specific NMDA inhibitor) or the α_2-agonist clonidine are added to the regimen (Figure III-54). Such multimodal concept in post operative pain management is based on the thinking that:

1. Non-opioid analgesics such as the NSAIDs can have an opioid sparing effect of up to 20%.
2. Spasmolytic agents (i.e. butylscopolamine) should be added for pain management after gynecological procedures because of spastic contractions of smaller muscle groups in the lower pelvis.
3. Always consider epidural analgesia with a local anesthetic (levopupivacaine, ropivacaine) as a safe method to selectively block the peripheral nerve not affecting the patients sensory system.
4. Consider adding ketamine in a low dose (0.2–0.4 mg/kg body weight) because it potentiates opioid analgesia.
5. Use the option of an α_2-agonist such as clonidine (180 μg/70 kg) as it binds to α_2-receptors, which are involved in the propagation of nociception within the spinal cord.
6. Think of the new antiepileptic agent gabapentine given preoperatively (600 mg/70 kg) as a choice to intraoperatively reduce opioid dose, and postoperatively have an opioid sparing effect.
7. Lastly, triple agent therapy has been suggested for optimization of postoperative pain control where aside from an opioid, and an NSAID, ketamine is given on-top [170].

A benzodiazepine, a neuroleptic or an antidepressant should not be administered together with an opioid, as this can induce respiratory depression

Last but not least it is imperative to outline the "analgesic effects" of the medical personal in the PACU, which reassures the patient that he/she is not left all by him (her) self (Figure III-55). This results in a major reduction in opioid use as demonstrated in several studies when using the patient controlled analgesia (PCA) system. Especially in the PACU the medical personnel should recognize the basic principles in postoperative pain management:

1. Choose the appropriate agent.
2. Titrate the agent to effect.
3. Give the agent intravenously, because it is the fastest way to the receptor.
4. Find the individual/maintenance dose.
5. Control on a short-term basis

    – Respiration
    – Blood pressure/heart rate
    – Vigilance
    – Blood loss

6. Regularly check the efficacy of your regimen using a non-rating scale such as the visual analogue scoring system (VAS).
7. Treat any side effects accordingly.
8. Use a multimodal concept for the alleviation of postoperative pain.

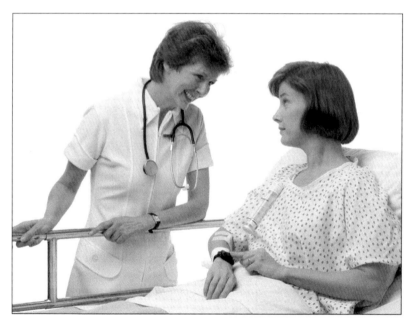

Figure III-55. Personal care in the PACU should not be underestimated when striving for an optimization in postoperative pain alleviation in patients

IMPLICATIONS OF AGONIST/ANTAGONISTS IN POSTOPERATIVE PAIN MANAGEMENT

While it had been demonstrated that this group of opioids when being used for postoperative pain management result in a lesser incidence of postoperative nausea and/or emesis (Figure III-56), from the clinical point of view it is important to note, that one should never mix a pure μ-type ligand such as morphine or hydrocodone with an agonist/antagonist such as pentazocine, nalbuphine or butorphanol.

This is because the latter agents induce an antagonistic effect at the opioid μ-receptor while they mediate their analgesic effect through interaction with the opioid κ-receptor (Figure III-57). Therefore, an agonist/antagonist given after a pure μ-type ligand is able to reverse analgesia resulting in an increase of pain [173].

It is because of this antagonistic potency that some mixed agonist/antagonists such as nalbuphine and butorphanol (Table III-17) can be used as reversal agents in an overhang of fentanyl-related respiratory depression [174, 175, 176]. At the same time these agents have a lesser spastic effect on the sphincter Oddi resulting in more favorable intrabiliary tract dynamics [177]. Last but not least, they have a lesser addiction liability, which is why they are scheduled as class IV agents, and not like morphine, need a special opiate prescription form.

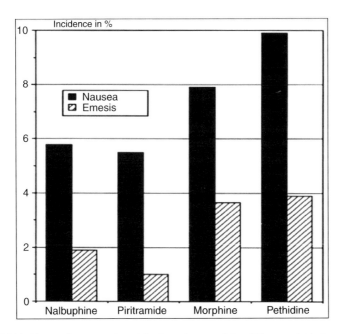

Figure III-56. Incidence of nausea and vomiting in patients receiving different opioids for postoperative pain management, using either nalbuphine (1086 patients), pethidine (234 patients), morphine (486 patients) and the fentanyl analogue piritramide (9756 patients) (Adapted from [171, 172])

Table III-17. Agonistic and antagonistic potency of various opioid agonist/antagonists and partial agonists, when compared to the pure agonist morphine (= 1) and the pure antagonist naloxone (= 1) respectively

Opioid	Company	Antagonistc profile	Agonistic profile	Analgesia ceiling (mg/70 kg)
Butorphanol	BristolMeyers	0.025	40	> 1.2
Buprenorphine	Reckitt Benckiser	0.5	30	2–4
Levallorphane	Roche	0.2	1	?
Naloxone	Watson	1	0	0
Morphine	Astra/Zeneca	0	1	0
Nalbuphine	Endo/Du Pont	0.5	0.8	240
Pentazocine	Watson	0.04	0.4	90
Meptazinol	Shire	0.02	0.15	100

In addition this group of opioids is characterized by a respiratory ceiling effect. In comparison to morphine, cumulative dosages do not result in a dose-dependant impairment of respiratory drive until total apnea. On the contrary, every agonist/antagonist has a specific dose where respiratory depression reaches a plateau, "the ceiling". Further increase in dosages even results in a reversal of respiratory impairment (Figure III-58).

However, similar to a respiratory "ceiling effect" there is also an analgesic ceiling effect [179, 180]. Depending on the product and the dose being administered there is no further increase in analgesia (Table III-18). It is because of this analgsic

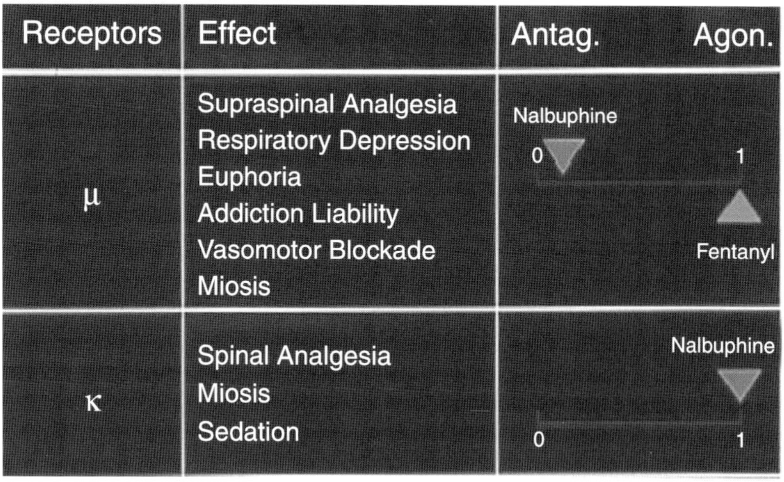

Figure III-57. Principal of mode of action of agonist/antagonists with an antagonistic effect at the µ- and the mediation of analgesia via the opioid κ-site

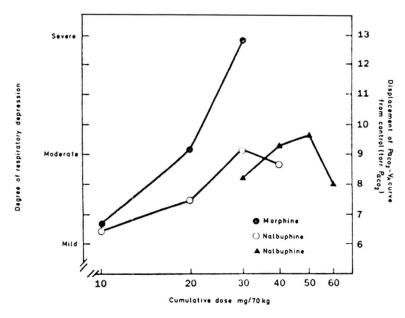

Figure III-58. Increasing doses of morphine result in a continuous impairment of respiratory drive. Contrary, increasing doses of the mixed agonist/antagonist analgesic nalbuphine, at a certain quantity, result in a "ceiling effect" where there is no further deterioration of respiration Adapted from [178]

"ceiling effect" that very intense postoperative pain is insufficiently treated with mixed narcotic analgesics.

The mixed narcotic agonist/antagonist butorphanol has been recommended for nasal application as a useful agent to block postoperative pain. Aside from its use as an "on-demand" type of spray by the patient, and similar to all other κ-ligands characterized by marked sedative effect, it was claimed to result in a reduced incidence of other side effects [181]. Due to the fast reabsorption via nasal soft tissue (high lipophilicity), there is an onset time within minutes with peak plasma levels after 1 h. It is because of this first-pass transfer that the liver is by-passed, resulting in an up to 70% bioavailability. Also, because of the by-pass of the liver, lower doses than usual are needed, which is the cause of lesser

Table III-18. Suggested dosing of opioids in patient-controlled analgesia (PCA) and their respective lock-out times

Opioid	Bolus on-demand dose	Lockout time (min)
Morphine	1–2 mg	8–15
Buprenorphine	1 μg	30
Fentanyl	20–40 μg	5–8

Modified from [195]

side effects. With a mean duration of action between 4 and 5 h, the agent was able to induce sufficient to good pain relief in medium to intense nociception following orthopedic procedures, cesarian section, hernia repair [181, 182] or in post episiotomy pain [183]. It should be noted that there is little or no irritation of nasal soft tissue even after prolonged use [184]. The nasal preparation of butorphanol (Stadol® NS) has also been tested positive in migraine headache and/or cluster pain [185, 186]

In comparison to the mixed narcotic analgesics, the partial agonist meptazinol has an interesting pharmacodynamic profile. With an analgesic potency, similarly to that of pethidine (meperidine, USP), when given in equipotent dosages (100 mg/70 kg) it does have a lesser respiratory depressive and a lesser sedative effect than pentazocine (60 mg/70 kg) or pethidine (100 mg/70 kg). Especially in obstetrics, when any agent given for the alleviation of pain should not affect the neonate, it has a larger margin of safety resulting in higher APGAR-scores when compared to pethidine [187]. And when compared with morphine in the management of postoperative pain, it resulted in a lesser impairment of respiration [188]. This drug therefore should be considered as a true alternative especially in obstetrics but also in the aging patient population with a frail cardiovascular system, who because of preexisting respiratory problems is more sensitive in developing an opioid–related respiratory impairment.

PATIENT-CONTROLLED ANALGESIA (PCA) FOR POSTOPERATIVE PAIN THERAPY

Patient-Controlled Analgesia (PCA) has become an acceptable and highly effective means of relieving post-operative pain. PCA is a medication-dispensing unit equipped with a pump attached to an intravenous line, which is inserted into a blood vessel in the patient's hand or arm (Figure III-59). By means of a simple push button mechanism, the patient is allowed to self-administer doses of pain relieving medication (narcotic) on an 'as need' basis. Prior to release from the hospital, the patient is weaned from the PCA and given oral medication to control pain. Before surgery, the anesthesiologist and/or doctor will discuss postoperative pain and how it can be controlled. Patients who are given options feel more confident, comfortable, and reassured about their surgical outcomes.

Patient-controlled analgesia is a technique of parenteral drug administration in which the patient controls a pump that delivers bolus doses of an analgesic, delivery rate and the physician presets a lock-out time. Use of a patient-controlled analgesia device allows the patient to titrate the opioid dose to his/her individual needs. The rational for use of such a pump is the fact that every patient has a different level of pain intensity and need of analgesics in the postoperative period. Fixed amounts of opioids often result in under- or even an overdose of the narcotic analgesic. Since the patient by himself is more able to tell when he needs a drug for alleviation of pain, the technique of "patient-controlled analgesia" seems a rational approach in order to have a content and pain-free individual. By pressing a button two times

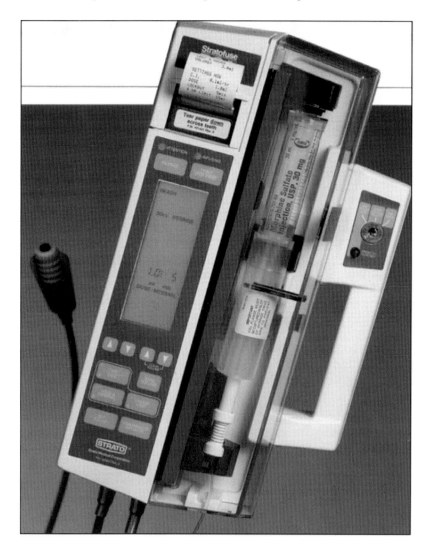

Figure III-59. View of the computerized programmable PCA-system with the preloaded syringe on the right-hand side

a fixed dose of a solution containing the opioid will be delivered via a motor-pump into his vein, permitting a reliable, fast and individual titration according to his/her need (Figure III-60). A prerequisite for such a procedure is a computerized small "on-demand" machine, connected to an intravenous line, whereby the medical personnel can preprogram the dose, the lock-out time and the interval.

Absolute contraindications for such an "on-demand" device are a respiratory insufficiency or a pre-existing hypovolemia. A relative contraindication exists in the

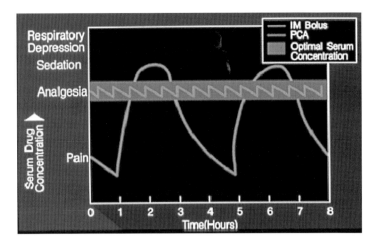

Figure III-60. Principle of patient-controlled analgesia (PCA) using an on-demand system. By the push of a button the preset dose of a narcotic analgesic is released into an intravenous line. This results in more constant blood plasma levels and a continuous occupation of opioid binding sites avoiding the conventional heights and lows of plasma concentrations with intramuscular dosing

elderly patient population, who is not able to operate an on-demand device [189]. Although there has been much controversy on the mechanical malfunctions and the use of an on-demand system that patient care will be neglected, that machine malfunction had led to an overdose with respiratory arrest, a patient lying in bed with severe pain in spite of him pressing the button, or visitors changing the setting of the machinery [190, 191, 192], this technique has made its way into the PACU being used by a number of institutions, thus reducing staff hours and manning of the ward with experienced personnel, which eventually reduces overhead costs.

A constant low-dose background infusion during "on-demand analgesia" for alleviation of postoperative pain has no advantages over the pure "on-demand" technique [193]. However, similar as in any other chronic pain therapy, patient-controlled analgesia does not have to be administered via an IV line. Similar beneficial results were attained with a subcutaneous on-demand system, because there is a nearly 100% bioavailability, while at the same time reducing possible complications of an IV line. The PCA can be used effectively to evaluate the efficacy of various opioid ligands in postoperative pain relief. In a double-blind controlled study design in patients following gynecological operations, similar to other short-acting opioid analgesics such as fentanyl and alfentanil, analgesics with a long duration of action, however, with a much lesser potency, were also able to sufficiently obtund postoperative pain (Figure III-61).

Before starting to use a PCA device several questions have to be answered, all of which relate to the clinical utility of an on-demand system:
1. Choose the optimal narcotic.
2. Determine the concentration of the opioid in the reservoir.

3. Choose a lock-out time where the patient is unable to retrieve the opioid.
4. Determine the dose of the bolus.
5. Make the decision if a basal-infusion rate is necessary.

As there is no real advantage of one opioid analgesic over the other, one should use the agent with the most experience. The short-acting opioids such as alfentanil, fentanyl, sufentanil and remifentanil, although having a sufficient potency, are more difficult to titrate in a PCA setting. It is because of this drawback that these agents are not recommended for PCA use. Aside from the selection of the appropriate agent, it is of utmost importance to choose the right bolus dose in order to have a satisfactory analgesic effect when using PCA. While small doses result in insufficient pain relief, too large doses might result in severe side effects, especially respiratory impairment. The bolus-dose, therefore, should have a quantity where the patient senses pain relief, however at the same time does not experience any side effects (Table III-18).

In summary, the advantages of PCA are:
1. The patients feel less apprehensive about pain following surgery because they know they have control in their hand by simply pushing a button.
2. The physician determines the amount (dosage) based on the patient's weight to prevent an overdose.
3. A narcotic addiction can be avoided because the drug is taken on a short-term controlled basis.
4. The pain relief is available around the clock. There is no need to wait for a nurse to deliver pain medication.
5. The medication does not need to be swallowed or injected.
6. The PCA unit is 'programmed' to control the dosage. The unit 'locks out' if the dosing frequency is exceeded.

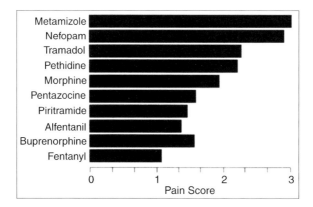

Figure III-61. Mean pain scores in patients following abdominal hysterectomy using a patient on-demand system for pain control with different agents. Note that a peripheral acting agent (metamizole) results in the least pain relief, while patients having access to a narcotic analgesic like, alfentanil fentanyl and buprenorphine were able to titrate their pain

7. The patient is assured they are receiving the correct medication and dose prescribed by their physician.
8. The doses are smaller and available more frequently, which helps prevent sleepiness and weakness.
9. Pain is more consistently controlled.
10. A dosing at regular intervals reduces the overall amount of medication needed to control pain.
11. Prior to expected activity (e.g. physical therapy, getting out of bed) the patient can self-dose to control pain during movement.
12. Most adults and children can use PCA. Overall, PCA can help patients to a quicker recovery.
13. Patients who are given control over their pain ambulate sooner, which promotes circulation and healing.

Opioids On-Demand, Without Use of a PCA System

If, however, one wants to achieve sufficient postoperative analgesia without the use of an additional mechanical device, the opioid has to be administered when the patient develops an increase in pain and demands the first dose. Followed by the immediate and intravenous titration of the analgesic until significant alleviation using a non-rating scale such as VAS < 3.0 (visual analogue scale where 0 denotes no pain and 10 reflects unbearable pain). Between titration, every 10th minute VAS is evaluated, in order not to overdose but at the same time administer the proper and individual quantity for pain relief. By use of the intravenous route of administration, the fastest way of the opioid agent is chosen in order to reach the specific receptor sites in the CNS. This results in an analgesic effect within minutes, and at the same time, give the medical personnel an objective sign when to stop or consider a second or even a third dose.

Such procedure is safe since because once the patient still experiences pain after the opioid medication, respiratory depression will not to be expected.

> **The most effective antagonist of opioid-related respiratory impairment is a nociceptive stimulus**

Individual non-verbal pain rating (using a non rating scale between 0 and 10) is a necessity in order to document sufficient pain relief in the patient's chart. In addition, subtle vegetative signs of sufficient/insufficient pain relief are recorded at fixed intervals:
- Heart rate, which increases with pain
- Blood pressure, which increases with pain
- Respiratory rate, which also increases if the patient has pain
- Perspiration, a definite sign of insufficient analgesia.

Once the individual dose has been established in the PACU, this amount is recommended for use in the ward at an interval, which closely matches with the half-life of the agent. Using this practice, time-contingent dosing is possible, thus avoiding breakthrough pain, which otherwise would result in a delay of recovery and impose an unnecessary stress reaction in the patient. The individual opioid requirement in the PACU can be used to determine future analgesic requirement on the ward. A Canadian group conclusively demonstrated, that when morphine is titrated intravenously (3–6 mg) to a VAS below 3.0 in the PACU, 2.2 times of that dose is needed every 4 h in order efficient to obtain sufficient postoperative analgesia in the majority of patients [196].

The necessary dose of an opioid differs in each patient, it therefore should be titrated to effect. Depending on the individual dose in the PACU a recommendation is given for future treatment in the ward

---

In summary there are several points, which have to be considered in order to attain a sufficient post-operative pain therapy:
1. Consider individual dosing a necessity.
2. Discuss with the patients the different modalities of postoperative analgesia during the premedicaton visit.
3. Give sufficient doses of a medium to potent opioid when necessary.
4. Establish a close surveillance of efficacy during dosing intervals for adapting to patients need.
5. Regularly record pain VAS, and any potential side effects.
6. Consider a multimodal approach (i.e. COX_2 inhibitor such as parecoxib plus an opioid, or ketamine plus an opioid, or a regional technique plus an opioid).
7. Immediately start with a potent opioid after upper abdominal operation or after thoracotomy, because postoperative pain will be intense.
8. Never mix a pure μ-type ligand like morphine, or hydromorphone with a mixed narcotic analgesic such as butorphanol or nalbuphine.

For medium type of pain, especially in the elderly patient population the combination of a fixed dose of tramadol together with an NSAID and an antiemetic, clinically has demonstrated an advantage.

First, there is a negligible respiratory depressive effect; second, analgesia is potentiated by the simultaneous use of a peripherally acting analgesic; third, the emetic effect of the opioid is counteracted by the additional antiemetic. And lastly, there is little consequence on the otherwise brittle cardiovascular system, which after the use of potent opioids may induce hypotension

This combination of an infusion of 500 cc of Ringers with tramadol consists of:
- 400 mg tramadol
- 5.0 g metamizole
- 25 mg trifluopromazine

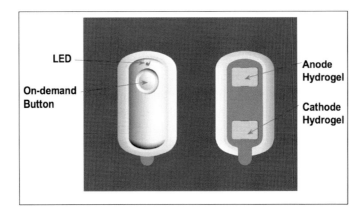

Figure III-62. Ionsys® system features where the opioid fentanyl is propelled through the skin using an electrical current LED = light emitting diode

Following an initial bolus dose of 100 cc of the solution, this is followed by a steady drip of 2 ml/h via an infusion pump [197] resulting in a total dose of 18 mg/h of tramadol and 200 mg/h of the NSAID.

> **Presently there is no ideal opioid for postoperative pain therapy; therefore a multimodal approach is advocated resulting in dose-reduction of each agent, thus avoiding potential side effects**

NEW TECHNIQUES FOR POSTOPERATIVE PAIN MANAGEMENT

Patient-controlled modalities using intravenous or epidural routes have dramatically improved postoperative pain management. However, acute post-operative pain continues to be undermanaged. Intravenous patient-controlled analgesia (PCA), the current standard of care for acute postoperative pain management, requires the patient to be attached to a staff-programmed pump apparatus via an intravenous catheter and tubing, rendering it invasive and mobility limiting. An innovative, needle-free, iontophoretic, fentanyl-HCl patient-controlled, transdermal system (PCTS; Figure III-62) is being marketed for acute postoperative pain management. Fentanyl-HCl PCTS is a compact, self-contained system that is easily applied to the upper outer arm or chest. It provides pain relief therapeutically equivalent to that of a standard regimen of morphine intravenous PCA, with pharmacokinetics similar to those of intravenous fentanyl infusion. Fentanyl HCl PCTS may be an effective, non-invasive alternative to currently available PCA modalities

The E-TRANS Iontophoresis is a method of transdermal administration of drugs in which the ionized form of a drug is propelled through the skin by an externally applied electric field. Sweat gland ducts and hair follicles provide the pre-existing aqueous pathways that potentially allow the passage of water-soluble molecules across the skin upon the application of low voltages. The permeation flux achieved with low voltages, however, is often much smaller than is desirable. For transdermal drug delivery through human skin, the use of high voltage pulses, resulting in transdermal voltages greater than 50 volts, is sufficient to cause electroporation within the stratum corneum. This results in new aqueous pathways that facilitate ionic and molecular transport across the skin. E-TRANS (Alza Corporation and J&J company), an electrotransport transdermal system, uses low-level electrical energy to deliver drugs that would not normally diffuse across the skin. It has been used for the transdermal delivery of the analgesic fentanyl in a patient-controlled transdermal system. Compared to standard intravenous PCA, the patient-controlled transdermal system has the advantage of being needle-free, potentially reducing interruptions in pain relief stemming from I.V. problems, and without the cumbersome PCA pump (Figure III-63). This self-contained and disposable system adheres to the skin and is approximately the size of a credit card. Occasionally, a temporary minor skin discoloration may occur at the electrode surface.

In a study with 636 adults having major surgical procedures, three hundred and sixteen patients were titrated to comfort with incremental doses of the opioid and then randomized to treatment groups. The PCTS delivered $40\,\mu g$ of fentanyl on demand over 10 min up to 6 times per hour, while the I.V.-PCA delivered 1 mg morphine bolus with a 5-min lockout, up to a maximum of 10 mg/h. Visual analogue scale (VAS) pain intensity scores were measured over 72 h. All efficacy end points had comparable outcomes between treatment groups. Patient global assessments for pain control of excellent or good were reported for 75.5% of the PCTS group versus 79.1% of the I.V.-PCA morphine group (p = 0.18). Similarly, physician global assessments of excellent or good were reported for 80.3% of the PCTS group versus 82.9% of the I.V.-PCA morphine group (p = 0.26). Outcome variables measured also included discontinuation of treatment after 3 h of inadequate pain relief, discontinuation for any reason, and last measured VAS pain score. No significant differences were noted between treatment groups for any of these variables. One serious episode of respiratory depression was reported in the I.V.-PCA group but none in the PCTS group [198].

Other adverse effects were as expected with systemic opiate therapy. Mild application site reactions occurred in 54% of patients in the PCTS group. The investigators considered PCTS and I.V.-PCA to be comparable for the treatment of acute postoperative pain.

SELECTIVE OPIOID ANTAGONISTS
FOR POSTOPERATIVE REVERSAL OF OPIOID
SIDE EFFECTS

An opioid antagonist that is selective for peripheral opioid receptors would be useful to treat two of the most common adverse effects of opioids: opioid bowel dysfunction and pruritus. Although constipation may be treated with the use of bowel

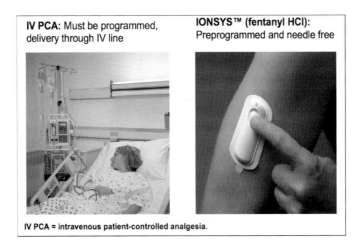

Figure III-63. Compared to PCA the needle free Ionsys® system in situ, placed on the upper arm. By pushing a button, fentanyl iontophoretically is driven through the skin where it migrates into the capillaries

regimens and pruritis with antihistamines, these agents are sometimes ineffective, are themselves associated with adverse effects, and often require the use of multiple agents. A recent comprehensive review examined available data for opioid antagonists, and concluded that peripherally acting agent's show the greatest promise because of their ability to reverse opioid-induced constipation and pruritus without compromising centrally mediated pain control. A potential advantage of opioid antagonists is the use of a single agent for the treatment of multiple adverse effects, which offers advantages of decreased drug costs and nursing time, improved drug compliance, and ease of administration [199]. Postoperative ileus, a serious side effect of opioid therapy, occurs commonly in patients undergoing lower abdominal surgery. Inhibition of gut motility occurs through activation of peripheral μ-opioid receptors in the gastrointestinal tract. Available opioid antagonists (e.g., naloxone) are not useful clinically to prevent this effect because they are readily absorbed, cross the blood-brain barrier, and act centrally to reverse analgesia.

Alvimopan (Adolor Corporation; Figure III-64) is a recently developed opioid antagonist that, like methylnaltrexone, has pharmacologic activity restricted to peripheral opioid receptors, and has shown the ability to reverse opioid-induced bowel dysfunction without reversing analgesia [200]. Alvimopan, being a moderately large, polar molecule, does not cross the blood-brain barrier [201].

Alvimopan may prove useful clinically as a selective inhibitor of gastrointestinal opioid receptors, thereby decreasing the incidence of postoperative ileus [202]. In normal volunteers, the prolongation of gastrointestinal transit time observed after administration of i.v. morphine (0.05 mg/kg) was prevented by oral administration of Alvimopan (4 mg). While morphine prolonged gastrointestinal transit time from 69 ± 33 to 103 ± 37 min ($p = 0.005$), this was prevented by Alvimopan ($p = 0.004$; Figure III-65).

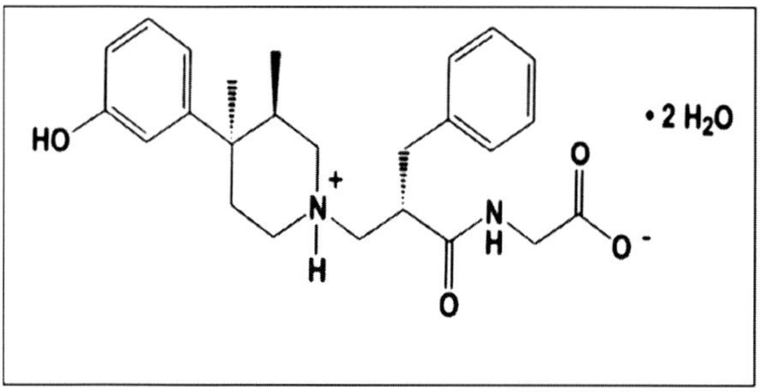

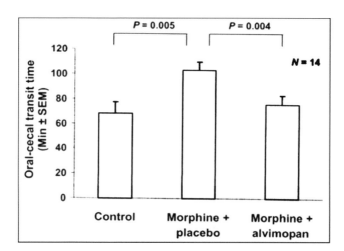

Figure III-64. Molecular structure of the selective peripheral opioid antagonist Alvimopan. Being a piperdine derivative with high affinity to the opioid μ-receptor, due to its large molecular size, cannot cross the blood-brain barrier

A randomized, controlled study of 78 patients who underwent lower abdominal surgery (15 patients, partial colectomy; 63 patients, total hysterectomy) evaluated its effect on recovery of gastrointestinal function. Patients received one capsule containing 1 mg or 6 mg of Alvimopan or an identical-appearing placebo 2 h before surgery and then twice daily until the first bowel movement or until hospital discharge. All patients received opioids for postoperative analgesia. Compared to the control group, the group that received 6 mg Alvimopan experienced significantly faster median times to passage of first flatus (49 h versus 70 h; p = 0.03), first bowel movement (70 h versus 111 h; p = 0.01), and time to discharge (68 h versus 91 h; p = 0.03) [203]. In addition to the reversal of constipation alvimopan was also able to reduce the incidence of postoperative nausea and vomiting (PONV) in patients having received an opioid for postoperative pain (Figure III-66).

Figure III-65. Prevention of morphine-induced delay in oral-cecal transit times, using the lactulose hydrogen breath test (Adapted from [201])

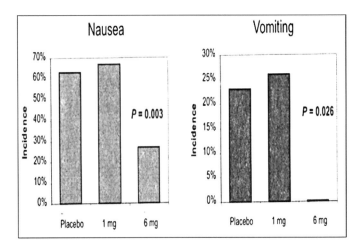

Figure III-66. Reduction of PONV in patients after hysterectomy and colectomy with the peripheral opioid antagonist alvimopan (Adapted from [204])

Another compound, which may be of interest to anesthesiologists and pain specialists and recently was approved by the FDA, is methylnaltrexone (Progenics Pharmaceuticals). Methylnaltrexone is the quaternary derivative of the opioid antagonist naltrexone [205].

It was originally developed by Leon Goldberg for use in cancer patients with opiate-induced constipation (Figure III-67), and now is indicated in all patients receiving opioids for acute and chronic pain.

In a subsequent randomized, double-blind, placebo-controlled study in human volunteers, single *oral* doses of methylnaltrexone (ranging from 0.64 to 19.2 mg/kg) acted quite similarly. Oral methylnaltrexone prevented the morphine-induced delay in oral-cecal transit time in a dose dependent manner without affecting analgesia

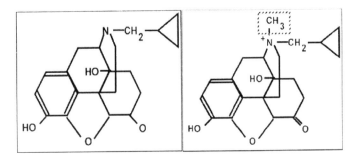

Figure III-67. Molecular structure of opioid antagonist naltrexone (**left**) and its derivative methylnaltrexone (**right**), a selective peripheral antagonist, which is not able to cross the blood-brain barrier

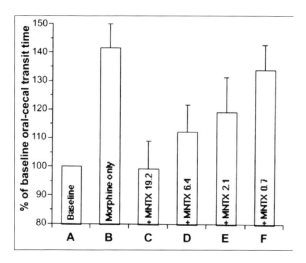

Figure III-68. Dose-related response with and without methylnaltrexone (MNTX 0.7, 2.1, 6,4 and 19.2 mg/kg respectively) on oral-cecal transit time in volunteers after morphine 0.05 mg/kg when normalized to control (= 100) (Adapted from [206])

(Figure III-68). Pharmacokinetic data revealed the effects primarily in the gut itself, not in response to systemic absorption of the drug [206]

Although the acute effects of opiates on GI motility proved to be completely reversible by methylnaltrexone, the efficacy of methylnaltrexone as a therapy in opiate-tolerant individuals represented a more complex problem of dose titration. To resolve this problem, a double-blind, placebo-controlled, randomized clinical trial was performed in 22 subjects undergoing chronic methadone maintenance therapy for addiction [207]. Normally, patients on methadone maintenance programs laxate only infrequently, sometimes only once or twice per week, and have a marked reduction in oral-cecal transit. Subjects in the study received methylnaltrexone intravenously on an ascending dose schedule. Both oral-cecal transit time and laxation were recorded and signs of withdrawal were monitored. Although oral-cecal transit time was normalized with methylnaltrexone, no subject showed psychological or physical signs of opiate withdrawal. In the 11 subjects in the placebo-treated group laxation response was not affected, whereas 10 of the 11 subjects in the methylnaltrexone-treated group evacuated on day 1, and all 11 evacuated on day 2.

In preliminary human studies, administration of small doses of morphine (averaging 3–5 mg) to volunteers slowed GI transit (as measured by oral-cecal transit time) by 50%. When subjects were treated with small doses of methylnaltrexone (0.4 mg/kg intravenously) this opiate-induced change in motility was almost completely reversed. Importantly, the cold pressor test demonstrated that morphine analgesia was intact with methylnaltrexone. This represented the first demonstration of separation of the central and peripheral effects of opiates on GI motility in humans [208]. Laxation occurred within 1 min of injection of the drug. The GI

motility of methadone maintenance patients was exquisitely sensitive to methylnaltrexone (5 times more sensitive in the chronic opiate users than in the volunteers).
Goldberg reasoned that a charged molecule with opiate antagonist properties would
not penetrate the blood-brain barrier, thus preserving central analgesia when given
with opiates. In the in vitro studies of human and guinea pig gut, methylnaltrexone
had one-third the potency of naloxone in reversing morphine-induced inhibition of
contraction. In these studies, 97% of morphine's effect on gastric motility could
be reversed by methylnaltrexone and the effect was luminal. Similar effects were
noted with *oral* methylnaltrexone in 12 methadone maintenance subjects. In another
study, oral methylnaltrexone reversed hypomotility and bowel movement in 5 h at
the highest dose (Figure III-68). The route of administration may be significant.
Laxation occurred immediately after IV administration of methylnaltrexone but
several hours after oral administration. After subcutaneous administration, changes
in oral cecal transit time occurred over a period of about 15 min [205]. Thus, the
several routes for administration, oral, intravenous, or subcutaneous, have various
onset and duration times.

POSTOPERATIVE OPIOIDS – SUMMARY AND OUTLOOK

In clinical practice today, analgesia is administered throughout the perioperative
period, beginning preoperatively, and continuing intraoperatively and postoperatively. Pain management protocols at many institutions use some form of multimodal therapy, incorporating combinations of a variety of agents, such as local
anesthetics, opioids, nonsteroidal anti-inflammatory drugs (NSAIDs), selective
COX-2 inhibitors, acetaminophen, and α_2-agonists. Ketorolac injection, NSAIDs,
administered orally (in patients who can take drugs by mouth) or local anesthetics
infiltrated into the wound are techniques often used as a part of multimodal analgesia
therapy. Use of NSAIDs as co-analgesics can reduce the need for opioids in the
postoperative period. Pharmacologically, improved analgesia is achieved through
interruption of nociceptive impulses at multiple sites, central and peripheral, of the
pain transmission pathway. With epidural analgesia, if side effects with use of a drug
mixture containing local anesthetic and opioid (e.g., sedation, nausea, hypotension,
numbness) are excessive, addition of a coanalgesic may allow a reduction in the
infusion rate.

Newer continuous drug delivery systems allow the delivery of opioid analgesic
drugs through more convenient modalities, which provide consistent analgesia and
other therapeutic advantages. Often, analgesia is facilitated significantly with the
use of multimodal therapy. Novel therapeutic agents under development will likely
provide important adjuncts to current treatment protocols and, in some cases, may
supplant currently available treatments. In anesthesiology practice, a new formulation DepoMorphine has evolved, which provides the benefit of a catheter-free,
less labor-intensive epidural technology compatible with anticoagulation therapy
(see below). This may allow the use of epidural analgesia in a wider patient

population and could potentially provide a useful replacement for current infusion pump and epidural catheter technology. At the same time, certain patient populations may continue to benefit from currently available treatment modalities. While it is expected that newer continuous drug delivery systems will provide greater convenience for patients and staff, optimal postoperative pain management is still best achieved through frequent, periodic assessment and reassessment of the patient's comfort level and side effects. Although continuous delivery systems may allow a reduced locus on issues related to pump and catheter maintenance, surveillance of the patient remains the principal issue in optimizing postoperative analgesic outcome. New compounds are also being identified that will specifically target the side effects of opioid analgesics. Agents like Alvimopan and methylnaltrexone should provide useful means for treating common side effects of opioid analgesia. It is anticipated that new drugs and new technologies will ultimately find their place in treatment as a part of multimodal treatment protocols for postoperative pain management.

Neuraxial Administration of Opioids for Pain Therapy

Aside from the intermittent or continuous local neural blockade, such as intercostal nerve blockade or infusion of a local anesthetic through an interpleural catheter, spinal/epidural analgesia is an effective technique to be used in postoperative pain therapy. Neuraxial drug administration describes techniques that deliver drugs in close proximity to the spinal cord, i.e. intrathecally into the cerebrospinal fluid (CSF) or epidurally into the fatty tissues surrounding the dura, by injection or infusion. This approach was initially developed in the form of spinal anesthesia over 100 years ago. Since then, neuraxial drug administration has evolved and now includes a wide range of techniques to administer a large number of different drugs to provide anesthesia, but also analgesia and treatment of spasticity in a variety of acute and chronic settings. This is usually done using an epidural opioid and/or local anesthetic injected intermittently or infused continuously.

> **Use of spinal analgesia, neural blockade or the infusion of local anesthetic through interpleural catheters require special expertise and well-defined institutional protocols and procedures for accountability. Administration of regional analgesia is best limited to specially trained and knowledgeable staff, typically under the direction of an acute or postoperative pain treatment service**

Rationale for application of opioids into the epidural/intraspinal space is opioid receptors, which are not only found in the supraspinal area. They are also found in the dorsal horn of the spinal cord (lamina I and the deep layers V–VI; Figure III-69),

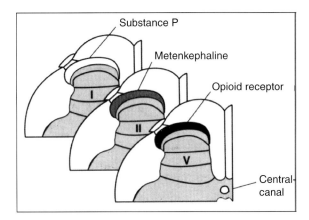

Figure III-69. Localization of substance P, metencephaline and opioid receptors in lamina I and II in the substantia gelatinosa of the spinal cord, where 90% are μ-receptors, 7% are δ-receptors and 3% are κ-receptors. Within the central canal, receptor distribution is 65% for the μ-, 33% for the δ- and 2% for the κ-type (Adapted from [209])

being responsible for the mediation of an analgesic effect. There nociceptive afferences are transmitted via interneurons to the spinothalamic, which projects to higher cortical areas such as the brain stem (medulla, pons), and to midbrain areas, which synapse to the ventroposterior and intrathalamic nuclei of the thalamus. Projections from the thalamus finally terminate in the primary somatosensory cortex (S1 and S2 region).

At the level of the spinal cord, nociceptive impulses can be modulated by afferent signals from peripheral touch receptors. Within the spinal cord, nociceptors release glutamate and substance P in layers I and II (substantia gelatinosa) and III where they stimulate both excitatory NMDA, AMPA, glutamate and neurokinin NK1 receptors (Figure III-70). At the same time the substantia gelatinosa is the site, where endogenous opioids are being released, which regulate the release of excitatory transmitters.

As a consequence of NMDA receptor activation, two potent mediators of pain, nitric oxide (NO) and adenosine are released. If, however, opioids are applied in that area they are able to reduce the release of pain mediators resulting in an inhibition of afferent activity. Neuraxial opioids are able to produce a sufficient analgesic effect in both surgical and non-surgical pain. Contrary to the sole application of local anesthetics for the treatment of pain, injection of an opioid close to the spinal cord results in lesser sensory, sympathetic or motor inhibition. As a consequence there is lesser orthostatic hypotension and there is no risk in loss of motor coordination.

The advantage of a neuraxial application of an opioid especially is of benefit in patients with preexisting pulmonary, cardiovascular disease, the extreme obese patient, and the elderly patient population undergoing major operations [210]. The neuraxial opioid application, contrary to an intramuscular or an intravenous dose, is characterized by a longer duration of action and a lesser dose, necessary for blockade

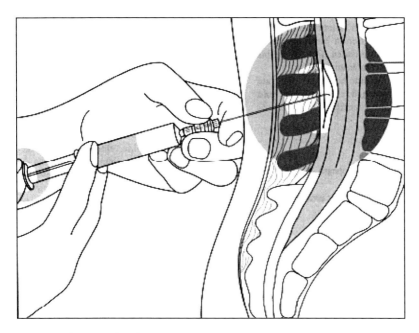

Figure III-70. Following peridural application, opioids diffuse to the lamina V where opioid receptors are unevenly distributed with 70% for the μ-, 20% for the δ- and 2% for the κ-type

of nociception. However, when compared to intravenous or intramuscular mode of application, there is no proof for superior quality of analgesia following epidural or intrathecal opioids. Also, possible neurotoxicity and incompatibility of the agent with the cerebrospinal fluid has to be anticipated. This is why the neuraxial application of an opiate like opium and an opioid like remifentanil is banned [211, 212].

The major indication for use of neuraxial opioids is postoperative pain following orthopedic, intraabdominal, and thoracic or perineal operations. In the intensive care situation a patient with a flail chest as well as the polytraumatized patient, where repetitive evaluation of consciousness is of importance, analgesia by means of an epidural catheter is an advantage when compared to systemically-induced analgesia and sedation [213].

The benefits of adding an epidural opioid for alleviation of pain are as follows:
• a highly selective blockade of noiceptive afferences
• a maintenance of motor control, no loss of deep sensory and temperature sensations
• a long duration of action
• a potentiation of action when applied with a local anesthetic
• a regional distribution
• a lesser dose for efficacy (20%–25%) when compared to systemic application
• a lesser incidence of side effects.

There are following indications for neuraxial opioids in acute and chronic pain syndrome:
1. Terminal tumor pain
2. Excessive dosages for pain relief with oral opioids
3. Inefficiency of oral opioids
4. Severe side effects during oral opioid
5. Prolonged postoperative pain therapy.
6. Cesarean section
7. Visceral pain during the first stage of labor
8. Potentiation of peridural analgesia with a local anesthetic
9. Prolongation in duration of action of local anesthetics.

Opioids suitable for a neuraxial application (Table III-19) should have the following physicochemical and pharmacokinetic properties [214]:
1. A high affinity to the opioid receptor site with concomitant high analgesic potency.
2. High lipophilicity, which enables the drug to quickly pass the dura mater and accumulate in the spinal cord tissue.
3. A low hydrophilic property with a lesser time of stay in the cerebrospinal fluid.
4. A high molecular weight with increased absorption in the surrounding tissue [215].
5. A long duration of receptor binding, with a concomitant long duration of action.
6. A low incidence in the development of tolerance followed by low habituation.

Due to the different physicochemical properties, there is a different mode of action of opioids following neuraxial application. Since the diffusion rate from epidural space into the spinal tissue and the blood stream mostly depends on lipophilicity, fentanyl has a faster onset of action than the hydrophilic compound morphine. However, at the same time, the duration of action of fentanyl is much shorter. This is because morphine has hydrophilic properties, which results in a delayed diffusion into spinal cord tissue and at the same time demonstrate a slowed rediffusion out of the spinal cord (Figure III-71).

While the long duration of action of morphine is due to its hydrophilic property, the long duration of action of buprenorphine is due to its intense receptor binding.

Table III-19. Summary of opioids used for neuraxial application

Opioid generic name	Opioid trade name	Mean epidural dose (mg/70 kg)
Buprenorphine	Buprenex	0.15–03
Diamorphine	Heroin	5
Fentanyl	Sublimaze	0.1–0.35
Hydromorphone	Dilaudid	1
Methadone	Polamidone	5
Pethidine	Meperidine	100–210
Morphine Sulfate	Morphine	2–5
Sufentanil	Sufenta	0.01–0.05

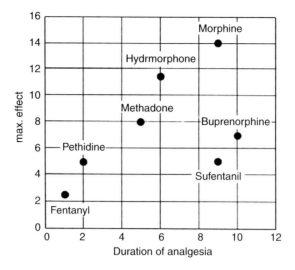

Figure III-71. Comparison of onset time and duration of action of different opioids used for peridural analgesia (Adapted from [214, 216])

This results in a slow dissociation from its binding site. Morphine when being injected into the cerebrospinal fluid with a physiologic pH, 75% is present as morphine-hydrochloride showing little tendency to diffuse into spinal tissue. The residual 25% are present as a base, which rapidly diffuses through the dura mater and into the substantia grisea of the spinal cord, the genuine site of action. Following diffusion equilibrium is established. Since the hydrophilic morphine hydrochloride very slowly diffuses out of the liquor, it stays within the epidural space where it acts as a reservoir, contributing to the long duration of action (Figure III-72).

> **Only morphine and sufentanil are legitimated for epidural or intrathecal use. If other opioids are utilized for neuraxial application this is done under the sole responsibility of the physician**

SIDE EFFECTS OF EPIDURAL OPIOIDS

The following side effects, which seldom are of hazardous magnitude, are observed after neuraxial opioid application:
1. Drop of blood pressure in about 11.5% of patients
2. Bradycardia in 1.6% of patients
3. Muscle relaxation in 7% of patients
4. Late (> 8 h) respiratory depression

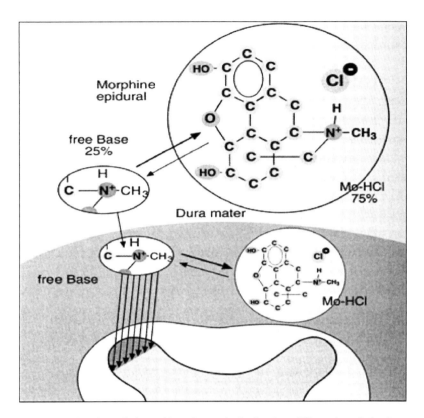

Figure III-72. Peridurally applied morphine where only the free base diffuses through the dura mater and into spinal cord tissue (lamina I and II)

The late respiratory depression is a common and most dangerous side effect, which occurs with a neuraxial opioid. It is often observed after morphine use, because after epidural injection this agent slowly spreads to the respiratory center, located at the floor of the IVth cerebral ventricle. This delay in onset of respiratory impairment is due to the cephalic migration of the opioid within the cerebrospinal fluid, which needs about 6–10 h in order to reach the IVth cerebral ventricle following intrathecal application [217] [218].

Due to the greater hydrophilic characteristic of morphine, a greater portion of the agent remains in the cerebrospinal fluid, migrating rostrally to the respiratory center, from where the impairment in respiratory drive is triggered. Such depression clinically is most relevant in patients with excessive blood loss and hypovolemia [219]. In general, the time at which the opioid-related respiratory depression is established depends very much on the route of application. Following an intravenous injection this side effect is seen within 5 min, and when the opioid is given peridurally and/or intrathecally there is a delay of 4–12 h (Table III-20) [220].

Table III-20. The onset of respiratory depression following different routes of application

Route of application	Onset of Respiratory depression
Intravenous	2–5 min
Intramuscular	> 30min
Epidural	> 8h
Intrathecal	> 8h

Adapted from [220, 221, 222]

Contrary to morphine, the opioid buprenorphine with its high lipophilicity, results in an accumulation of the agent within spinal cord tissue. Therefore epidural application of this opioid is not accompanied by a potential risk of late respiratory impairment. This is because the administered dose binds for a long time to the receptor site, resulting in a deep and long analgesic effect [223, 224, 225]. Due to the high affinity to the opioid receptor, epidural sufentanil or fentanyl also demonstrates a fast onset. Although it had been acclaimed that compounds with a high lipophilic property result in a lesser incidence of respiratory depression, this deleterious side effect has also been observed after epidural application of the lipophilic agent fentanyl [225]. Such observation suggest that other components are relevant for the induction of respiratory impairment, where the applied dosage seems to have a significant impact (Table III-21):

If, however, *respiratory depression* clinically becomes evident after an epidural/intrathecal opioid, this can be reversed rapidly by a bolus injection of the opioid antagonist naloxone (0.1–0.2 mg i.v.) or by an infusion (5–10 mg/h). In addition, the mixed narcotic analgesic nalbuphine (5–10 mg i.v.) or the potent antagonist naltrexone (3–6 mg oral) can also be used for the same purpose [226, 227]. The low dosages of the antagonists/mixed agonist antagonist are sufficient to restore spontaneous respiration without reversing the analgesic effect of the epidural

Table III-21. Summary of reasons resulting in increase/decrease of side effects following epidural opioid application

Augmentation of side effects	– increased dosage
	– repetitive injections
	– additional parenteral administration
	– high age
	– low lipophilicity of opioid
	– aortic cross clamping
	– supine position
	– upright position
Decrease of side effects	– hyperbaric solution
	– high lipophilicity of opioid
	– dose reduction
	– volume reduction

opioid. However, a reduction in duration of analgesic action has to be anticipated. Occasionally, a repetitive injection of naloxone may become necessary in order to maintain a long-term sufficient respiration.

Another often observed side effect of neuraxial opioids is *pruritus*, which is observed in 5%–50% of all patients. It is of vegetative origin being caused by the irritation of sensory nerve fibers within the upper cervical ganglia. Because after epidural application opioid-related pruritus has a late onset time, histamine is not the cause of itching [228]. Also, similar to respiratory depression, opioid-induced pruritus can be reversed by the antagonist naloxone given in titrated doses (0.2–0.8 mg/70 kg body weight). This can be considered as conclusive evidence for the participation of opioid receptors. For the attenuation of itching also dyphenhy-dramine or propofol (10 mg/70 kg i.v.) is advocated.

Urinary retention is another side effect observed after neuraxial opioids and is observed in 14% of all patients receiving an epidural or intrathecal opioid [229]. As a cause of this side effect an opioid-receptor related inhibition of acetylcholine release from efferent postganglionic ganglia is discussed. This is because Ach (Acetylcholine) is an important mediator innervating urinary bladder musculature [230]. For the reversal, naloxone (titrated dosages of 0.2–0.8 mg/70 kg body weight) or the α_2-agonist clonidine has been shown to be effective in reversing urinary retention.

Other side effects following neuraxial opioids are *nausea/emesis*, whereby the opioid reaches the chemoreceptor trigger zone in the medulla, and activates the vomiting center. The time of manifestation closely correlates with the rostral spread of the opioid via the cerebrospinal fluid [228] (Figure III-73). Also, these side effects can be reversed with a intravenous low dose of naloxone without affecting analgesia [231]. Alternatively, a low dose of a neuroleptic (for instance haloperidol 5.0 mg/70 kg body weight), or a transdermal scopolamine patch can be effective for reversal [232].

Other side effects are often observed after epidural use of local anesthetics, are less likely to turn up.

In summary, after epidural opioids the following side effects can be seen clinically. However, the incidence and the severity is much less than after an intravenous injection [224, 233, 234, 225, 235, 236]:

1. Rostral spread after application

   – Late respiratory depression

2. By "remorphinisation"

   – Vertigo
   – Head ache
   – Pruritis
   – Urinary retention
   – Dysuria
   – Euphoria, disorientation

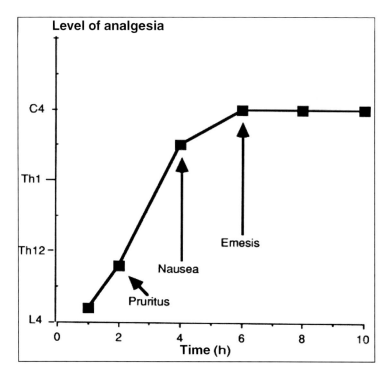

Figure III-73. Time-related rostral spread of the pain free area following epidural morphine and the time and incidence of side effects (Adapted from [218])

– Muscular rigidity
– Somnolence
– Nausea/vomiting.

Lipophilic or Hydrophilic Opioids for Neuraxial Use

While there is a close relation between lipophilicity and the onset of action of epidurally applied opioids (Figure III-74), there is the connotation that lipophilic opioids for neuraxial use are much safer in regard to a possible respiratory impairment. This implication, however, is not sufficiently substantiated by clinical results. This is because:

1. Pruritus as well as nausea can be observed after the lipophilic fentanyl as well as after the hydrophilic morphine.
2. Fentanyl can be detected in the cervical cerebrospinal fluid following lumbar application. Clinical studies have identified conclusively a high concentration in the cervical cerebrospinal fluid 30 min after the injection of lumbar fentanyl [225].
3. The incidence of respiratory depression is about the same with a lipophilic agent as with the hydrophilic morphine. There is a reported case following a continuous epidural analgesia with fentanyl for 5 h (125 μg/h), where late respiratory depression developed after 17 h [237].

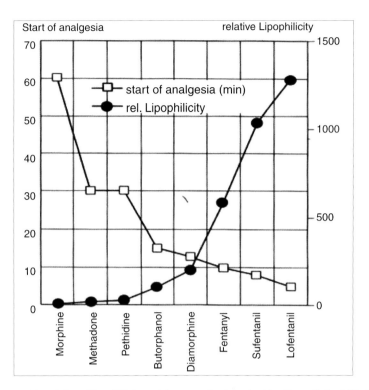

Figure III-74. The relation of lipophilicity and the onset of action of epidurally applied opioids (Adapted from [214, 238])

Because of the above results there is the following requirement:

Following epidural application of the lipophilic opioids fentanyl as well as sufentanil, respiration has to be monitored

---

   The incidence of respiratory depression after a lipophilic agent is around 0.6% [237]. Although the mechanism of action of the migration of the opioid to the rostral area cannot be explained conclusively, such clinical data suggest that similar to the findings in the classical study of Bromage and coworkers with morphine [218], there is also a rostral spread of the lipophilic opioid fentanyl, with the possibility of respiratory depression. One likely cause for this side effect is the higher dosage of lipophilic agents, necessary for initiating a sufficient level of analgesia. When compared to morphine the relation of an intravenous to an epidural dose for analgesia is more in favor of the hydrophilic opioid (Figure III-75). The presumed advantage of lipophilic agents not to induce respiratory impairment when used in neuraxial analgesia, in reality does not exist. There is a much higher

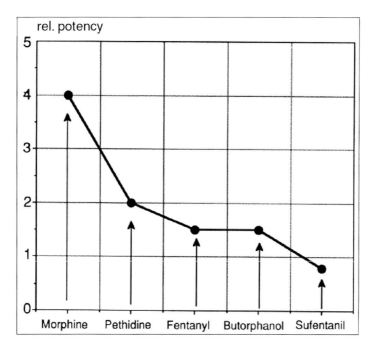

Figure III-75. Relative potencies of epidural versus intravenous dosages of different opioid analgesics. The hydrophilic opioid morphine demonstrates an optimal relation of sufficient antinociception and dose (Adapted from [232])

reduction of the required dose of the hydrophilic morphine when used for epidural analgesia. Both, the significantly reduced dose of the epidural opioid, essential for the induction of a sufficient analgesic level and the concomitant reduced incidence in side effects are in favor of the hydrophilic morphine. Such effects have been demonstrated in the animal, where morphine and other hydrophilic agents such as dihydromorphine induced a better analgesic level with lower dosages than fentanyl [239]. Such findings are also be corroborated by clinical data where relatively higher dosages of fentanyl are necessary for the induction of a similar level of analgesia [232].

Because of the lesser dose-related potency of lipophilic opioids of epidural when compared to systemic use, several possible explanations are being discussed:

1. Unspecific binding of the lipophilic opioid to peridural fat which acts like a depot. This may be one explanation why the dose of the lipophilic opioid sufentanil relatively has to be high, being around 30–50 μg for a bolus injection.
2. Lipophilic opioids demonstrate a fast diffusion through the dura mater into the spinal fluid and into the gray matter. At the same time there is also a fast re-diffusion out of the spinal cord tissue.
3. Contrary to the intense interaction with opioid receptors in the supraspinal areas, there is lesser binding of lipophilic agents with opioid receptors in the spinal cord.

4. Due to the systemic reabsorption of epidural opioids into the systemic circulatory system, there is additional supraspinal binding. For fentanyl, such additional binding is only of additive nature while morphine demonstrates a synergistic effect.
5. Aside from binding of lipophilic compounds to epidural fat, there is also unspecific binding to the substantia grisea, resulting in less available drug for receptor interaction (Figure III-76).

EXTENDED-RELEASE EPIDURAL MORPHINE FOR POSTOPERATIVE PAIN

DepoMorphine (Endo Pharmaceuticals) is a novel sustained release injectable formulation of morphine for the control of postoperative pain, and is approved by the FDA. It utilizes morphine suspended in a liposomal sustained-release epidural delivery system (DepoFoam, SkyePharma PLC). DepoFoam consists of microscopic spherical particles composed of numerous nonconcentric internal aqueous chambers containing morphine (Figure III-77).

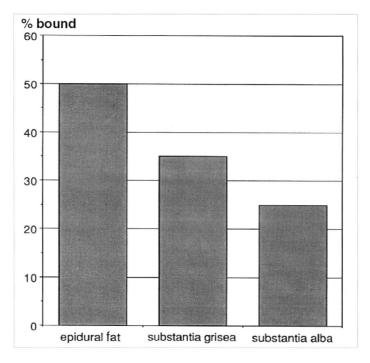

Figure III-76. Unspecific portions of fentanyl bound to epidural fat, substantia grisea and alba of the spinal cord respectively

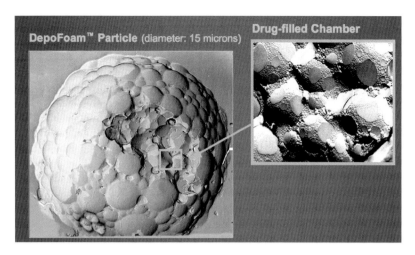

Figure III-77. Principle of liposomes containing morphine for sustained-release in the epidural space

Each chamber is separated from its neighbor by a single bilayer lipid membrane. In a physiologic milieu, the chambers break down and slowly release the drug contained within [240]. DepoMorphine is given as a single epidural injection before surgery, and clinical studies have shown that the formulation provides pain relief for 48 h, at which time a transition to an oral agent may be appropriate for many patients. This delivery system bypasses the need for an indwelling epidural catheter and infusion pump, thereby avoiding potential problems, which may be associated with these devices. A randomized, double-blind, placebo-controlled study in 194 hip arthroplasty patients evaluated the reduction in postoperative i.v. fentanyl requirement in patients who received a single epidural injection (15 mg, 20 mg, 25 mg) of DepoMorphine (Figure III-78). Patients were administered the test drug or placebo before induction of general or intrathecal anesthesia for surgery. Postoperatively, fentanyl was provided via I.V. PCA pump. Fentanyl consumption, the primary outcome measure, was markedly reduced for the data collection period, extending to 48 h after surgery. The time to first fentanyl request also showed a strong dose-dependent relationship and was significantly longer for the aggregate test group ($p < 0.0001$). Furthermore, patient and physician satisfaction scores for pain control were improved for the test group compared to the control group. In this study, DepoMorphine provided extended, dose-related analgesia for 48 hours during the postoperative period. Adverse events were not significantly different between study groups. The investigators concluded that DepoMorphine might offer an effective and safe alternative to the use of an indwelling epidural catheter. Side effects were as expected with systemic opioid therapy, and were readily managed [241]. Another double-blind, randomized study in 75 patients undergoing Caesarean section showed similar results with regard to postoperative analgesia. A combined spinal/epidural technique was utilized in which patients received spinal anesthesia

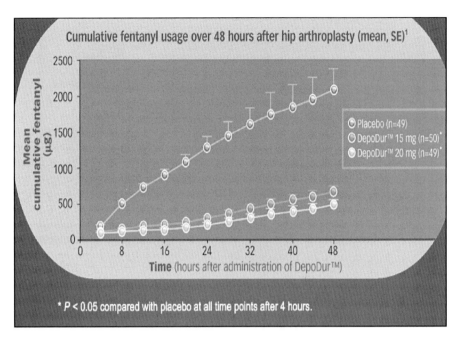

Figure III-78. Significant reduction of additional fentanyl postoperatively in patients having received epidural DepoDur preoperatively

(bupivacaine 12–15 mg intrathecally and fentanyl 10 μg). After clamping of the umbilical cord, a single epidural dose of either 5 mg of conventional morphine sulfate or 5 mg, 10 mg, or 15-mg DepoMorphine was administered. Postoperatively, patients received oral or i.v. opioids as needed. Rescue analgesic usage was converted to i.v. morphine equivalents for purposes of analysis. Throughout the 48-h postsurgical period, opioid analgesic use was significantly reduced for patients who had received DepoMorphine.

Functional ability scores at 24 and 48 h were also significantly improved. The authors of this study suggested that DepoMorphine is a promising new epidural analgesic for the long-term management of pain after cesarean section [242]. Surgeons who participated in these studies noted a consistent level pain of relief throughout the 48-h postoperative period, when pain intensity is most severe. A single injection consistently maintained analgesia, with minimal need for rescue medication, low analgesic gaps, and no catheter or pump maintenance issues. Clinical benefits were noted in that, unlike epidurals delivering local anesthetics, intermittent adjustment of medication levels was not needed. In addition, incidence of hypotension was rare. Epidural DepoMorphine analgesia was compatible with anticoagulation therapy, and this was considered an important benefit for orthopedic surgery populations. Postoperative ileus was not found to be a problem in abdominal surgery patients, as no difference was noticed with respect to the return of normal bowel function. Also, the absence of an additional pump and an i.v. pole with extra tubing, which can sometimes limit the patient's ambulation, clinically is advantageous.

COMBINATION OF AN EPIDURAL OPIOID WITH A LOCAL ANESTHETIC

When opioids alone are used in obstetric anesthesia, adequate analgesia is only achieved in the treatment of visceral pain in the first stage of labor. Somatic pain in the second stage is more difficult to manage. Nowadays because of the faster onset of action, especially in obstetrics, the rapidly acting lipophilic opioids sufentanil and fentanyl, which have a duration of effect of 2–3 h, have replaced the more hydrophilic morphine (duration of effect 8–24 h). The agents of choice are low-dose sufentanil or fentanyl in combination with low-dose bupivacaine in the form of an epidural infusion. This results in advantages with a faster onset, and a longer duration of analgesia, it lowers the total dose of a local anesthetic and opioid by about 20–25%, and reduces motor block, which is commonly seen after the sole epidural use of a local. In addition, there are lesser significant side effects for the mother and child when using such co-administration. The following combinations of an opioid with a local anesthetic are recommended:

1. Sufentanil and ropivacaine. After administering a test dose and incremental bolus administration of 15 mL 0.1% ropivacaine and 1–2 μg/mL sufentanil (10–20 μg), the continuous infusion can be started: 0.1% ropivacaine and 0.2–0.3 μg/mL sufentanil using a speed of 10 ml/h.
2. Fentanyl and ropivacaine. After administering a test dose and incremental bolus administration of 15 mL 0.1% ropivacaine and 30 μg fentanyl, the continuous infusion can be started: 0.1% ropivacaine and 2 μ/ml sufentanil, using a speed of 10–12 ml/h.
3. Sufentanil and bupivacaine (levobupivacaine). After administering a test dose and bolus administration of 10 mL 0.125–0.0625% bupivacaine (0.125–0.0625% levobupivacaine) and 1–2 μg/ml sufentanil (10–20 μg), the continuous infusion can be started after about 30 min: 0.0625–0.125% bupivacaine (0.0625–0.125% levobupivacaine) and 0.2–0.3 μg/ml sufentanil, using a speed of 6–10 ml/h.
4. Fentanyl and bupivacaine (levobupivacaine). After administering a test dose and bolus administration of 10 ml 0.25% bupivacaine (0.25% levobupivacaine) and 50 μg fentanyl, the continuous infusion can be started after about 30 min: 0.0625% bupivacaine (0.0625% levobupivacaine) and 1–2 μg/ml fentanyl, using a speed of 10 ml/h.

Epinephrine is added mostly in obstetrical anesthesia where it has both alpha-adrenergic and beta-adrenergic effects. Adding epinephrine causes a dose-dependent reduction in uterine activity and leads to a delay in delivery. If there is an inadvertent intravascular injection of a local anesthetic with epinephrine, adverse circulatory reactions can occur both in the mother (hypertonia, cardiac arrhythmia) and in the child (reduced placental perfusion due to vasoconstriction). Any addition of epinephrine in obstetrics must therefore be strictly indicated.

When a cesarean section is to be performed, lumbar catheter epidural anesthesia for pain control can be used. The spread of the injected local anesthetic must reach segments T4–T6. The higher the spread of the local anesthetic, the greater the risk of severe hypotension. Segments L5, S 1 and S2 are not always adequately anesthetized and there is often a delay in anesthesia in this area.

When using a *Patient-controlled epidural analgesia* (**PCEA**) the opioid is combined with a local anesthetic [243]. The following combinations have been shown to be of clinical relevance:

1. Sufentanil and ropivacaine. 0.1% ropivacaine and 1 μg/ml sufentanil. Speed: 5–10 ml/h. Bolus dose: 5 mL. Lockout period: 10–20 min.
2. Fentanyl and ropivacaine. 0.1% ropivacaine and 2 μg/mL fentanil. Speed: 10 ml/h. Bolus dose: 10 ml. Lockout period: 10–20 min.
3. Sufentanil and bupivacaine (levobupivacaine). After administering a test dose with a bolus administration of 5–10 ml, 0.125% bupivacaine (0.125% levobupivacaine) and 10–30 μg/ml sufentanil, the continuous infusion can be started: 0.0625% bupivacaine (0.0625% levobupivacaine) and 1 μg/mL sufentanil. Basic setting: Speed 5 ml/h (5 μg sufentanil) Bolus dose 5 mL (5 μg sufentanil) Lockout period: 20 min.
4. Fentanyl and bupivacaine (levobupivacaine). After administering a test dose and bolus administration of 6–10 mL, 0.125–0.25% bupivacaine (0.125–0.25% levobupivacaine), and 10 μg fentanyl, incremental, doses until segment T10 is reached. Now the continuous infusion can be started: 0.125% bupivacaine (0.125% levobupivacaine) and 0.0001% fentanyl. Basic setting: Speed 4 ml/h Bolus dose 4 mL Lockout period: 20 min.

CONTINUOUS-INFUSION EPIDURAL ANALGESIA (CIEA)

This technique is selectively used in parturients and in chronic pain patients because it results in the following advantages [243, 244]:

1. Long-term antinociception with a preserved sensitivity for pressure and position.
2. Block of nociceptive afferents is confined to selective neural segments.
3. Central effects of opioids like sedation and/or respiratory depression are avoided.
4. Analgesia is prominent, and there is a long duration of action.
5. Due to the continuous administration of an opioid with a low flow rate the risk of respiratory depression is very low.

In order to benefit from this technique, careful selection of patients is imperative. Therefore the patients:

- where pain cannot be managed by the conventional (oral) way,
- where systemic administered opioids induce substantial side effects,
- where patients present pain on both sides of their body,

The opioid is being administered via an external or internal (subcutaneous pouch) reservoir with a pump system, from which an epidural catheter runs to the epidural space through a subcutaneous tunnel [245]. The catheter is placed at the appropriate dermatome, close to the origin of pain (Figure III-79). Individual dosing is done with the help of the pain questionnaire using an individual flow rate, which results in a significant reduction of pain. Flow rate can be adjusted to patients need and the reservoir has to be refilled every 2–3 weeks, depending on the flow rate.

When using an external pump, the relatives of the patients or the health care personnel should be instructed how to appropriately fill the reservoir. Especially when using the port system, the subcutaneously placed epidural catheter is attached to a subcutaneous port, being connected via puncture with the externally carried small-sized pump. Such port systems increase the mobility of patients, result in lesser visits at the doctors office, and the patients can be treated in an outpatient department.

The selection of the appropriate pump system depends on life expectancy of the patient. If this is $> 1/2$ year and a previously stationary patient, due to pain relief, now becomes mobile, an implantable pump system is recommended. When using the percutaneous pump system, there is a potential incidence of secondary contamination of catheter and pump. However, on the other side, the higher costs for an implantable pump system and the necessity of a surgical procedure have to be considered.

INTRATHECAL USE OF OPIOIDS

The intrathecal application of an opioid presents a more direct way to administer the opioid close to its site of action, the substantia gelatinosa at the dorsal column

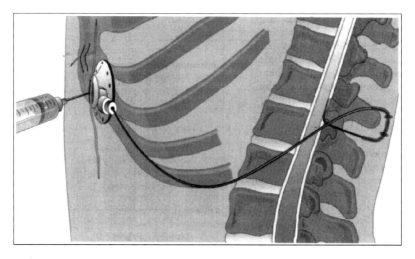

Figure III-79. Example of an external pump system with a subcutaneous port for continuous infusion epidural analgesia

of the spinal cord. Aside from the lack of diffusion through the dura mater, the usual migration of the opioid within the cerebrospinal fluid and the unspecific binding of the opioid to epidural fat tissue as well as the vascular reabsorption through the venous plexus within the epidural space is avoided [246]. From such consideration it can be concluded that the activity of intrathecal use of opioids is far better foreseeable, is more intense, and results in a longer duration of action. This for instance has been demonstrated for sufentanil and morphine given in obstetric anesthesia during the first stage of labor where the analgesic dose was 10 μg and 1 mg respectively, resulting in a duration of action lasting 1–2 h (Figure III-80). Such low doses are incapable to induce sufficient analgesia when using the epidural or the intravenous route [247].

Several studies however have documented that the highly lipophilic opioids (e.g. sufentanil, fentanyl, alfentanil, butorphanol, pethidine) demonstrate little dose reduction when comparing the intravenous with the intrathecal mode of application [248]. When comparing the intrathecal with the epidural mode, clearly there is an advantage for the intrathecal route, and in order to achieve similar cerebrospinal concentrations, the epidural dose has to be increased 5fold [249]. For morphine and fentanyl there are similar dose differences, whereby morphine 0.3 mg or fentanyl 25 μg in combination with bupivacaine results in a good analgesic level during labor pain. In spite of such encouraging results, and contrary to the peridural use of opioids, there are only few controlled studies. In order to give general recommendations and definitively outline the putative advantage of an intrathecal use of opioids, additional studies are needed. Since the known side effects, as

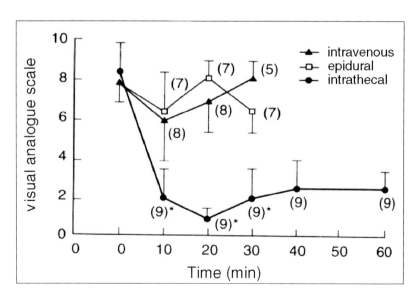

Figure III-80. Visual analogue scale (VAS) in patients using different routes and dosages of sufentanil for treatment of labor pain (*p < 0.01)

they are observed after epidural application (i.e., respiratory depression, pruritis) very likely appear shortly following application [250]. In case of an inadvertent respiratory depression, low-dose naloxone is the agent of choice to reverse this side effect without significantly affecting the analgesic level [251].

In summary the followed advantages of intrathecal versus peridural application of an opioid are obvious:

1. Lower systemic reabsorption.
2. Lower non-specific absorption via peridural fat tissue.
3. Lower dosages, resulting in a reduced incidence in side effects.
4. Pronounced selection of the analgesic level [252].

However, there are several considerations why presently, contrary to intrathecal use, the epidural route is still considered to have a major advantage [230, 253]:

1. The necessary catheter technology is not fully developed.
2. Lipophilic opioids necessarily do not result in a longer duration of action than the hydrophilic morphine.
3. There is a higher potential risk in incidence of side effects, especially of respiratory depression.
4. The question of a possible neurotoxicity of agents has not been answered adequately.

MIXED AGONIST/ANTAGONISTS AND α_2-AGONISTS FOR NEURAXIAL USE

Since κ-receptors have also been localized in the spinal cord theoretically mixed agonist analgesics (nalbuphine, pentazocine, butorphanol) should also induce an analgesic effect when administered epidurally/intrathecally. First results with 10 mg nalbuphine in the epidural space were promising as a postoperative pain relief was achieved for over 15 h, and compared to morphine, patients experienced lesser side effects [254]. However, since this opioid is diluted in a solvent, which may have neurotoxic properties, its peridural application is not recommended. In addition, results of a multicenter study in Canada, nalbuphine when given peridurally was inadequate for postoperative pain alleviation. Although other agonist/antagonists analgesics like pentazocine [255] or butorphanol [254] demonstrated mixed results when used epidurally for postoperative pain, the general use of this group of narcotic analgesic for epidural use has not gained wide acceptance.

Other agents, which have been tested for epidural use in chronic pain therapy are the α_2-agonist clonidine, benzodiazepines, and somatostatin. Although co-administration of an opioid like morphine with a benzodiazepine, somatostatin, ketamine or the κ-ligand dynorphin resulted in a potentiation of action and a prolongation in the duration (Figure III-81), their epidural use is not recommended because of potential neurotoxicity [256]. One promising candidate for epidural use is the potent opioid lofentanil, which demonstrated a high specificity and selectivity for the opioid μ-receptor resulting in an optimal dose-response relationship [238]. Although it has an optimal pharmacological profile for epidural use, Janssen

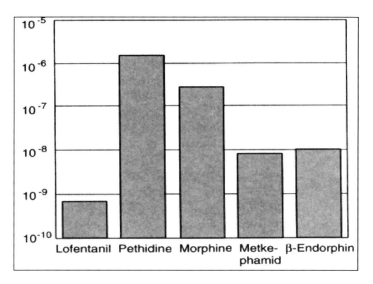

Figure III-81. Different magnitude in antinociceptive action (shock titration test in the monkey) of various agents applied epidurally (mol/l) (Adapted from [246])

Company has made no effort to market that agent. Another compound, however, has made its way from preclinical tests into the clinical field for treatment of chronic pain. Co-administration of the opioid morphine (2 mg) with the α_2-agonist clonidine (450 µg/24 h) epidurally has become an accepted method in chronic pain treatment. Even when administered by itself or with a local anesthetic, and using a dose of 75–150 µg in 6–7 cc saline solution as a single shot into the epidural space or by continuous epidural infusion (750 µg in 50 ml saline), analgesia is induced through activation of α_2-receptors in the substantia gelatinosa of the spinal cord. When used for the postoperative period, this resulted in fewer side effects, a potentiation and a prolongation of analgesia [257, 258, 57]. For chronic pain patients the addition of 50 µg/h of clonidine to an epidural dose of morphine induced a 45% increase in patient satisfaction [50] while in neuropathic pain the addition of clonidine resulted in a 56% increase in patients who gained total pain mitigation [51]. For the treatment of postoperative and chronic pain, epidural clonidine has been approved by the FDA [49].

References

1. Geddes, I.C. and T.C. Gray, *Hyperventilation for the maintenance of anaesthesia.* Lancet, 1959, **2**: pp. 4–6.
2. Laborit, H. and P. Huguenard, *L'hibernation artificielle par moyens pharmacodynamiques et physiques.* Presse Med, 1951, **59**: pp. 1359–1365.
3. De Castro, G. and P. Mundeler, *Anesthésie sans sommeil: "Neurolpetanalgésie".* Acta Chir Belg, 1959, **58**: pp. 689–693.

4. De Castro, J., P. Viars, and J.C. Leleu, *Utilisation de la Pentazocine comme antimorphinique et analgesique dans une technique d'anesthesie analgesique sequentielle*, in *Utilisation de la Pentazocine en anesthesie-reanimation*, J. De Castro, P. Viars, and J.C. Leleu, Editors, 1969, Ars Medici: Bruxelles. pp. 33–36.

5. Flacke, J.W., W.E. Flacke, and G.D. Williams, *Acute pulmonary edema following naloxone reversal of high dose morphine anesthesia*. Anesthesiology, 1977, **47**: pp. 376–378.

6. Gasparetto, A. and G. Giron, *Clinical value of vitamin anesthesia: Thiamine algosynaptolysis according to De Castro and Mundeleer*. Acta Anaesthesiol, 1964, **15**: pp. 699–710.

7. Freye, E. and H. Agoutin, *The action of vitamin B1 (thiamine) on the cardiovascular system of the cat*. Biomedicine, 1978, **28**: pp. 315–319.

8. Freye, E. and E. Hartung, *The potential use of thiamine (Vit.B1) in patients with cardiac insufficiency*. Acta Vtaminol Enzymol, 1982, **4**: pp. 285–290.

9. Lobera, A. and J.L. Renaud-Salis, *General anesthesia in major cancer surgery of the upper respiratory and digestive tracts. Significance of a fentanyl-thiamine combination*. Ann Anesthesiol Fr, 1976, **17**: pp. 621–627.

10. Lagler, F., et al., *Toxikologische Untersuchungen mit Tramadol, einem neuen Analgetikum*. Drug Res, 1978, **28** (I): pp. 164–172.

11. Cookson, R.F., *Carfentanil and lofentanil*. Clin & Anaesthesiol, 1983, **1**: pp. 156–158.

12. Leysen, J.E., W. Gommeren, and C.J.E. Niemegeers, *3H-sufentanil, a superior ligand for the mu-opiate receptor: binding properties and regional distribution in rat brain and spinal cord*. Eur J Pharmacol, 1983, **87**: pp. 209–225.

13. Niemegeers, C.J.E. and P.A.J. Janssen, *Alfentanil (R 39 209) – a particularly short-acting narcotic analgesic in rats*. Drug Dev Res, 1981, **1**: pp. 83–88.

14. De Castro, J., *Association des analgésiques centraux et des neuroleptiques en cours d'intervention*, in *Les analgésiques et la douleur. Influences pharmacologiques diverses exercées sur morphiniques*, G. Vourch, et al., Editors, 1971, Masson: Paris. pp. 185–194; 383–403.

15. De Castro, J., S. Andrieu, and J. Boogaerts, *Buprenorphine: a review of its pharmacological properties and therapeutical uses*. New Drug Series, ed. J. De Castro (Eds) Vol. 1. 1982, Kluwer: Antwerpen NVM & ISA. 180.

16. Bovill, J.G., et al., *The pharmacokinetics of alfentanil (R 39209): a new opioid analgesic*. Anesthesiology, 1982, **57**: pp. 439–443.

17. Sebel, P.S., et al., *Effects of high dose fentanyl anesthesia on the electroencephalogram*. Anesthesiology, 1981, **55**: pp. 203–211.

18. Stanley, T.H. and S. de Lange, *Comparison of sufentanil-oxygen and fentanyl-oxygen anesthesia for mitral and aortic valvular surgery*. J Cardiothoracic Anesth, 1988, **2**: pp. 6–11.

19. De Lange, S., et al., *Comparison of sufentanil-02 and fentanyl-02 for coronary artery surgery*. Anesthesiology, 1982, **56**: pp. 112–118.

20. Tolksdorf, W., et al., *Adrenalin-, Noradrenalin-, Blutdruck- und Herzfreqenzverhalten während der Intubation in Abhängigkeit unterschiedlicher Fentanyl-Dosen*. Anästh Intenivther Notfallmed, 1987, **22**: pp. 171–176.

21. Stark, R.D., et al., *A review of the safety and tolerance of propofol (Diprivan™)*. Postgrad Med J, 1985, **61**: pp. 152–156.

22. Grant, I.S. and N. MacKenzie, *Recovery following propofol (Diprivan) anaesthesia-a review of three different anaesthetic techniques*. Postgrad Med J, 1985, **61**: pp. 133–137.

23. Cockshott, I.D., *Propofol (Diprivan) pharmacokinetics and metabolism-an overview*. Postgrad Med J, 1985, **61**: pp. 45–50.
24. Becker, L.D., et al., *Biphasic respiratory depression after fentanyl-droperidol or fentanyl alone used to supplement nitrous oxide anesthesia*. Anesthesiology, 1976, **44**: pp. 291–296.
25. Habib, A.S. and T.J. Gan, *Food and Drug Administration black box warning on the perioperative use of deoperidol: a review of the cases*. Anesth Analg, 2003, **96**: pp. 1377–1379.
26. Kissin, I., et al., *Alfentanil potentiates midazolam-induced unconsciousness in subanalgesic doses*. Anesth Analg, 1990, **71**: pp. 65–69.
27. Oldendorf, H., et al., *Clinical pharmacokinetics of midazolam in intensive care patients, a wide interpatient variability?* Clin Pharmacol Ther, 1988, **43**: pp. 263–269.
28. Geller, E., et al., *Risk and benefits of therapy with flumazenil (Anexate®) in mixed drug intoxications*. Eur Neurol, 1991, **31**: pp. 241–250.
29. Freye, E. and A. Fournell, *Postoperative Demaskierung einer überhängenden Vigilanzminderung nach Midazolameinleitung durch den Antagonisten Flumazenil (Ro 15–1788)*. Anaesthesist, 1988, **37**: pp. 162–166.
30. Freye, E., B. Neruda, and K. Falke, *Flumazenil (Anexate®) for the reversal of residual benzodiazepine activity*. Drugs Today, 1989, **25**: pp. 119–124.
31. Bergmann, S.A., et al., *GABA agonists enhancer morphine and fentanyl antinociception in rabbit tooth pulp and mouse hot plate test*. Drug Dev Res, 1988, **14**: pp. 111–122.
32. Tejwani, G.A., et al., *Inhibition of morphine-induced tolerance and dependence by a benzodiazepine receptor agonist midazolam in the rat*. Anesth Analg, 1993, **76**: pp. 1052–1060.
33. Luger, T.J., et al., *The spinal potentiation effect and the supraspinal inhibitory effect of midazolam on opioid-induced analgesia in rats*. Eur J Pharmacol, 1995, **275**: pp. 153–162.
34. Rosland, J.H., S. Hunskaar, and K. Hole, *Diazepam attenuates morphine antinociception test-dependently in mice*. Pharmacol Toxicol, 1990, **66**: pp. 382–386.
35. Luger, T.J., et al. *Mechanisms of the influence of midazolam on morphine antinociception at spinal and supraspinal levels in rats*. Eur J Pharmacol, 1994, **271**: pp. 421–431.
36. Luger, T.J., H.F. Hill, and A. Schlager, *Can midazolam diminish sufentanil analgesia in patients with major trauma? A retrospective study with 43 patients*. Drug Metab Drug Interact, 1992, **10**: pp. 177–184.
37. Michaels, I. and P.C. Barash, *Does nitrous oxide or a reduced FI02 alter the hemodanymic function during high dose sufentanil anesthesia?* Anesth Analg, 1983, **62**: p. 275.
38. Murphy, M.R. and C.C. Hug, *The enflurane sparing effect of morphine, butorphanol, and nalbuphine*. Anesthesiology, 1982, **57**: pp. 489–492.
39. Hall, R.I., M.R. Murphy, and C.C. Hug, *The enflurane sparing effect of sufentanil in dogs*. Anesthesiology, 1987, **67**: pp. 518–525.
40. Murphy, M.R. and C.C. Hug, *The anesthetic potency of fentanyl in terms of its reduction of enflurane MAC*. Anesthesiology, 1982, **57**: pp. 485–488.
41. Hecker, B.R., et al., *The decrease of the minimum alveolar anesthetic concentration produced by sufentanil in rats*. Anesth Analg, 1983, **62**: pp. 987–990.

42. Hartung, E., E. Freye, and H. Dehnen-Seipel, *Enflurane in cardiac surgery*. Acta Anaesth Belg, 1982, **33**: pp. 141–145.

43. Hartung, E. and E. Freye, *An open comparison of propofol and enflurane for prolonged abdominal operations*. Anaesthesia, 1988, **43**: pp. 105–107.

44. Ismaily, A.J., et al., *Die Auswirkungen einer Kombinationsanästhesie mit Fentanyl und Enfluran auf den Kreislauf und die unmittelbare postoperative Phase*. Anäst Intensivmed, 1987, **28**: pp. 216–220.

45. Hartung, H.J., *Klinische Erfahrungen mit Alfentanil zur "balanced anesthesia" bei Oberbauch-Eingriffen*. Anaesthesist, 1988, **37**: pp. 620–624.

46. Stanley, T.H., *Comparison of alfentanil with thiopental sodium for induction of anesthesia*. 1982, Janssen Pharmazeutika, Beerse, Belgien.

47. Smith, N.T., et al., *An electroencephalographic comparison of alfentanil with other narcotics and with thiopental*. J Clin Monit, 1985, **1**: pp. 236–244.

48. Redmond, D.E. and Y.H. Hwang, *The primate locus coeruleus and affects of clonidine on opiate withdrawal*. J Clin Psychiatr, 1982, **43**: pp. 25–31.

49. Eisenach, J.C., S.Z. Lysak, and C.M. Viscomi, *Epidural clonidine analgesia following sugery. Phase I*. Anesthesiology, 1989, **71**: pp. 640–646.

50. Eisenach, J.C., et al., *Epidural clonidine analgesia for intractable cancer pain. Phase I*. Anesthesiology, 1989, **71**: pp. 647–652.

51. Eisenach, J.C., et al., *The epidural clonidine study group: epidural clonidine analgesia for intractable cancer pain*. Pain, 1995, **61**: pp. 391–399.

52. Flacke, J.W., et al., *Reduced narcotic requirement by clonidine with improved hemody-namic and adrenergic stability in patients undergoing coronary bypass surgery*. Anesthesiology, 1987, **67**: pp. 11–19.

53. Ghignone, M., *Effects of clonidine on narcotic requirements and hemodynamic response during induction of fentanyl anesthesia and endotracheal intubation*. Anesthesiology, 1987, **67**: pp. 3–10.

54. Aantaa, R., A. Kallio, and R. Virtanen, *Dexmedetomidine, a novel alpha2-adrenergic agonist: A review of its pharmacodynamic profile*. Drugs Future, 1993, **18**: pp. 49–56.

55. Noyer, M., et al., *Mivazerol, a novel compound with high binding specificity for alpha2 adrenergic receptor: binding studies on different human and rat membrane preparations*. Neurochem Int, 1994, **24**: pp. 221–229.

56. McSPI-Europe, *Perioperative sympathicolysis. Beneficial effects of the alpha2-agonist mivazerol on hemodynamic stability and myocardial ischemia*. Anesthesiology, 1997, **86**: pp. 346–363.

57. Carabine, U.A., K.R. Milligan, and J. Moore, *Extradural clonidine and bupivacaine for postoperative analgesia*. Br J Anaesthesia, 1992, **68** (2): pp. 132–135.

58. Motsch, J., E. Gräber, and K. Ludwig, *Addition of clonidine enhances postoperative analgesia from epidural morphine; a double blind study*. Anesthesiology, 1990, **73**: pp. 1067–1073.

59. Gabriel, A.H., et al., *Clonidine: an adjunct in isoflurane N20/02 relaxant anaesthesia*. Anaesthesia, 1995, **50**: pp. 290–296.

60. Engelman, E., et al., *Effects of clonidine on anesthetic requirements and hemodynamic response during aortic surgery*. Anesthesiolgy, 1989, **71**: pp. 178–187.

61. Hoffmann, W.E., et al., *Dexmedetomidine improves neurologic outcome from incom-plete ischemia in the rat: reversal by the alpha2 antagonist atipamezole*. Anesthesi-ology, 1991, **75**: pp. 328–332.

62. Jarrot, B., et al., *Clonidine: understanding its disposition, sites and mechanism of action*. Clin Exp Pharmacol Physiol, 1987, **14**: pp. 471–479.

63. Bjoerkqvist, S.E., *Clonidine in alcohol withdrawal*. Acta Psychiat Scand, 1975, **52**: p. 256.

64. Kleber, H.D., et al., *Clonidine and naltrexone in the outpatient treatment of heroin withdrawal*. Am J Drug Alcohol Abuse, 1987, **13** (1, 2): pp. 1–17.

65. Vining, D.H., T.R. Kosten, and H.D. Kleber, *Clinical utility of rapid clonidine-naltrexone detoxification for opioid abusers*. Br J Addict, 1988, **63**: pp. 567–575.

66. Striebel, H.W., D. Koenigs, and T. Heil, *Clonidin – Stellenwert in der Anästhesie*. Anaesthesist, 1993, **42**: pp. 131–141.

67. Maze, M. and W. Tranquilli, *Alpha-2 adrenoreceptor agonists: defining the role in clinical anesthesisa*. Anesthesiology, 1991, **74**: pp. 581–605.

68. Cube von, B., et al., *Permeation morphinartiger Substanzen an den Ort der antinociceptiven Wirkung im Gehirn in Abhängigkeit von ihrer Lipoidlöslichkeit nach intravenöser und nach intraventrikulärer Applikation*. Naunyn-Schmiedebergs Arch Pharmacol, 1970, **265**: pp. 455–473.

69. Prys-Roberts, C. and C.E. Hug, *Pharmacokinetics of Anaesthesia*. 1984, Blackwell: Oxford Scientific Publications.

70. Hug, C.C.J., *Pharmacokinetics of new synthetic narcotic analgesics*, in *Opioids in Anesthesia*, F.G. Estafanous, Editor, 1984, Butterworth: Boston. pp. 50–60.

71. Westmoreland, C., et al., *Pharmacokinetics of remifentanil (GI87084B)*. Anesthesiology, 1993, **79** (3A): p. A372.

72. Hermann, D.J., et al., *Pharmacokinetic comparison of GI87084B, a novel ultra-short acting opioid, and alfentanil*. Anesthesiology, 1991, **75**: p. A379.

73. Taeger, K., et al., *Uptake of fentanyl by human lung*. Anesthesiology, 1984, **61**: p. A246.

74. Cube von, B., et al., *Permeation of morphine-like substances to their site of antinociceptive action in the brain after intravenous and intraventricular application and dependence on lipid solubility*. Arch Pharmacol, 1970, **265**: pp. 455–502.

75. Stanski, D.R. and C.C. Hug, *Alfentanil-a kinetically predictable narcotic analgesic*. Anesthesiology, 1982, **57**: pp. 435–438.

76. Schenk, H.D., F.B.M. Ensink, and M. Rhönisch, *Alfentanil – Porträt eines Opioids zur Anästhesie*. 1993, Urban & Schwarzenberg: München-Wien-Baltimore. 1–144.

77. Scott, J.G., J.E. Cooke, and D.R. Stanski, *Electroencephalographic quantitation of opioid effects: comparative pharmacodnamics of fentanyl and sufentanil*. Anesthesiology, 1991, **74**: pp. 34–42.

78. Michiels, M., R. Hendricks, and J. Heykants, *A sensitive radioimmunassay for fentanyl: plasma levels in dogs and man*. Eur J Pharmacol, 1974, **12**: p. 153.

79. Miller, R.D., *IV drug delivery systems*, in *Anesthesia*. 2000, Churchill Livingstone: Oxford. pp. 377–408.

80. Shafer, S.L. and S.R. Varvel, *Pharmacokinetics, pharmacodynamics, and rational opioid selection*. Anesthesiology, 1991, **74**: pp. 1136–1138.

81. Scott, J.C., K.V. Ponganis, and D.R. Stanski, *EEG quantification of narcotic effect: the comparative pharmacodynamics of fentanyl and alfentanil*. Anesthesiology, 1985, **62**: pp. 234–241.

82. Lemmens, H.J.M., et al., *The application of pharmacokinetics dynamics and computer simulations to drug development: A-3665 versus fentanyl and alfentanil*. Anesthesiology, 1992, **77** (3A): p. A456.

83. Ausems, M.E., D.R. Stanski, and C.C.J. Hug, *An evaluation of the accuracy of pharmacokinetic data for the computer assisted infusion of alfentanil.* Br J Anaesth, 1985, **57**: pp. 1217–1225.

84. Egan, T.D., et al., *The pharmacokinetics of the new short-acting opioid remifentanil (GI87084B) in healthy adult male volunteers.* Anesthesiology, 1993, **79**: pp. 881–892.

85. McDonnell, T.E., R.R. Bartowski, and J.J. Williams, *ED50 of alfentanil for induction of anesthesia in unpremedicated young adults.* Anesthesiology, 1982, **57**: p. A362.

86. Minto, C.F., T.W. Schnider, and S.L. Shafer, *Pharmacokinetics and pharmacodynamics of remifentanil. II-Model application.* Anesthesiology, 1997, **86**: pp. 24–33.

87. Hughes, M.A., P.S.A. Glass, and J.R. Jacobs, *Context-sensitive half-time in multicompartment pharmacokinetic models for intravenous anesthetic drugs.* Anesthesiology, 1992, **76**: pp. 334–341.

88. Egan, T.D., *Remifentanil pharmacokinetics and pharmacodynamics.* Clin Pharmacokinet, 1995, **29**: pp. 80–94.

89. Read, D.J.C., *A clinical method for assessing the ventilatory response to carbon dioxide.* Aust Ann Med, 1979, **16**: pp. 20–32.

90. Suttmann, H. and A. Doenicke, *Interim report on dose-establishment with alfentanil.* 1983, Janssen Pharmaceutica, Beerse, Belgium.

91. Freye, E., E. Hartung, and R. Buhl, *Alfentanil als letzte Dosis (on-top) in der Neuroleptanalgesie mit Fentanyl.* Anaesthesist, 1986, **35**: pp. 231–237.

92. Nauta, J., et al., *Anesthetic induction with alfentanil: a new short-acting narcotic analgesic.* Anest Analg, 1982, **61**: pp. 267–272.

93. Sebel, P.S., N. De Brujin, and W.K. Neville, *Median nerve somatosensory evoked potentials during anesthesia with sufentanil or fentanyl.* Anesthesiology, 1988, **69** (A312).

94. Kochs, E., et al., *Modulation of pain-related somatosensory evoked potentials by general anesthesia.* Anesth Analg, 1990, **71**: pp. 225–2230.

95. Freye, E. and B. Neruda, *Averaged somatosensory evoked potentials for intraoperative evaluation of analgesia in patients.* J Clin Monit, 1988, **4**: pp. 138–139.

96. Rundshagen, I., E. Kochs, and J. Schulte am Esch, *Surgical stimulation increases median nerve somatosensory evoked responses during isoflurane-nitrous oxide anaesthesia.* Br J Anaesth, 1995 (75).

97. Freye, E., *Somatosensorisch evozierte Potentiale (SEP) zur Algesiemetrie*, in *Alfentanil – Ein neues, ultrakurzwirkendes Opioid*, M. Zindler and E. Hartung, Editors, 1985, Urban & Schwarzenberg: München-Wien-Baltimore. pp. 17–23.

98. Minto, C.F., et al., *Influence of age and gender on the pharmacokinetics and pharmacodynamics of remifentanil. I.Model development.* Anesthesiology, 1997, **86**: pp. 10–13.

99. Crawford, M.W., et al., *Development of acute opioid tolerance during infusion of remifentanil for pediatric scoliosis surgery.* Anwesth Analg, 2006, **102**: pp. 1662–1667.

100. Guignard, B., et al., *Acute opioid tolerance: intraoperative remifentanil increases postoperative pain and morphine requirements.* Anesthesiology, 2000, **93**: pp. 409–417.

101. Albrecht, S., et al., *Postoperative pain control following remifentanil-based anaesthesia for major abdomional surgery.* Anaesthesia, 2000, **55**: pp. 315–322.

102. De Castro, J., et al., *Comparative study of cardiovascular, neurological, and metabolic side effects of eight narcotics in dogs.* Acta Anaesth Belg, 1979, **30**: pp. 5–99.

103. Van Bever, W.F.M., et al., *N-4-substituted 1-(2arylethyl)-4-piperidinyl-N-phenylpropanamides, a novel series of extremely poteut analgesics with unusually high safety margin.* Drug Res/Arzneimittelforsch, 1978, **26**: pp. 1548–1551.

104. Niemegeers, C.J.E., et al., *Sufentanil, a very potent and extremely safe intravenous morphine-like compound in mice, rats and dogs.* Drug Res/Arzneimittelforsch, 1976, **216**: pp. 1551–1556.

105. Janssen, P.A.J., *The development of new synthetic narcotics*, in *Opioids in Anesthesia*, F.G. Estafanous, Editor, 1984, Butterworth: Boston. pp. 37–44.

106. Tollenaere, J.P. and H. Moereels, *Atlas of the three-dimensional structure of drugs.* 1979, Amsterdam, New York, Elsevier: Oxford/North Holland Biomedical Press.

107. Magnan, J., et al., *The binding spectrum of narcotic analgesic drugs with different agonist and antagonist properties.* Naunyn-Schmiedebergs Arch Pharmacol, 1982, **319**: pp. 197–205.

108. Flacke, J.W., et al., *Comparison of meperidine, fentanyl and sufentanil in balanced anesthesia.* Anesth Analg, 1985, **64**: pp. 897–910.

109. De Lange, S., et al., *Antidiuretic and growth hormone responses during coronary artery surgery with sufentanil-oxygen and alfentanil-oxygen anesthesia in man.* Anesth Analg, 1982, **61**: p. 434.

110. De Lange, S., et al., *Catecholamine and cortisol responses to sufentanil-O2 and alfentanil-O2 anaesthesia during coronary artery surgery.* Can Anaesth Soc J, 1983, **30**: p. 248.

111. Bailey, P.L., et al., *Sufentanil produces shorter lasting respiratory depression and longer lasting analgesia than equipotent doses of fentanyl in human volunteers.* Anesthesiology, 1986, **65**: p. A493.

112. Bailey, P.L., et al., *Differences in magnitude and duration of opioid induced respiratory depression and analgesia with fentanyl and sufentanil.* Anesth Analg, 1990, **70**: pp. 8–15.

113. Spiegel, K. and G.W. Pasternack, *Meptazinol: a novel mu-1 selective opioid analgesic.* J Pharmacol Expt Ther, 1984, **228**: pp. 414–419.

114. Jaffe, J.H. and W.R. Martin, *Opioid analgesics and antagonists*, in *The Pharmacological Basis of Therapeutics*, A.F. Gilman, et al., Editors, 1990, Pergamon Press: New York. pp. 485–531.

115. Bovill, J.G., et al., *Electroencephalographic effects of sufentanil anaesthesia in man.* Br J Anaesth, 1982, **54**: pp. 45–52.

116. Bowdle, T.A. and R.J. Ward, *Induction of anesthesia with small doses of sufentanil or fentanyl: dose versus EEG response, speed of onset, and thiopental requirement.* Anesthesiology, 1989, **70**: pp. 26–30.

117. Hilgenberg, J.C., *Intraoperative awareness during high dose fentanyl-oxygen anesthesia.* Anesthesiology, 1981, **54**: pp. 341–343.

118. Mummaneni, N., T.L.K. Tao, and A. Montoya, *Awareness and recall during high-dose fentanyl-oxygen anesthesia.* Anesth Analg, 1980, **59**: pp. 948–949.

119. Freye, E. and E. Hartung, *Kardiovaskuläre und zentralnervöse Effekte unter Fentanyl versus Sufentanil bei der Intubation herzchirurgischer Patienten.* Anästhesie Aktuell, 1993, **9**: pp. 3–14.

120. Brian, S.E. and A.B. Seifen, *Tonic-clonic activity after sufentanil.* Anesth Analg, 1987, **66**: p. 481.

121. Freye, E., E. Hartung, and R. Buhl, *Die Lungencompliance wird durch die rasche Injektion von Alfentanil beeinträchtigt.* Anaesthesist, 1986, **35**: pp. 543–546.

122. Smith, N.T., et al., *EEGs during high-dose fentanyl, sufentanil-, or morphine-oxygen anesthesia.* Anesth Analg, 1984, **63**: p. 386.

123. Katz, R.I., et al., *Two instances of seizure-like activity in the same patient associated with two different narcotics.* Anesth Analg, 1988, **67**: p. 289.

124. Young, W.L., et al., *The effect of sufentanil on cerebral hemodyamics during carotid endarterectomy.* Anesthesiology, 1988, **69**: p. A591.

125. Keykhah, M.M., D.S. Smith, and C. Carlson, *Influence of sufentanil on cerebral metabolism and circulation in the rat.* Anesthesiology, 1985, **63**: pp. 274–277.

126. Werner, C., *Der Einfluß von Sufentanil auf die regionale und globale Hirndurchblutung und den zerebralen Sauerstoffverbrauch beim Hund.* Anaesthesist, 1992, **41**: pp. 34–38.

127. Milde, L.N., J.H. Milde, and W.J. Gallagiter, *Effects of sufentanil on cerebral circulation and metabolism in dogs.* Anesth Analg, 1990, **70** (2): pp. 138–146.

128. Weinstabl, C., et al., *Effects of sufentanil on intracranial pressure in neurological patients.* Anaesthesia, 1991, **46**: pp. 837–840.

129. Sperry, R.J., et al., *Fentanyl and sufentanil increase intracranial pressure in head trauma patients.* Anesthesiology, 1992, **77** (3): pp. 416–420.

130. Stephan, H., et al., *Einfluß von Sufentanil auf Hirndurchblutung, Hirnstoffwechsel und die C02-Reaktivität der menschlichen Hirngefäße.* Anaesthesist, 1991, **40**: pp. 153–160.

131. Freye, E., et al., *Slow EEG-power spectra correlate with hemodynamic changes during laryngoscopy and intubation following induction with fentanyl and sufentanil.* Acta Anaesth Belg, 1999, **50**: pp. 71–76.

132. Hull, R.I., R.I. Murphy, and C.C. Hug, *The enflurane sparing effect of sufentanil in dogs.* Anesthesiology, 1987, **67**: pp. 518–525.

133. Monk, J.P., R. Beresford, and A. Ward, *Sufentanil: A review of its pharmacological properties and therapeutic use.* Drugs, 1988, **36**: pp. 286–313.

134. Gravlee, G.P., F.M. Ramsey, and R.C. Roy, *Rapid administration of a narcotic and a neuromuscular blocker: a hemodynamic comparison of fentanyl, sufentanil, pancuronium, and vecuronium.* Anesth Analg, 1988, **67**: pp. 39–47.

135. Brizgys, R.V., R. Morales, and B. Owens, *Effects of thiopental requirements and hemodynamic response during induction and intubation.* Anesthesiology, 1985, **63**: p. A377.

136. Lappas, D.G., et al., *Filling pressures of the heart and pulmonary circulation of the patient with coronary artery disease after large doses of morphine.* Anesthesiology, 1975, **42**: p. 153.

137. Lappas, D.G., I. Placios, and C. Athanasiadis, *Sufentanil dosage and myocardial blood flow and metabolism in patients with coronary artery disease.* Anesthesiology, 1985, **63**: p. A58.

138. Becker, C.E., et al., *A quick guide to common drug interaction*, in *Patient Care*, J. Bigelow, Editor, 1974, Miller & Fink: Philadelphia. pp. 1–32.

139. Sifton, D.W., *Drug Interaction and Side Effects Index*™. 42 ed. *Physicians Desk Reference (PDR)*, ed. M. Trelewicz. 1988, Medical Economics Company Inc.: Oradell, N.Y. 1–787.

140. Coté, D., R. Martin, and J.P. Tétrault, *Haemodynamic interactions of muscle relaxants and sufentanil in coronary artery surgery.* Can J Anaesth, 1991, **38**(3): pp. 324–329.

141. Maurer, P.M. and R.R. Bartkowski, *Drug interactions of clinical significance with opioid analgesics.* Druf Safety, 1993, **8**: pp. 30–48.

142. Bovill, J.G., et al., *Electroencephalographic effects of sufentanil anaesthesia in man.* Br J Anaesth, 1982, **54**: pp. 45–52.

143. Helmers, J.H., L. Van Leuwen, and W. Zuurmond, *Sufentanil-Dosierungsstudie bei allgemeinen chrirurgischen Eingriffen.* Anaesthesist, 1989, **38**: pp. 397–400.

144. Gerwig, W.H., C.W. Thompson, and P. Blades, *Pain control following upper abdominal operations.* Arch Surg, 1951, **62**: pp. 678–682.

145. Morris, T. and J. Tracey, *Lignocaine: its effect on wound healing.* Br J Surg, 1977, **64**: pp. 902–903.

146. Dundee, J.W., *Problems associated with strong analgesics,* in *Pain. New Perspectives in Measurement and Management,* A.W. Harcus, R. Smith, and B. Whittle, Editors, 1977, Churchill Livingstone: Edinburgh, London, New York. pp. 57–62.

147. Ferrari, H.A., R.L. Fuson, and S.J. Dent, *The relationship of the anaesthetic agent to postoperative analgesic requirements.* South Med J, 1969, **62**: pp. 1201–1203.

148. Clark, N.J., et al., *Comparison of sufentanil-N2O and fentanyl-N2O in patients without cardiac disease undergoing general surgery.* Anesthesiology, 1987, **66**: pp. 130–135.

149. Suwatakul, K., et al., *Analysis of narcotic analgesic usage in the treatment of postoperative pain.* JAMA, 1983, **250**: pp. 926–929.

150. Koo, P.J., *Postoperative pain management with a patient-controlled transdermal delivery system for fentanyl.* Am J Health Syst Pharm, 2005, **62**: pp. 1171–1176.

151. Striebel, H., J. Hackenberger, and A. Wesel, *Beurteilung der postoperativen Schmerzintensität. Selbst- versus Fremdbeurteilung.* Schmerz, 1992, **6**: pp. 199–203.

152. Ripamonti, C., *Pain experienced by patients hospitalized at the National Cancer Institute of Milan: Research project "towards a pain-free hospital".* Tumori, 2000, **86**: pp. 412–418.

153. Strohbücker, B., H. Mayer, and G. Evers, *Schmerzprävalenz an den Unikliniken Köln: Vorkommen und Intensität von Schmerzen bei stationären Patienten. Unveröffentlichte Masterarbeit,* 2001, Institut für Pflegewissenschaft, Medizinische Fakultät, Universität Witten/Herdecke.

154. Marks, R.M. and E.J. Sachar, *Undertreatment of medical inpatients with narcotic analgesics.* Ann Int Med, 1973, **78**: pp. 173–181.

155. Angell, M., *The quality of mercy.* New Engl J Med, 1982, **306**: pp. 98–99.

156. Porter, J. and H. Hick, *Addiction rare in patients treated with narcotics.* New Engl J Med, 1980, **302**: pp. 123–126.

157. Taub, A., *Opioid analgesics in the treatment of chronic intractable pain of non-neoplastic origin,* in *Narcotic Analgesics in Anesthesiology,* L.M. Kitahata and J.G. Collins, Editors, 1982, Williams and Wilkins: Baltimore. pp. 199–208.

158. Portenoy, R.K. and K.M. Foley, *Chronic use of opioid analgesics in non-malignant pain: Report of 38 cases.* Pain, 1986, **25**: pp. 171–186.

159. Eide, W.K., *Wind-up and the NMDA receptor complex from a clinical perspective.* Eur J Pain, 2000, **4**: pp. 5–17.

160. Barsoum, M.W., *Comparison of the efficacy and tolarability of tramadol, pethidine and nalbuphine in children with postoperative pain.* Clin Drug Invest, 1995, **9**: pp. 183–190.

161. Quiding, H., et al., *Infants and young children metabolise codeine to morphine. A study after single and repeated rectal administration.* Br J Clin Pharmacol, 1992, **33**: pp. 45–49.

162. Moore, R.A. and H.J. McQuay, *Single-patient data meta-analysis of 3453 postoperative patients: oral tramadol versus placebo, codeine and combination analgesics.* Pain, 1997, **69**: pp. 287–294.

163. Lewis, J.W., *Buprenorphine*. Drug Alcohol Depend, 1985, **14**: pp. 363–372.
164. Heel, R.C., et al., *Buprenorphine: a review of its pharmacological properties and therapeutic efficacy*. Drugs, 1979, **17**: pp. 81–100.
165. Lewis, J.W. *Structure-activity relationships of opioids – a current perspective*. in *VIII. International Symposium on Medicinal Chemistry*. 1985, Stockholm: Swedish Pharmaceutical Press.
166. Krizanits-Weine, F., et al., *Präemptive Analgesie mit retardiertem Dihydrocodein bei Patienten mit elektiven Kniearthroskopien*. Schmerz, 1996, **10**: p. S54.
167. Steffen, P., et al., *Nichtinvasive perioperative Analgesie nach Allgemeinanästhesien. Kombination von Dihydrocodein ret. mit den Nichtopioidanalgetika Diclofenac und Metamizol*. Schmerz, 1996, **10**: p. S51.
168. Lotsch, J., et al., *Fatal respiratory depression after multiple intravenous morphine injections*. Clin Pharmacokinet, 2006, **45**: pp. 1051–1060.
169. Wen-Ying, C., et al., *Human opioid receptor A118G polymorphism affects intravenous patient-controlled analgesia morphine consumption after total abdominal hysterectomy*. Anesthesiology, 2006, **105**: pp. 334–337.
170. Good, P., et al., *Prospective audit of short-term concurrent ketamine, opioid and anti-inflammatory ('triple-agent') therapy for episodes of acute and chronic pain*. Intern Med J, 2005, **35**: pp. 39–44.
171. Saarne, A., *Clinical evaluation of a new analgesic piritramide*. Acta Anaesthesiol Scand, 1969, **13**: pp. 11–19.
172. Schmidt, W.K., et al., *Nalbuphine*. Drug Alcohol Depend, 1985, **14**: pp. 339–362.
173. Wood, P.L., *Kappa agonists analgesics: evidence for µ2 and delta opioid receptor antagonism*. Drug Dev Res, 1984, **4**: pp. 429–435.
174. Wermeling, D.P., et al., *Patient-controlled analgesia using butorphanol for postoperative pain control: an open label study*, in *Butorphanol Tartrate: Research Advances in Multiple Clinical Settings*, C.E. Rosow, Editor, 1986, S. Karger: Basel, Paris, London, New York, Singapore, Sydney. pp. 31–39.
175. Freye, E., L. Azevedo, and E. Hartung, *Reversal of fentanyl-related respiratory depression with nalbuphine; effects on the CO2-response curve of man*. Acta Anaesth Belg, 1985, **36**: pp. 365–374.
176. Magruder, M.R., R.D. DeLaney, and C.A. DiFazio, *Reversal of narcotic-induced respiratory depression with nalbuphine hydrochloride*. Anesthesiol Rev, 1982, **9**: pp. 34–37.
177. McCammon, R.L., R.K. Stoelting, and J.A. Madura, *Effects of butorphanol, nalbuphine, and fentanyl on intrabiliary tract dynamics*. Anesth Analg, 1984, **63**: pp. 139–142.
178. Romagnoli, A. and A.S. Keats, *Ceiling effect for respiratory depression by nalbuphine*. Clin Pharmacol Ther, 1980, **27**: pp. 478–485.
179. Herz, A., *Opiat-Partialantagonisten*, in *Pentazocin im Spiegel der Erfahrungen*, S. Kubicki and G.A. Neuhaus, Editors, 1981, Springer: Berlin-Heidelberg-New York. pp. 19–21.
180. Gal, T.J., C.A. Di Fazo, and J. Moscicki, *Analgesic and respiratory depressant activity of nalbuphine: a comparison with morphine*. Anesthesiology, 1982, **57**: pp. 367–374.
181. Abboud, T.K., et al., *Transnasal butorphanol: a new method for pain relief in post-cesarean section pain*. Acta Anaesthesiol Scand, 1991, **35**: pp. 14–18.
182. Wetchler, B.V., C.D. Alexander, and M.A. Uhll, *Transnasal butorphanol tartrate for pain control following ambulatory surgery*. Curr Ther Res, 1992, **52** (4): pp. 571–580.

183. Joyce III, T.H., et al., *Efficacy of transnasal butorphanol tartrate in postepisiotomy pain: a model to assess analgesia.* Clin Therap, 1993, **15** (1): pp. 160–167.

184. Shyu, W.C., et al., *Multiple-dose phase I study of transnasal butorphanol.* Clin Pharmacol Ther, 1993, **54**: pp. 34–41.

185. Couch, J., et al. *Evaluation of the efficacy and safety of Stadol® NS™ (transnasal butorphanol) in the treatment of acute migraine in outpatients.* in *7th World Congress on Pain.* 1993, Paris: ISAP Publications.

186. Diamond, S., et al., *Transnasal butorphanol in the treatment of migraine headache pain.* Headache Quat Curr Treat Res, 1992, **3** (2): pp. 164–171.

187. Morrison, C.E., et al., *Pethidine compared with meptazinol during labour; a prospective randomised double-blind study in 1100 patients.* Anaesthesia, 1987, **42**: pp. 7–14.

188. Jordan, C., *A comparison of the respiratory effects of meptazinol, pentazocine and morphine.* Br J Anaesth, 1979, **51**: pp. 497–501.

189. Keeri-Szanto, M., *Drugs or drums: what relieves postoperative pain?* Pain, 1979, **6**: pp. 217–230.

190. Eagen, K.J. and L. Ready, *Patient satisfaction with intravenous PCA or epidural morphine.* Can J Anaesth, 1994, **41**: pp. 6–11.

191. White, P.F., *Mishaps with patient-controlled analgesia.* Anesthesiology, 1987, **66**: pp. 81–83.

192. Thomas, D.W. and H. Owen, *Patient-controlled analgesia – the need for caution.* Anaesthesia, 1988, **43**: pp. 770–772.

193. Parker, R.K., B. Holtmann, and P.F. White, *Patient-controlled analgesia: does a concurrent opioid infusion improve pain mangement after surgery?* JAMA, 1991, **266** (14): pp. 1947–1952.

194. Lehmann, K.A., *Neue Möglichkeiten zur Behandlung akuter Schmerzen.* Drug Res Arzneimittelforsch, 1984, **34**: pp. 1108–1114.

195. Ginsberg, B., et al., *The influence of lockout intervals and drug selection on patient-controlled analgesia following gynecological surgery.* Pain, 1995, **62**: pp. 95–100.

196. Butscher, K., J.Y. Mazoit, and K. Samii, *Can immediate opioid requirements in the post-anaesthesia care unit be used to determine analgesic requirements on the ward?* Can J Anaesth, 1995, **42**: pp. 461–466.

197. Krimmer, H., et al., *Die kombinierte infusionsanalgesie – Ein alternatives Konzept zur postoperativen Schmerztherapie.* Chirurg, 1986, **57**: pp. 327–329.

198. Viscusi, E.R., et al., *Non-invasive, patient-controlled, fentanyl HCl analgesia: comparison of safety and efficacy to intravenous morphine pump for the treatment of postoperative pain after major surgery: a randomized, multi-center trial.* Anesth Analg, 2002, **94**: p. S. 224.

199. Friedman, J.D. and F.A. Dello Buono, *Opioid antagonists in the treatment of opioid-induced constipation and pruritus.* Am Pharmacother, 2003, **35**: pp. 85–91.

200. Kurz, A. and D.I. Sessler, *Opioid-induced bowel dysfunction; pathophysiology and potential new therapies.* Drugs, 2003, **63**: pp. 649–671.

201. Liu, S.S., et al., *ADL 8-2698, a trans-3, 4-dimethyl-4-(3-hydroxyphenyl) piperidine, prevents gastrointestinal effects of intravenous morphine without affecting analgesia.* Clin Pharmacol Ther, 2001, **69**: pp. 66–71.

202. Holte, K. and H. Kehlet, *Prevention of postoperativ ileus.* Minerva Anesthesiol, 2002, **68**: pp. 152–156.

203. Taguchi, A., et al., *Selective postoperative inhiibition of gastrointestinal opioid receptors*. N Engl J Med, 2001, **345**: pp. 935–940.

204. Schmidt, W.K., *Alvimopan* (ADL 8-2698) is a novel peripheral opioid antagonist*. Am J Surg, 2001, **182**: pp. 27S–38S.

205. Yuan, C.S. and J.F. Foss, *Methylnaltrexone: investigation of clinical applications*. Drug Dev Res, 2000, **50**: pp. 133–141.

206. Yuan, C.S., et al., *The safety and efficacy of oral methylnaltrexone in preventing morphine-induced delay in oral cecal transit time*. Clin Pharmacol Ther, 1997, **61**: pp. 1–9.

207. Yuan, C.S. and J.F. Foss, *Oral methylnaltrexone for opioid-induced constipation*. JAMA, 2000, **284**: pp. 1383–1384.

208. Yuan, C.S., et al., *Methylnaltrexone prevents morphine-induced delay on oral-cecal transit time without affecting analgesia: a double-blind randomized placebo-controlled trial*. Clin Pharmacol Ther, 1996, **59**: pp. 469–475.

209. Stevens, C.W., et al., *Biochemical characterization and regional quantification of mu, delta, and kappa opioid binding sites in rat spinal cord*. Brain Res, 1991, **550**: pp. 77–85.

210. Rawal, N., *Klinischer Einsatz der rückenmarknahen Opioidanalgesie, Teil 1*. Der Schmerz, 1996, **10**: pp. 176–189.

211. Börner, U., et al., *Epidurale Opiatanalgesie – Gewebe und Liquorverträglichkeit der Opiate*. Anaesthesist, 1980, **29**: pp. 570–571.

212. Bürkle, H., S. Dunbar, and H. van Aken, *Remifentanil: a novel, short-acting, μ-opioid*. Anesth Analg, 1996, **83**: pp. 646–651.

213. Rawal, N. and B. Tandon, *Epidural and intrathecal morphine in intensive care units*. Intensive Care Med, 1985, **11**: pp. 129–135.

214. De Castro, J. and L. Lecron, *Peridurale Opiatanalgesie: Verschiedene Opiate – Komplikationen und Nebenwirkungen*, in *Peridurale Opiatanalgesie*, M. Zenz, Editor, 1981, G. Fischer: Stuttgart, New York. pp. 103–107.

215. Moore, R.A., et al., *Dural permeability to narcotics: in vitro determination and application to extradural administration*. Br J Anaesth, 1982, **54**: pp. 1117–1127.

216. Leicht, C.H., et al., *Evaluation and comparison of epidural sufentanil citrate and morphine sulfate for analgesia after cesarean section*. Anesthesiology, 1986, **65**: pp. A 365.

217. Camporesi, E.M., C.H. Nielsen, and P.R. Bromage, *Ventilatory CO_2 sensitivity after intravenous and epidural morphine in volunteers*. Anesth Analg, 1983, **62**: p. 633.

218. Bromage, P.R., et al., *Rostral spread of epidural morphine*. Anesthesiology, 1982, **56**: pp. 431–436.

219. Johnson, A., et al., *Influence of intrathecal morphine and naloxone intervention on postoperative ventilatory regulation in elderly patients*. Acta Anaethesiol Scand, 1992, **36** (5): pp. 436–444.

220. McCaughey, W. and I.L. Graham, *The respiratory depression of epidural morphine: time course and effect of posture*. Anaesthesia, 1982, **37**: pp. 990–994.

221. Jaffe, J.H. and W.R. Martin, *Opioid analgesics and antagonists*, in *The pharmacological Basis of Therapeutics*, A.G. Gilman, et al., Editors, 1993, McGraw Hill: New York. pp. 485–531.

222. Glynn, C.I., L.E. Mather, and M.E. Cousins, *Spinal narcotics and respiratory depression*. Lancet, 1979, **2**: p. 356.

223. Cohen, S.E., S. Tan, and P.F. White, *Sufentanil analgesia following cesarean section: epidural versus intravenous administration.* Anesthesiology, 1988, **68**: pp. 129–134.

224. Davies, G.K., C.L. Tolhurst-Cleaver, and T.L. James, *Respiratory depression after intrathecal opiates.* Anaesthesia, 1980, **35**: p. 1080.

225. Gourlay, G.K., et al., *Pharmacokinetics of fentanyl in lumbar and cervical CSF following lumbar epidural and intravenous administration.* Pain, 1989, **38**: pp. 253–259.

226. Chalmer, P.C., C.M. Lang, and B.B. Greenhouse, *The use of nalbuphine in association with epidural narcotics.* Anesthesiol Rev, 1988, **15**(2): pp. 21–27.

227. Cheng, E.Y. and J. May, *Nalbuphine reversal of repiratory depression after epidural sufentanil.* Crit Care Med, 1989, **17**: pp. 378–379.

228. Bromage, P.R., Camporesi, E.M., and P.A.C. Durant, *Nonrespiratory side effects of epidural morphine.* Anesth Analg, 1982, **61**: p. 490.

229. Rawal, N., K. Möllefors, and K. Axelsson, *Naloxone reversal of urinary retention after epidural morphine.* Lancet, 1981, **2**: p. 1411.

230. Cousins, M.J. and L.E. Mather, *Intrathecal and epidural administration of opioids.* Anesthesiology, 1984, **61**: pp. 276–310.

231. Rawal, N. and M. Wattwil, *Respiratory depression after epidural morphine – an experimental and clinical study.* Anesth Analg, 1982, **63**: p. 8.

232. Eisenach, J.C., *Epidural and spinal narcotics*, in *ASA Refresher Courses in Anesthesiology*, P.G. Barash, Editor, 1992, Lippincott: Philadelphia. pp. 1–4.

233. Bailey, D.R. and B.E. Smith, *Continuous epidural infuson of fentanyl for postoperative analgesia.* Anesthesiology, 1980, **42**: p. 538.

234. Gjessing, J. and P.J. Tomlin, *Postoperative pain control with intrathecal morphine.* Anaesthesia, 1981, **36**: p. 268.

235. Kitahata, L.M. and J.G. Collins, *Spinal action of narcotic analgesics.* Anesthesiology, 1981, **54**: p. 153.

236. Rutter, D.V., D.G. Skewes, and M. Morgan, *Extradural opioids for postoperative analgesia: a double blind comparison of pethidine, fentanyl and morphine.* Br J Anaesth, 1981, **53**: p. 915.

237. Weightman, W.M., *Respiratory arrest during epidural infusion of bupivacaine and fentanyl.* Anaesth Int Care, 1991, **19**: pp. 282–284.

238. Waldvogel, H.H., and M. Fasano, *Extradural administration of lofentanyl for balanced postoperative pain.* Anaesthesist, 1983, **32**: pp. 256–257.

239. Herz, A. and H.J. Teschemacher, *Activities and site of antinociceptive action of morphine-like analgesics.* Adv Drug Res, 1971, **6**: pp. 79–119.

240. Howell, S.B., *Clinical application of a novel sustained-release injectable drug delivery system DepoFoam technology.* Cancer J, 2001, **7**: pp. 219–227.

241. Viscusi, E.R., et al., *EREM Study Group: fourty-eight hours of postoperativ pain relief following total hip arthroplasty with a novel, extend-release epidural morphine formulation.* Anesthesiology, 2005, **102**: pp. 1014–1022.

242. Carvallo, B., E. Riley, and G. Manvelian, *Phase II study of long-acting encapsulated epidural morphine for postoperative pain after cesarean section.* Reg Anesth Pain Med, 2004, **29**: p. A37.

243. Gambling, D.R., et al., *A compararive study of patient controllled epidural analgsia (PCEA) and continuous infusion epeidural analgesia (CIEA) during labour.* Can J Anaesth, 1988, **35**: pp. 249–254.

244. Velickovic, I. and G. Leicht, *Patient-controlled epidural analgesia for labor and delivery in parturient with chronic inflammatory demyelating polyneuropathy*. Reg Anesth and Pain Med, 2001, **27**: pp. 217–219.

245. Zenz, M., S. Piepenbrock, and M. Tryba, *Epidural opiates: long-term experiences in cancer pain*. Klin Wochenschr, 1985, **63**: pp. 225–229.

246. Durant, P.A.C. and T.L. Yaksh, *Epidural injections of bupivacaine, morphine, fentanyl, lofentanil, and DADL in chronically implanted rats: a pharmacologic and pathologic study*. Anesthesiology, 1986, **64**: pp. 43–53.

247. Camann, W.R., et al., *A comparison of intrathecal, epidural, and intravenous sufentanil for labor analgesia*. Anesthesiology, 1992, **77**: pp. 884–892.

248. McQuay, H.J., et al., *Intrathecal opioids, potency, and lipophilicity*. Pain, 1989, **36**: pp. 111–115.

249. Hansdottir, V., et al., *The CSF and plasma pharmacokinetics of sufentanil after intrathecal administration*. Anesthesiology, 1991, **74**: pp. 264–269.

250. D'Angelo, R., et al., *Intrathecal sufentanil compared to epidural bupivacaine for labor analgesia*. Anesthesiology, 1994, **80**: pp. 1209–1215.

251. Jones, R.D.M. and J.G. Jones, *Intrathecal morphine: naloxone reverses respiratory depression but not analgesia*. Br Med J, 1980, **281**: pp. 645–646.

252. Meignier, M., et al., *Continuous intrathecal opioids and bupivcaine for the management of intractable cancer pain in children*. Anesth Analg, 1993, **76**: p. S259.

253. Brown, D.V. and R.J. McCarthy, *Epidural and spinal opioids*. Curr Opinion Anaesth, 1995, **8**: pp. 337–341.

254. Mok, M.S., et al. *Analgesic effect of intrathecal stadol, nubain, meperidine, morphine and fentanyl, a comparative study*. in *VIII. World Congress of Anaesthesiologists*. 1984, Manila/Philippines.

255. Kalia, P.K., et al., *Epidural pentazocine for postoperative pain relief*. Anesth Analg, 1983, **62**: p. 949.

256. Malinovsky, J.M., et al., *Ketamine and midazolam neurotoxicity in the rabbit*. Anesthesiology, 1991, **75**: pp. 91–97.

257. Wilcox, G.L., et al., *Mutual potentiation of antinociceptive effects of morphine and clonidine on motor and sensory responses in rat spinal cord*. Brain Res, 1987, **405**: pp. 84–93.

258. Ossipov, M.H., L.J. Suarez, and T.C. Spaulding, *Antinociceptive interactions between alpha2-adrenergic and opiate agonists at the spinal level of rodents*. Anesth Analg, 1989, **68**: pp. 194–200.

Part IV

Use of Potent Opioids for Chronic Pain Management

Contents

Long-Term Management of Chronic Pain

If during the therapy of chronic pain, sufficient attenuation of nociception can not be achieved with a peripheral analgesic (i.e., acetaminophen, NSAIDs), an opioid has to be added in order to reach the therapeutic goal (Figure IV-1). However, it is also possible to start with opioid therapy in those patients who complain of intense tumor-related pain or in patients with other severe painful symptoms. In such cases, one immediately can start with an opioid Step 3 of the analgesic ladder (Table IV-2). Such strategy has to be carefully weighed in particular if pain is due to the extension or the progression of the underlying disease, where peripheral analgesics and/or weak opioids are insufficient in action.

The extent to which pain responds to opioid analgesics varies depending on both patient and pain characteristics. No pain is predictably unresponsive to opioids. Neuropathic pain can respond to opioids, although the response may be incomplete. All patients with moderate to severe cancer pain should have a trial of opioid analgesia, using the following paradigm (Figure IV-2):

1. A patient's treatment should start at the step of the WHO analgesic ladder appropriate for the severity of the pain.
2. Prescribing of primary analgesia should always be adjusted as the pain severity alters.
3. If the pain severity increases and is not controlled on a given step, move upwards to the next step of the analgesic ladder. Do not prescribe another analgesic of the same potency.
4. All patients with moderate to severe cancer pain, regardless of etiology, should receive a trial of opioid analgesia. Chronic pain in patients with cancer is usually

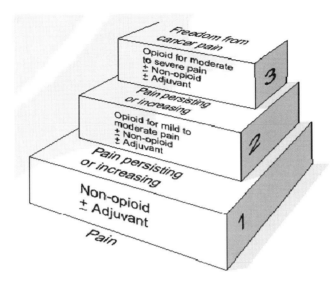

Figure IV-1. The three-step analgesic ladder, being part of the WHO guidelines for the management of pain

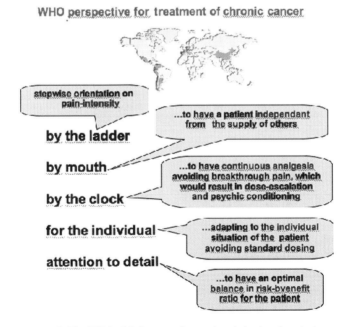

Figure IV-2. The WHO global perspectives and goals in chronic pain therapy

continuous and therapeutic plasma levels of analgesics must be maintained. This only can be achieved when the drug is given regularly at correct intervals according to the pharmacokinetic and pharmacodynamic profile of the drug:

5. Analgesia for continuous pain should be prescribed on a regular basis, not as required (pro re nata).
6. It should be explained to the patient with chronic cancer pain that pain control medication must be taken regularly to gain optimal results.

In such patients, treatment should start immediately in order to achieve rapidly sufficient analgesia and potent opioids should be administered from the start.

As it is the case with all modalities in opioid therapy, rigid dosing has to be rejected in chronic pain therapy. Dosages have to be increased to a point of sufficient pain relief. Such dogma especially is necessary in the therapy of chronic pain because a continuous analgesic effect is only possible by continuous occupation of the opioid receptor, a principle. This can be achieved only by constant plasma level using a controlled release formulation.

In summary, when initiating opioid therapy the following factors have to be considered:

• Severity of pain
• Setting in which the regimen will be started
• Whether patient is opioid-naïve
• Prior medication exposure and experience

Then start titration of the opioid keeping in mind:

1. Start at lowest acceptable dose
2. Adjust dose for pain relief with acceptable side effects
3. Use a titration rate depending on opioid half-life

Table IV-1. Classification of opioid analgesics into agonists, partial agonists, agonist/antagonists and antagonists

Agonists	Partial agonists
Morphine	Buprenorphine
Codeine	Meptazinol
Oxycodone	
Dipipanone	Agonist/antagonists
Dihydrocodeine	Butorphanol
Oxymorphone	Nalbuphine
Pethidine	Dezocine
Levorphanol	Pentazocine
Hydromorphone	
Methadone	Antagonists
Fentanyl	Naloxone
Dextropropoxyphene	Naltrexone
Diamorphine (heroin)	Nalmefene
Tramadol	
Phenazocine	
Dextromoramide	

4. There is no analgesic ceiling to single-entity opioid agonists
5. Use a maximum dose of the opioid in *combination* with a nonopioid *within dose limits* (e.g., acetaminophen 4 g/d).

When administering opioids for the alleviation of pain the following principles have to be considered.

The group of agonists (e.g., codeine, morphine, meperidine, fentanyl) has to be strictly separated from the group of the partial agonists (buprenorphine, meptazinol) and from the mixed agonist/antagonists (nalbuphine, pentazocine, butorphanol, dezocine; Table IV-1).

Defining the Different Type of Opioids

AGONISTS

An agonist is a drug that has affinity for and binds to cell receptors to induce changes in the cell that stimulate physiological activity. The agonist opioid drugs have no clinically relevant ceiling effect for analgesia. As the dose is raised, analgesic effects increase in a linear fashion, until either analgesia is achieved or dose-limiting adverse effects occur. Efficacy is defined by the maximal response induced by administration of the active agent. In practice, this is determined by the degree of analgesia produced following dose escalation through a range limited by the development of adverse effects. Potency, in contrast, reflects the dose–response relationship, and is influenced by pharmacokinetic factors (i.e. how much of the drug enters the body's systemic circulation and then reaches the receptors and by affinity to the drug receptors).

ANTAGONISTS

Antagonist drugs have no intrinsic pharmacological action but can interfere with the action of an agonist. Competitive antagonists bind to the same receptor and compete for receptor sites, whereas non-competitive antagonists block the effects of the agonist in some other way.

MIXED AGONIST–ANTAGONISTS

The mixed agonist–antagonist drugs produce agonist effects at one receptor and antagonist effects at another. Pentazocine is the prototype agonist–antagonist: it has agonist effects at the κ-receptors and weak antagonist actions at the μ-receptors. Thus, in addition to analgesia, pentazocine may produce κ-receptor mediated psychotomimetic effects not seen with full or partial agonists. When a mixed agonist–antagonist is administered together with an agonist, the antagonist effect at the receptor can generate an acute withdrawal syndrome. Therefore, when prescribing opioids, pure agonists and agonist/antagonists should never be given in an alternating or a sequential fashion. Such an approach has to be avoided in the therapy of post operative and especially in chronic pain management. This paradigm is underlined by the fact that the analgesic effect of both groups is mediated by means of interaction with different opioid receptors. Thus, attenuation of pain by the mixed agonist/antagonists, may even reduce the analgesic effect of the pure agonist ligands [1]. Exception to this rule are the partial μ-receptor agonists, buprenorphine and meptazinol. Because of their different mode of action, especially buprenorphine with its high receptor affinity, a small number of opioid receptors only needs to be occupied, resulting in sufficient pain relief. Because of the necessary lower dosages for therapeutic efficacy, there is the possibility of a switch or even the co-administration of another pure opioid agonist such as morphine, oxycodone (OxyContin®), or hydromorphone (Palladone®). Such effect is due to a sufficient receptor reserve as the partial agonist will not occupy all available binding sites.

The WHO Guidelines for Pain Therapy

In the past, WHO guidelines have been developed for the treatment of pain and the therapeutic armamentarium [2], recommended for use in a stepwise fashion (three-step analgesic ladder), includes three types of analgesics, which are the cornerstone in pain therapy:

1. Nonopioid analgesics include agents such as acetaminophen, aspirin, or other NSAIDs (nonsteroidal anti-inflammatory drugs). Use of nonopioid analgesics, however, is limited by a ceiling of analgesic effect beyond which increase of dosage produce no further relief but may increase side effects. If a non-opioid is ineffective or poorly tolerated than Step 2 comes into effect.
2. Weak opioid analgesics are used in mild-to-moderate pain. Weak opioids are codeine, hydrocodone, pentazocine, butorphanol, dezocine and nalbuphine. Some of these agents are used in a fixed combination with a non-opioid analgesic. If pain persists or increases the third step in the analgesic ladder is employed.
3. Potent opioids will have to be included in the therapeutic strategy in severe painful conditions. Among the known classical opioid morphine, other potent opioids such as oxycodone, hydromorphone, oxymorphone, methadone, levorphanol, methadone, fentanyl or buprenorphine can be used.

Although pain first should be treated with a non-opioid, certain cases with severe pain, especially in cancer pain management, a medium or even a strong opioid analgesic should be used as the first-line drug. This is because no time should be lost in order to find the appropriate analgesic as intense pain should be treated immediately with a potent opioid.

In summary, the following principles in pain pharmacotherapy and especially when using opioids should be observed:

• There are three main analgesic classes (non-opioids, opioids, co-analgesics).
• Select the agents based on advantages/disadvantages for different pain types.
• Consider non-pharmacologic therapy.

In addition, when using opioid therapy, the following essentials must be considered:
- Evaluate the patient
- Construct a treatment plan
- Use informed consent and agreement for treatment
- Consider periodic review
- Instruct the patient on repetitive consultation
- Use medical records
- Comply with controlled substances laws and regulations.

Oral analgesic drugs are usually the first line agents for treating severe cancer pain. The choice of analgesic should be based on the severity of the pain rather than the stage of the patient's disease. Analgesics should be taken regularly and the dose gradually increased, as necessary (Table IV-2). The World Health Organization [3] issued guidelines that involve the treatment of cancer pain. The guidelines are presented in a ladder formation and are referred to as the "analgesic ladder". The steps of the WHO ladder are described as follows:

Step 1: The first step involves treatment of mild to moderate pain with acetaminophen, aspirin, or another non-steroidal anti-inflammatory drug (NSAID). Medications should be administered as needed, or around-the-clock and dosing should be titrated upwards when necessary. Adjuvant analgesics, or medications that are not generally used for pain, but can have an enhancing effect on other analgesics, also may be used.

Step 2: The second step involves adding an opioid for pain that persists beyond treatment in Step 1. An opioid, often codeine or oxycodone, is added to the regimen at this step (the NSAID or acetaminophen should be retained). If the pain is persisting or worsening despite Step 1, then a mild opioid such as codeine should be added (not substituted). Examples are combination preparations including Co-proxamol®, a combination of two active ingredients, paracetamol and dextropropoxyphene, Co-codamol®, which contains two active ingredients, paracetamol and codeine phosphate and/or Vicodin® a combination of acetaminophen plus hydrocodone.

Step 3: When higher doses of opioid are necessary, the third step is started. At this step an opioid for moderate to severe pain is used, e.g. morphine. The dose of the stronger opioid can then be titrated upwards, according to the patient's pain as there is no ceiling dose for morphine. The third step involves treatment with an opioid on a continuous, round-the-clock basis for persistent pain. Morphine is generally the agent of choice, however, depending on the underlying disease (i.e. renal insuffinecy) another opioid with lesser pharmacological active metabolites (e.g. hydromorphone) should be given. Short-acting opioids are often prescribed as needed for pain as a supplement to a "background dose" of long-acting opioids. This type of dosing is called "rescue" or "breakthrough" and is given for exacerbations of pain that occur beyond the constant, background pain. Whenever possible, the same type of opioid should be given for background and breakthrough treatment.

Table IV-2. Type of analgesics in Step 3 in the analgesic ladder for treatment of tumor-related chronic pain, as defined by the World Health Organization (WHO)

Step 1: Acetaminophen, acetylsalicylic acid or metamizole recognizing dose limits and contraindications

- in case of insufficient pain relief additional administration of an antidepressive and/or an antiepileptic and/or transfer to
- controlled release diclofenac 100–200 mg or
- ibuprofen 300–400 mg or
- piroxicam 20–40 mg or
- naproxen 500 mg.

Step 2: In case of insufficient pain relief

- continuation of the antidepressive/antiepileptic plus
- codeine 30–50 mg or
- tramadol (Ultram®) 50–100 mg every 4–6 h or
- propoxyphene 65 mg (Darvon®) every 4–6 h.

Step 3: If previous therapy is insufficient

- continuation of the peripheral analgesics and the antidepressive/antiepileptic
- replace codeine/tramadol by morphine. Dose titration with an immediate release morphine preparation (MSIR solution 20 mg/ml, 10 mg/5 ml, 20 mg/5 ml, capsules 15/30 mg, tablets 15/30 mg) or suppositories (Roxamorph RMS® 5/10/20/30 mg) q 4 h until effective analgesic dose is reached, or
- buprenorphine sublingual tablets (Buprenex® 03–0.6 mg) every 6–8 h thereafter conversion to oral controlled/sustained release
- morphine sustaimed rekease (MS Contin®) 15/30/60/100/200 mg, or Oramorph SR® (30/60/100 mg) every 8–12 h or
- fentanyl TTS (Duragesic®) patch every 3 days or
- controlled morphine release MST Continus® caps (30/60/100/200 mg) every 12 h or
- sustained morphine release (Kadian®) 20/30/50/60/100 mg every 18–24 h or
- buprenorphine TDS (TranstecPro®) patch every 3 days or
- methadone 5–10 mg every 6–8 h or
- extended release morphine sulfate (Avinza®) 30/60/90/120 mg once daily or
- controlled release oxycodone (OxyContin®) 10/20/40/80/160 mg every 12 h or
- controlled release hydromorphone (Palladone®) 4/8/16/24 mg every 12 h.

DOSING OF OPIOIDS IN TUMOR PAIN

In the treatment of acute pain after trauma or for the elimination of pain after surgery, central analgesics usually are given parenterally. This is in contrast to chronic pain, e.g. in tumor related pain, where the oral administration is advocated. This method relieves the physician from the necessity to inject the analgesic, it results in autonomous and self-regulation of the patient, it is cheaper and guarantees a stable blood plasma concentration, with the consequence of constant receptor occupancy [4]. New galenic preparations with a controlled release or extended release formulation are available, which result in a constant release of the pharmacologically active agent and a long lasting concentration of the active compound in the blood plasma, e.g. controlled release morphine sulfate (MS Contin® tablets 105/30/60/100/200 mg, Oramorph® 30/60/100 mg, Kadian® 20/30/50/60/100 mg, Ainza® 30/60/90/120 mg) extended release oxycodone hydrochloride (OxyContin® SR 10/20/40 mg) or extended release hydromorphone hydrochloride (Palladone® SR 4/8/16/24 mg). In addition, there is a long lasting sublingual preparation of buprenorphine (Buprenex® 4/8 mg) all of which possess the advantage that the analgesic has to be given only twice or even once a day.

While the mean dose of buprenorphine is one sublingual tablet every 8 h, MS Contin 30 it should be take one tablet every 8–12 h. However, when using Morphine long acting 30 mg, the dose is one tablet every 12 h, and when taking MS Contin, 60 mg every 24 h.

An even longer duration of action is possible through the use of a transdermal opioid patch where the active compound is administered transdermally over a period of 72 h, e.g. the fentanyl transdermal therapeutic system (fentanyl TTS; Duragesic®) or the buprenorphine transdermal therapeutic system(buprenorphine-TDS; TranstecPro®).

The following recommendations are given when titrating the individual dose of an opioid to effect:

- Use only oral, controlled/sustained-release formulations of the agent. This results in long-lasting and stable plasma concentrations, a long-lasting occupation of the opioid receptors, which is followed by a long-lasting blockade of nociceptive afferents (Table IV-3).
- Titrate to the desired analgesic effect by increasing the dose 25%–50% and not by a reduction in the dosing interval (Fig. IV-3).
- The correct dose is reached, once the patient has sufficient pain relief.
- The dose of the opioid therefore has to be increased until pain subsides, or significant side-effects like sedation or a decline in respiratory rate below 12/min should prevent the physician from further dose increase. In the latter the dose and the type of the opioid have to be re-evaluated.
- Give the opioid only orally (*administration by the mouth*).
- Choose the opioid according to its pharmacokinetic half-life using a prescription with fixed time intervals (i.e. every 6 h, 12 h, or 24 h – *around the clock medication*).
- Evaluate efficacy by using a non-verbal rating scale for pain intensity, for instance the VAS (visual analog scale where 0 denotes no pain and 10 reflects unbearable, excruciating pain).
- Choose an opioid for initial treatment that is related to the intensity of pain. For instance, pain rating with a visual analgesic score of > 7.0 demands an opioid of Step 3 in the analgesic ladder (*WHO recommendation*).
- In addition, always prescribe a laxative with the opioid since all opioids induce constipation.
- Inform the patient on the possibility of breakthrough pain. Such pain episodes are best treated by the additional "rescue medication" of a fast acting compound such as morphine immediate release (MSIR tablets 15/30 mg, MSIR capsules

Table IV-3. Opioid analgesics (pure agonists and partial agonists) used for the treatment of chronic pain

Morphine like opioids	Equi-analgesic doses	Half-life (h)	Peak effect (h)	Duration of action (h)	Oral bio-availability (%)
Morphine	10 s.c.	2–3	0.5–1	3–6	20–30
	20–60 p.o.	2–3	1.5–2	4–7	
Sustained-release morphine	20–60 p.o.	2–3	3–4 Twice daily administration	8–12	20–30
Controlled-release morphine	20–60 p.o.	2–3	4–6 Once-a-day administration	24	20–30
Hydromorphone	7.5 p.o.	2–3	1–2	3–4	35–80
Oxycodone	20–30	2–3	1	3–6	60–90
Sustained-release oxycodone	20–30	2–3	3–4	8–12	60–90
Oxymorphone	10 s.c. No oral formulation available	–	0.5–1	3–6	20–30
Meperidine (pethidine) Not used for cancer pain due to toxicity in higher doses and short half-life	75 s.c.	2–3	0.5–1	3–4	30–60
Diamorphine	5 s.c. Analgesic action due to metabolites,	0.5	0.5–1	4–5	Same as morphine

Drug						
Levorphanol	4 p.o.	With long-half-life; accumulation accurs after beginning	12–16	0.5–1	4–6	Same as morphine
Methadone	20 p.o.	Risk of delayed toxicity due to accumulation; useful to start dosing on p.r.n.	12– > 150 High interindividual variability	0.5–1.5	4–8	60–90
Codeine	200 p.o.	Usually combined with non-opioid	2–3	1.5–2	3–6	60–90
		Propoxyphene HCl or napsylate, toxic metabolite may accumulate, combined with non-opioid	12	1.5–2	3–6	40
Hydrocodone		Only available in combination with acetaminophen	2–4	0.5–1	3–4	20–30
Dihydrocodone		Only available combined with aspirin or paracetamol in some countries	2–4	0.5–1	3–4	20
Fentanyl buccal	100–800 μg		—	6	15 min	65% bioavailabity
Fentanyl-transdermal	ratio oral morphine: transdermal fentanyl of 100:1		13–22	—	48–72	90
Buprenorphine-transdermal	ratio oral morphine: transder. buprenorphine 100:1		13–22	—	48–72	90

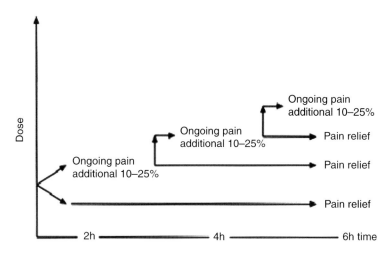

Figure IV-3. Algorithm for titration of the individual dose of an opioid necessary for the alleviation of pain

25/30 mg, MSIR solution 20 mg/ml, 10 mg/5 ml, 20 mg/5 ml) or oxycodone immediate release (OxyIR 5 mg). In addition oral transmucosal fentanyl citrate (OTFS) lozenge can be advocated (Actiq® 200, 400, 600, 800, 1200, 1600 µg), which acts via rapid absorption through buccal mucosal membranes.

- In chronic pain management always start with the lowest available dose of an immediate release formulation. Thereafter, the dose is titrated to effect (Table IV-3). If, however, prior to therapy, the patient had been exposed to an opioid with low potency (i.e., meperidine, codeine) or an agonist/antagonist (i.e., pentazocine, butorphanol), the starting dose is 5 mg morphine immediate release. In case of insufficient pain relief 50% of the previous dose is added to the subsequent one. If, however, the patient is pain free after the first dose, the next dose should be reduced by 50%.
- Because of their short duration of action, opioids such as fentanyl, alfentanil or sufentanil, should be omitted as a basic opioid medication since their application interval is between 15 and 30 min. This is in contrast to breakthrough pain, where a fast-acting and short-lasting opioid is given by an alternating route. For administration of a fast-acting opioid, the following alternatives are possible: transmucosal fentanyl lozenge, fentanyl effervescent buccal tablets, inhalation of liposome encapsulated fentanyl, inhalation of dry power fentanyl, or inhalation of morphine by means of a breath activated inhaler. All these newer techniques ideally can be used to counteract painful episodes of breakthrough pain (see more in chapter new developments in chronic pain therapy; page 380ff).
- Unless monitored by means of pulse oximetry and/or continuous surveillance, potent opioids should not be given intravenously in order to titrate to the desired analgesic effect, as respiratory depression often is seen immediately after an i.v. injection [5].

- Opioids such as codeine, oxycodone, morphine and merperidine on the average have to be given at in interval of 2–3 h, while pentazocine (Talwin®) is given every 4 h. Contrary, controlled release morphine (MS Contin®) as well as buprenorphine (Buprenex®) are given every 8–10 h. Especially the buccal mode of administration of buprenorphine is of advantage, since the first-pass effect through the liver is by-passed resulting in a lesser rate of metabolism, a higher bioavailability and lesser amounts of the active agent.

By using a special retarded technology, the administration interval of oral morphine slow release (MS Contin®) or morphine sulfate slow release capsules (Oramorph® 30/60/100 mg), which usually is between 8–12 h, can be prolonged by using the morphine sulfate sustained release capsules (Kadian® 20/30/50/60/100 mg). Dosing intervals can be extended once every 18–24 h, while use of extended release morphine sulfate formulation results in a one dose per 24 h.

Another opioid, methadone because of its specific pharmacokinetic profile, also inherits a long duration of action. While the levorotatory enantiomer (l-methadone) is about twice as potent as the racemic d,l-methadone, it is not available in the US, where the racemic mixture can only be prescribed (Dolophine® 10 mg). Because of its high volume of distribution the agent has the longest duration of action being > 24 h with a plasma half-life of up to 55 h [6]. The latter is related to its accumulation in the peripheral storage sites (skin, muscle, fat, connecting tissue), which act like a reservoir and from which the opioid is being released into the central blood compartment in a continuous fashion. However, due to its large volume of distribution, this opioid is difficult to handle, which is why it is not considered as the first agent of choice. Because titration to effect is only be achieved after 2–3 days this easily results in an overdose. Also, due to the large individual variability in plasma half-life between 8 and 80 h, methadone is not regarded as the analgesic of choice when an opioid-naïve patient is given the drug for the first time. It however, has the highest cost-effectiveness and represents a valid alternative, if tolerance to morphine or to transdermal fentanyl (Duragesic®) develops or when the patient has neuropathic pain. This latter implication is derived from the fact that methadone also inherits a small, but clinically relevant antagonistic action at the excitatory N-methyl-D-aspartate (NMDA) receptor, which results in a reduction of the usual high dosages of other first-line opioids.

It should be noted that aside from morphine, other opioids, due to their specific pharmacokinetic profile, present a valid alternative to the historically oldest opioid morphine. Characterized by a long duration of action, the controlled-release formulation of oxycodone (OxyContin®) and the controlled-release preparation of hydromorphone (Palladone®) have potential advantages when compared to morphine:

1. Contrary to morphine, oxycodone has an oral bioavailability of 60%–80% and hydromorphone a bioavailability of 40% (Table IV-3). Such higher fractions of an administered dose of the medication that reach the systemic circulation results in lesser doses necessary for pain relief.
2. Both opioids are characterized by minor quantities of pharmacologically active metabolites followed by less important side effects (Fig. IV-4). This is in

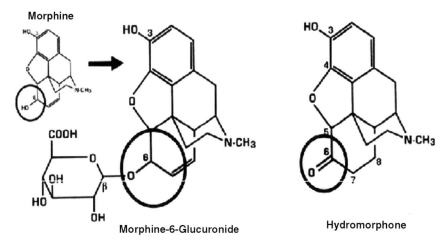

Figure IV-4. Metabolism of morphine via glucuronisation at the sixth position of the molecule. Due the double binding metabolism of hydromorphone is not possible resulting in lesser metabolites

contrast to morphine, where hallucinations, nausea, vomiting, and/or marked sedation regularly are observed with increasing dosages, necessary for pain relief, resulting in a limitation of the administered dose.
3. Both agents have a short onset of action averaging between 1 and 2 h which is in contrast to controlled-release morphine which needs at least 3 h to reach peak effects.

CO-ANALGESICS (ADJUVANTS) FOR LONG-TERM PAIN THERAPY WITH OPIOIDS

Co-analgesics are agents, which actually do not belong to the group of analgesics. In selective situations, however, they result in pain-modifying and opioid-additive/potentiating/opioid-sparing effects. In addition, co-analgesics are indicated whenever the pain is caused by a functional deficit in the descending pain-inhibitory pathways, or when basic suffering attains an important meaning for the patient. But most of all adjuvant therapy is related to the potential side effects of chronic opioid therapy (Table IV-4).

Co-analgesics, also termed adjuvants, rank as follows:

Corticosteroids – These non-selective co-analgesics have a major indication in case of nerve compression, cephalgia due to increased intracraniel pressure, spinal cord compression, bone metastases, plexus invasion, soft tissue swelling due to tumor invasion, lymphoedema, osteoarthritis and/or cartilage distruction. The general recommended agent is dexamethasone (Decadron®, Dexamethasone®) with an initial dose of 8–32 mg/day; followed by a slow reduction of the daily dose of up to 2–4 mg/day.

Table IV-4. Summary and incidence of possible side effects following pain therapy with an opioid (TCA=tricyclic antidepressant)

Side effect	Incidence (%)	Dose-dependent	Tolerance development	Therapy
Constipation	90–100	Yes	No	Laxatives
Nausea, emesis	20–40	No	5–7 days	Antiemetics
Sedation	2–10	Yes	3–4 days	Stimulants
Dizziness	2–5	Yes	No	Dose-reduction, opioid rotation
Hallucination	1–5	No	No	Haloperidol
Pruritus	1–5	No	Yes	Antihistamine
Urinary retention	0.5–1	No	No	Discontinuation TCAs

Antiepileptics – Their main indication is the lancinating-like spontaneous pain of neuropathic origin, which is seen in trigeminal neuralgia, post herpetic neuralgia, in tumor and phantom pain, as well as in pain of central origin (thalamic evoked pain following stroke). The most frequently used agent is carbamazepine (Tegretol®, Epitol®) or phenytoine sodium, which are given in combination with an opioid in doses of 800–1200 mg/day. Newer agents of the second generation of antiepileptics such as gabapentin, lamotrigine or topiramate often are used in pain of various origin and present an important part in the therapeutic armamentarium. Especially gabapentin (Neurontin®), due to its compatibility and few side-effects, has entered the core in pain therapy, whereby doses of up to 3200 mg/day can safely be administered.

Tricyclic antidepressants (TCA) – They are the mainstay in painful peripheral neuropathies, in pain with hyper-, dys-, or paresthesia and allodynia, which often are seen in diabetic patients, in herpetic neuralgia, and in tumor pain where nerve fibers are damaged or infiltrated by the underlying disease. The most frequently used compound of this class is amitriptyline (Elavil®, Enovil®), which induces a psychomotor sedation and increases the activity of the descending inhibitory nociceptive pathways. The initial dose amounts to 10–25 mg/day. When combining an opioid with amitriptyline, a single dose of 50–75 mg/day, because of its sedative properties, should be given before bedtime. Contrary, imipramine (Tofranil®, Janimine®), which also results in an increase in vigilance, the daily dose has to be given in the morning. The initial dose is 25–50 mg titrated to effect. When combined with an opioid, the dose should not exceed 50–100 mg/day. The rationale for use of an antidepressant is the fact that pain has its morphologic base in brain areas responsible for the emotional and the affective component of nociception, the limbic system. Apart, opioids also induce a euphoric-like feeling, which adds to the action of antidepressants. It is suggested that the antineuralgic properties of TCAs are independent of their antidepressant activity, and present research suggests that they activate the descending pain inhibitory system.

Neuroleptics and tranquilizer – Because chronic pain patients often present a jerky, provocative, and affect-unstable attitude with a disturbed sleep pattern while at the same time being tired and underpowered, sedative tranquilizers are often necessary to calm the patient down [7]. Based on their different profile in action, specific neuroleptic agents have to be chosen individually, using certain combinations in order to handle special psychological behavior patterns. Neuroleptics therefore are used in the context of a combination with an opioid, particularly when patients experience tumor-related pain. For combination of the opioid with a neuroleptic, haloperidol (Haldol®) 2–5 mg/day is recommended as this agent also prevents emesis. Although the nociceptive afferents are not affected, neuroleptics act indirectly by interfering at the nigrostriatal and the limbic system. Thus, they have an effect on the somatomotor and the emotional component of pain, resulting in tranquillization and an indifferent attitude. Especially, because of their potent antiemetic effect, neuroleptics present an important part in pain-related therapy with opioids (Table IV-5).

Contrary to pharmacological effects of neuroleptics at the monoaminergic, the serotoninergic, the noradrenergic, the dopaminergic and/or the cholinergic system, tranquilizers such as diazepam (Valium®, Diazepam®) or midazolam (Versed®) act at the g-amino butyric acid (GABA) receptor of the interneuronal inhibitory system of the spinal cord. By increasing interneuronal activity at the endorphinergic system, the analgesic effect of opioids is potentiated. At the same time the pain-mediating excitatory neurotransmitters such as glutamate and substance P, are inhibited particularly in the dorsal horn of the spinal cord [7]. While antidepressants activate the descending pain-inhbitory serotinergic and noradrenergic pathways via activation at the dorsal horn of the spinal cord, neuroleptics act as antagonists at the dopamine receptor, and potentiate tricyclic antidepressants indirectly (Fig. IV-5).

Laxatives – Parallel with any long-term administration of an opioid, control of constipation is mandatory (Table IV-4). Therefore, regular intake of a laxative like a stool softener (Docusate sodium), lactulose (Dupholax®), Sennosid B, bisacodyl (Dulcolax®) or sodium-picosulfate (Laxoberal®) is mandatory. Such co-medication

Table IV-5. Adjuvant therapy using TCAs in chronic pain treatment with different modes of action

Neuroleptics	Anxiolytics, antipsychotics
Pain with anxiety disorders	
Desipramine	Zolpidem
Levopromazine	Buspirone
Haloperidol	Fluphenazine
Promethazine	Doxepin
Prochlorperazine	Amitriptyline
Pain with depressive disorders	
Fluoxitine	Imipramine
Fluphenazine	Mianserine
Trazodone	Trimipramine
Thioridazine	Maprotiline
Paroxetine	Melitracen

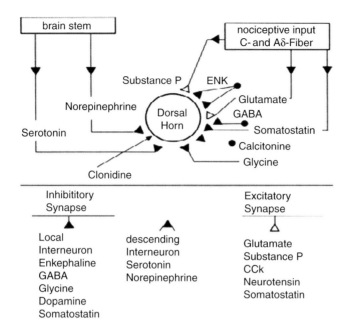

Figure IV-5. Schematic representation of the transmitter systems and agents involved the propagation and procession of pain impulses in the dorsal horn of the spinal cord, resulting in either both inhibition or potentiation of nociceptive afferents via neurotransmitter release (GABA = γ-aminobutyric acid; CCK = cholecystokinine; CGRP = calcitonine gene-related peptide; ENK = enkephalin)

should accompany each opioid, since opioid-related constipation may become a severe obstacle in opioid therapy, which may even become more difficult than the actual pain therapy. In cases with conventional resistent constipation, two selective peripheral opioid-antagonists, i.e., methylnaltrexone (0.1–0.3 mg/kg s.c.) [8] and alvimopan (6 mg oral) [8, 9] available. Since both agents do not penetrate the blood-brain barrier, centrally-mediated analgesia is preserved.

Antiemetics – When opioids induce nausea and/or emesis, administration of an antiemetic is indicated. For such purposes one should start with metoclopramide (Reglan®) and then change to more potent ones: the neuroleptic haloperidol (Haldol®) or domperidone (Motilium®), which act via dopamine-receptors in the chemoreceptor trigger zone (CTZ) within the medulla. Aside from a neuroleptic, a selective serotonine subreceptor inhibitor, which acts directly at the 5-HT$_3$ (5-hydroxytryptamine) binding site located in the chemoreceptor trigger zone (CTZ), ondansetron (Zofran®) should be considered. Since opioid-related nausea and emesis, because of tolerance development, are rather short-lived phenomena, the need for antiemetics is only within the first days in the opioid-naïve patient.

Analeptics – Sufficient pain therapy with central acting opioids often results in marked sedation. While this is seen predominantly with the start of opioid therapy, this side effect is characterized by the development of tolerance in the later period. If, however, side effects persists and if a dose reduction does not lead to desired reduction, analeptics such as caffeine, methylphenidate (Ritalin®), pemoline (Cylert®), dextroamphetamine (Dexedrine®) or modafinil (Provigil®) are indicated, resulting in an increase of vigilance.

Sodium channel blockers – Especially in nerve injury with ongoing ectopic activity and possible cross talk to spared nerves neuropathic pain develops. In such instances Na^+-channel blockers may be advantageous since they reduce the spontaneous ongoing activity which is perceived as continuing pain, resulting in central hyperexcitability and upregulation of voltage dependent Ca^{++}-channels within the spinal cord. Because there is loss of inhibitory interneurons (e.g. GABA), mexiletine (Mexitil®) or local anesthetics such as bupivacaine (Marcaine®, Sensorcaine®) or lidocaine (Xylocaine®, Lidocaine®) present attractive adjuvants, because spontaneous discharge in injured nerves and hyperactive collateral fibers is reduced.

Buprenorphine – Opioid with Unique Receptor Kinetics for Chronic Pain

Different opioids used in the therapy of chronic pain demonstrate a preference of binding to a different receptor population, which results in distinct pharmacodynamic effects, but also in the incidence of side effects (Table IV-6). In this regard buprenorphine (Buprenex®, Transtec®), due to its specific interaction with

Table IV-6. Summary of co-analgesics in chronic tumor-related pain therapy

Type of pain	Co-analgesics	Alternative therapy
Bone metastasis or infiltration	NSAIDs, steroids biphosponate agents	Local radiotherapy, radionucleoids
Nerve compression, infiltration	Cortocosteroids, antiepileptics, neuroleptics, antidepressants	Radiotherapy, neurolytic-sympathetic block
Increased intracranial pressure	Corticosteroids, diuretics, antiepileptics	Radiotherapy, head up positioning
Lymphoedema	Corticosteroids, diuretics	Sympathetic block, compression, lymph drainage
Muscle spasms, soft tissue infiltration	Corticosteroids, NSAIDs, centrally acting muscle relaxants	Physiotherapy, therapeutic local blocks, relaxation therapy
Distention pain (liver, spleen)	Corticosteroids	Radiotherapy, neurolytic block of coeliac plexus,
Bone related metastatic disorders	Biphosphonate agents (Clodronate, Etodronate, Palmidronate) Antiepileptics,	Radionucleotides
Postherpetic neuralgia	Antiepileptics	Sympatholysis, lidocaine patch 5%
Par-, dysesthesia	Antidepressants, neuroleptics,	Local anesthetic agents
Muscle spasticity	baclofen	NMDA-antagonists, gabapentin

Adapted from [10]

the opioid receptor site and contrary to the other opioids, is characterized by the following features:

1. It has a very slow association rate to the receptor site, which clinically results in a slow onset of action. Thus it can be expected that maximum efficacy is seen after 60 min.
2. Once having bound to the receptor site, binding is very intense which results in little or no displacement by other opioids.
3. Buprenorphine shows high affinity to the receptor site. This is of advantage in the clinical setting as small dosages already result in marked conformational changes of the serpentine loops (Fig. IV-6), resulting in an intense analgesic effect.
4. Buprenorphine exhibits a slow dissociation from the receptor site, which clinically results in a long duration of action.
5. Because of its high potency lesser opioid receptors have to be occupied in order to achieve a sufficient analgesic affect. Thus, there is a sufficient receptor reserve, which clinically can be used for the co-administration of or the switch to another opioid.

Due to the unique receptor kinetics, use of buprenorphine in general practice is characterized by the following features:

1. A long onset of action. When using a sublingual tablet, 60 min may elapse until the drug shows maximal analgesic effect, and after intravenous administration a time span of 30 min has to be expected until the patient achieves total pain relief.

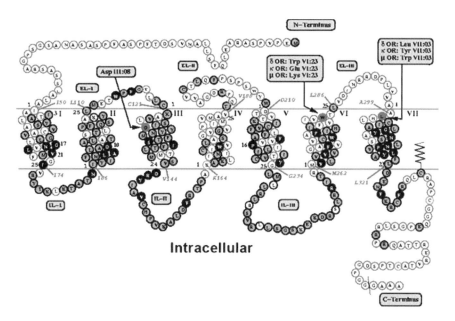

Figure IV-6. The opioid μ-receptor with the typical seven transmembrane serpentine loops, the site of binding of buprenorphine

Because of this apparent time lag, one has to wait before administering a second dose of the opioid. In particular, early repetitive doses of buprenorphine should be avoided in the elderly as this may result in respiratory depression (μ-receptor interaction!).

2. Because binding of buprenorphine to the opioid receptor is very intense, pure antagonists in doses higher than usually administered are necessary to displace the ligand from its receptor site [11]. If, however, respiratory depression gets to a clinical relevant degree, it can be antagonized by repetitive and higher doses of the potent antagonist naloxone (sometimes up to 10 mg of naloxone). When starting antagonism, the intravenous dose of naloxone should be titrated against vital parameters such as respiratory rate, blood pressure and behavior pattern. In order to avoid an acute abstinence syndrome, a starting dosage of 0.4–0.8 mg is given, followed by tapering up to 2.0 mg. Because of the short half-life of naloxone, an infusion of 5 mg/h should be administered in the following 24 h accompanied by the simultaneous surveillance in an intensive care environment. Such precautions are necessary in order to prevent a reoccupation of the receptors by buprenorphine [12], which otherwise would result in a late re-occurence of respiratory depression. Another specific opioid antagonist, nalmefene (Revex®) seems to be a more favorable agent for antagonists, because it has a higher receptor specificity and affinity, which results in a longer half-life than naloxone [12]. As an alternative, the nonspecific analeptic agent doxapram (Dopram®) can be used in order to reverse respiratory depression via stimulation of pressor receptors in the glomus caroticus. Such practice has the advantage that the analgesic effect of buprenorphine is not antagonized while at the same time reversing the depressed respiratory drive.

   Because of the respiratory depressive ceiling effect of buprenorphine, a clinical relevant impairment of respiration is rarely seen in patients while this often is due to the co-administration of a sedative or a hypnotic.

3. The intensive and long receptor binding results in a long duration of the analgesic effect. Besides controlled release morphine (MS-Contin®) or controlled release oxycodone (OxyContin®), it has the longest duration of action among opioids being used in medicine [13]. Therefore repetition may only be necessary every 8–9 h, which in chronic pain patients is advantageous. By using the new trans-dermal matrix technology of buprenorphine (BuTrans®), duration of analgesia may even be prolonged further up to 96 h, resulting in more comfort for and compliance by the patient.

4. The slow dissociation rate of buprenorphine from the receptor site results in limited physical dependency and a lesser likelihood in the development of tachyphylaxis. Since tachyphylaxis is accompanied by the necessity to increase the dose in order to achieve a similar effect, long-term administration of this opioid over weeks and months is characterized by little or no tolerance development. Tolerance development to an opioid is due to a decrease in binding affinity of the ligand to the receptor, it has been termed as "down-regulation" [14]. In addition long-term application is also linked to sequestration of receptors into the cell also termed internalization. Such an effect can be seen with morphine

and fentanyl while buprenorphine, due to its partial μ-agonistic potency does not show such a characteristic, since receptors demonstrate rapid re-emergence at cell surface [21] .

5. Because of the high affinity of buprenorphine at the receptor site, small doses (0.3–0.6 mg/70 kg i.v.) already induce a sufficient deep analgesic effect.

6. Also, because of the high affinity to the binding site and its potency (40× morphine) only a small number of receptors need to be occupied for mediating a sufficient analgesic effect. Such a characteristic has the advantage that pain relief can be increased by the additional application of a fast release buccal buprenorphine or by a morphine fast release tablet. Such a strategy is only possible through unbound, available receptor sites, termed receptor reserve, which enables additional binding (Fig. IV-7).

7. Since only a small number of receptors have to be occupied in order to induce a potent analgesic effect, opioid rotation from buprenorphine to oral extended release morphine or vice versa, is possible. Due to this receptor reserve (fig. IV-8) a change from one opioid to another, such as slow release oxycodone, hydromorphone or morphine, can be performed without any problem, whereby equianalgesic doses should be used [15]. Transformation is accomplished by multiplying the total daily buprenorphine dose by 70, thus receiving the total appropriate daily dose of morphine, which is distributed over 24 h, necessary for a sufficient blockade of nociceptive afferents with no gap in pain therapy [10].

8. The putative analgesic ceiling effect of buprenorphine so far has only been demonstrated in the animal when using extremely high doses, which clinically are above the therapeutic range [17] (Fig. IV-9).

9. In the clinical setting use of therapeutic doses of up to 10 mg/day, buprenorphine behaves like a pure μ-type ligand and no analgesic ceiling effect can

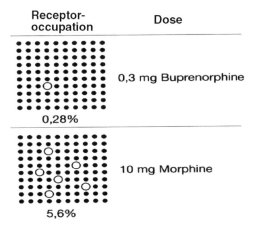

Figure IV-7. Proportional occupation of receptors by buprenorphine and morphine. Because of such receptor reserve, a switch from buprenorphine to morphine is possible as a sufficient number of non-occupied receptors are available for additional binding

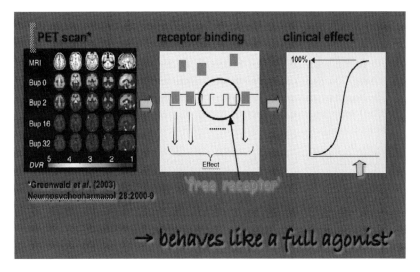

Figure IV-8. As demonstrated in PET scan studies, complete occupation of all binding sites with buprenorphine is only accomplished by very high doses of the agent >16mg [16]. In pain patients, lower dosages are commonly used and buprenorphine behaves like a full agonist, resulting in available receptors sites for binding with another opioid

be demonstrated [19]. Contrary to other potent opioids, however, there is a respiratory ceiling as demonstrated in human volunteers (Fig. IV-10).

10. Because of its high affinity, buprenorphine has a wide therapeutic margin of safety (LD_{50}/ED_{50}), which results in little or no cardiovascular depression

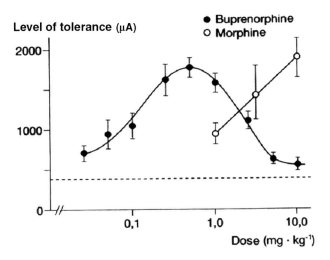

Figure IV-9. Analgesic ceiling-effect of buprenoprhine when compared to morphine in the animal using the shock titration test. Adapted from [18]

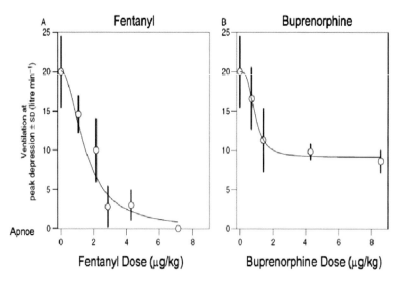

Figure IV-10. Contrary to fentanyl there is a respiratory ceiling-effect following increasing doses of buprenorphine. Adapted from [20]

(Fig. IV-11). Even inadvertent overdose, except respiratory depression, results in no negative side effects such as marked hypotension or a depression of myocardial contractility.

11. For signal transduction buprenorphine interacts with a subset of the intracellular transmitter system, the G-protein (Fig. IV-12). It is because of this difference in

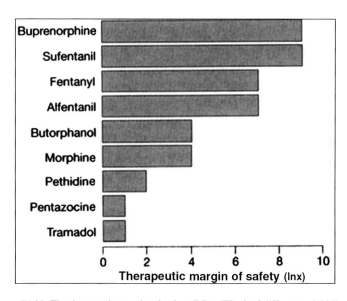

Figure IV-11. The therapeutic margin of safety (LD_{50}/ED_{50}) of different opioid ligands

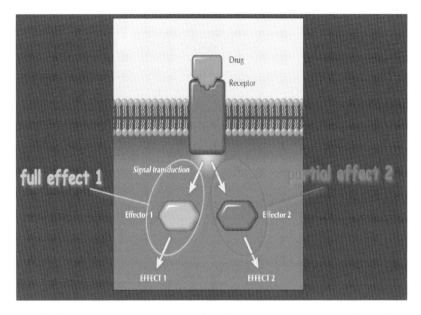

Figure IV-12. Following drug binding at the cell surface the message is conveyed intracelluarly via the G-protein. Contrary to other opioids a subset of G-proteins is activated by buprenorphine. Adapted from [21]

   the mode of action, that a low incidence in tolerance development is observed. This is in contrast to other pure agonists such as morphine or fentanyl, where long-term application for chronic pain treatment often results in the gradual increase of the necessary dose.
12. Compared to other opioids buprenorphine exhibits a simultaneous κ-antagonistic effect (Table IV-7). Because of this feature the ligand demonstrates a lesser incidence of dysphoria, especially when given in higher doses.

Table IV-7. Receptor interaction of different opioids and their prototype ligands used in chronic pain therapy

Opioid	Agonistic activity	Antagonistic activity
Pure μ-type agonist, e.g. morphine	μ, κ, δ	None
Pure antagonist, e.g. naloxone	None	μ, κ, δ
Mixed agonist/antagonist e.g. nalbuphine	κ	μ, δ
Partial agonist, e.g. buprenorphine	μ	κ

Adapted from [22]

Transdermal Patches for Use in Chronic Pain – Fentanyl TTS and Buprenorphine TDS

Opioid therapy can adequately relieve pain in more than three quarters of cancer patients [23]. This extraordinary success rate justifies the widely held view that long-term opioid therapy is the first-line approach to moderate or severe cancer pain. While it is now commonly accepted that opioids present an integrated part in chronic pain especially for the alleviation of cancer pain, new modes of application present attractive alternatives, especially when oral intake is not possible.

RATIONALE FOR THE USE OF TRANSDERMAL SYSTEMS

While the oral route (tablet, liquid) is commonly used and the preferred mode of application for patients who can take oral medication, the continuous subcutaneous (s.c.), epidural, intramuscular (i.m.) or intravenous (i.v.) mode of administration provide a faster onset, however, with a shorter duration of action. Therefore patients requiring continuous opioid analgesia and who do not experience intolerable side effects from parenteral dosing, the oral route of opioid administration is the most effective. If, however, nursing support is not possible, it may result in an inconsistent level of analgesia when the infusion rate is not controlled appropriately, or when weekly change of the infusion pump is not done in time. Contrary, the intramuscular mode of administration results in a slow absorption resulting in less variable plasma levels than the subcutaneous route, resulting in a long duration of action. However, patients who cannot take oral medication (e.g. emesis or GI obstruction) maintenance of effective drug levels over a longer period of time can be achieved by rectal suppositories. Such a mode of application presents an attractive alternative, because in contrast to the oral way, a lesser amount of the drug will be metabolized during the first-pass effect through the liver, resulting in a reduction of the dose necessary for pain alleviation (Fig. IV-13). Contrary, rectal administration is inappropriate for patients with diarrhea, anal/rectal lesions, mucositis, and patients with thrombocytopenia or neutropenia or patients who are physically unable to place the suppository in the rectum. In addition, certain cases where systemic opioids result in marked side effects such as sedation, nausea, emesis and/or severe constipation, the intrathecal route may be a useful alternative. This is because lower dosages can be administered to the site of action resulting in lesser or a marked reduction of side effects. On the other hand the addition of a local anesthetics or of an α_2-agonist such as clonidine can be used to potentiate the analgesic effect of opioids.

Because the half-life of most oral opioids is less than 6 h, repetitive intake of the opioids by the clock is necessary. In order to circumvent this drawback, several products have entered the market, which due to their controlled release preparation result in sustained liberation with sufficient plasma levels over a long period of time.

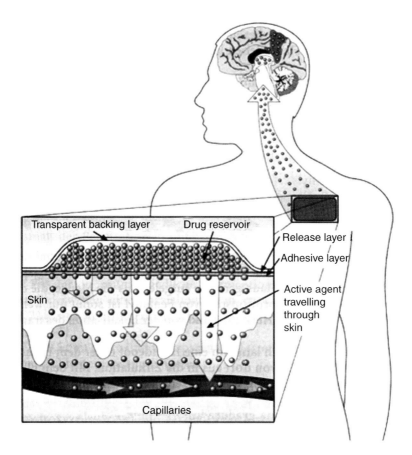

Figure IV-13. The basic mechanism of the therapeutic transdermal system where the drug enters the skin from a rate controlled patch. From depots in the upper layers of the skin the opioid diffuses into deeper layers where it is taken up by the blood stream of the capillaries and transported to the site of action within the CNS

Thus, morphine (MS Contin™, Oramorph™ SR), controlled/sustained release oxyco-done (OxyContin®) or hydromorphone (Palladone®SR) are available reducing the oral intake by one tablet/12–24 h.

The mode of application which however represents the least burden of drug intake for the patient is that of transdermal application where the opioid containing formulation offers a 48–72 h dosing interval (Fig. IV-13). First introduced in 1986 it presents a mode of delivery for those patients:

1. Who present a relative stable pain level where rapid increase or decrease in pain intensity is less likely to develop.
2. Who are unable to swallow or present malabsorption of an oral administered opioid.
3. Where the compliance presents a problem in daily drug intake.

4. Who present severe constipation, which purportedly is significantly less in transdermal application [24] or sublingual application [25].
5. Who want to gain more independence from regular oral drug intake resulting in
   an increase in quality-of-life as the patch needs only to be replaced every 96 h.

Pharmacokinetics of Opioids Used in Transdermal Systems

Two transdermal patches presently are avaiable to the treatment of chronic pain,
fentanyl TTS (Duragesic®) and buprenorphine TDS (TranstecPro®; BuTrans®).
A comparison of the physicochemical properties of the two opioids fentanyl and
buprenorphine illustrate some of the prerequisites of the potential candidate, for
transdermal application (Table IV-8). Because the skin acts like an anorganic phase
the partitioning of the opioid between the skin and the dermal reservoir has to
be in favor of a highly lipophilic drug. Compared to morphine, both fentanyl
and buprenorphine are much more lipophilic than morphine, a property which is
reflected in the difference of the partition coefficient in the oil phase compared to
the aqueous phase, the octanol/water coefficient (Table IV-8).

Because of the larger differences in lipophilicity, as reflected in the partition
coefficient, both fentanyl and buprenorphine present a favorable transdermal flux
through the skin than morphine. Also, because of the much higher potency of
fentanyl and buprenorphine when compared to morphine (Table IV-8) these two
opioids are preferable drug candidates for transdermal delivery because smaller
amounts of the drug have to cross the skin to attain similar analgesic effects. By
using a saturated solution this results in a continuous transdermal delivery rate.

This, however, relies upon the skin as the sole determinant of drug delivery
rate. As there is a variation in permeability among patients, and between different

Table IV-8. Pharmacokinetic properties of the opioids fentanyl and buprenorphine when compared
to morphine

Physicochemical properties	Morphine	Fentanyl	Buprenorphine
Analgesic potency	1	100–200	30–40
Antagonistic potency to naloxone = 1	0	0	0.7–1.0
Molecular weight	336.5	285.3	504.1
Heptane/water coefficient	1.4	860	2320
Non-ionized (%)	23	8.5	9
Protein binding (%)	30	84.4	96
Volume of distribution (Vd; L/kg)	3.0–4.0	4.0	2.7

Adapted from [26, 27, 28]

skin sites in different persons, a rate-controlling membrane is used in the opioid patch in order to provide a steady release of the drug into the skin (Fig. IV-14). In addition, the opioid patch also has an absorption enhancer (i.e. alcohol), which augments skin permeability resulting in an increase in drug flux into the skin. First being marketed, the fentanyl therapeutic transdermal reservoir system (fentanyl TTS) was introduced, which later was further developed into a transdermal patch where the active ingredient is bound in a matrix for transdermal delivery. Similar to the buprenorphine patch, it consists of a polymer where the saturated opioid is imbedded in a matrix serving both as a rate-controlling reservoir and as an adhesive to the skin (Fig. IV-14).

In both patches, the amount of fentanyl and buprenorphine release from a system is proportional to the surface area yielding fluxes of 25, 50, 75 and $100\,\mu g/h$ in the fentanyl patch and 35, 52.5 and $70\,\mu g/h$ in the buprenorphine patch, respectively.

SPECIFICITY OF TRANSDERMAL BUPRENORPHINE

Buprenorphine is an opioid analgesic administered sublingually or by injection for the treatment of moderate to severe pain. Transdermal buprenorphine (BuTrans®, Napp Pharmaceuticals) is formulated as a matrix patch and is licensed for the treatment of moderate to severe cancer pain and severe pain not responding

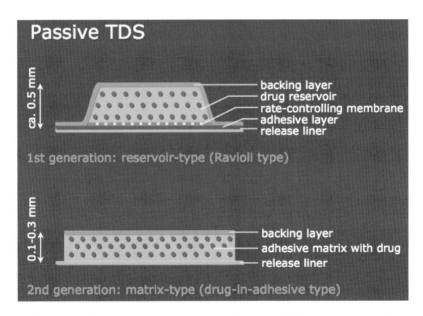

Figure IV-14. Composition of the two transdermal opioid systems (TDS) used in chronic pain therapy, the former Ravioli type and the available matrix type, both of which are marketed as fentanyl TTS and buprenorphine TDS

to non-opioid analgesics. BuTrans® ptaches (Napp Pharmaceuticals-UK; Purdue Pharma-USA) are available in three different strengths delivering 5, 10, 20 μg/hr over 96 h. The starting dose is determined by the dose and type of previous analgesic. Patients not previously taking an analgesic, or taking a non-opioid analgesic, should begin with a dose of 10 μg/hr. The patch should be replaced every 96 h and at least 7 days should elapse before a new patch is applied to the same area of skin. Sublingual buprenorphine should be available to treat break-through pain; if 0.4–0.6 mg/day is regularly required, the next patch strength should be used. Blood levels of buprenorphine increase slowly after application of the first patch. Therefore, additional analgesia may be required for the first 24–48 h. The commonest adverse events reported in clinical trials were nausea (17% of patients), erythema (17%), pruritus (15%), vomiting (9%), dizziness (7%), tiredness (6%) and constipation (5%).

The use of any transdermal systems is limited by the cost, the difficulties involved in delivering high doses, and the need for an alternative route to provide supple-mental doses for breakthrough pain. In addition, these delivery systems are not preferred for therapy titration of opioid doses in the setting of severe pain since there is a lag of up to 14 h until sufficient high concentration of the opioid have been attained in the plasma (Fig. IV-15). Also, fever spikes, a problem affecting some patients with AIDS, and heat sources potentially may lead to an unstable or

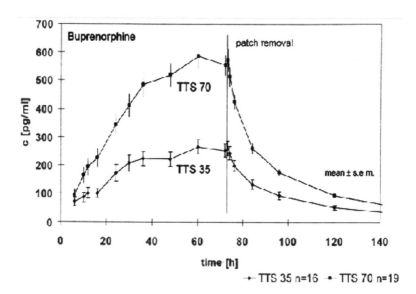

Figure IV-15. Representative example of increasing plasma concentrations over time using a buprenor-phine patch with a concentration of 35 (*n* = 11) or 70 (*n* = 17)μg/h respectively. Note, after patch removal there is a gradual decay of plasma concentration because of the opioid depot still being present in the skin

an increase of absorption from the transdermal system, resulting in higher concentrations than necessary.

It is important to follow carefully the instructions that have been given with this medicine.

1. BuTrans® patches should be applied to a clean, dry, non-hairy, non-irritated area of skin, preferably on the upper outer arm, upper chest, upper back, or the side of the chest. Avoid areas with large scars. If you need to clean the skin before sticking on the patch use only water, not soap or other cleansers. If hair needs to be removed before applying the patch it should be cut with scissors, not shaved. The patch should not be stuck on immediately after a hot bath or shower, one should wait for the skin to cool down first, and not use talc, creams or moisturisers before applying the patch as they may prevent it sticking. The patch is stuck on immediately after removing it from the pouch and pressed firmly into place with the palm of the hand for 30 s.
2. The patches should not be divided, cut or damaged in any way.
3. One should not wear more patches than told by the physician. No more than two patches should be worn at any one time.
4. While wearing a patch one can swim, bathe and shower as normal, but one should avoid exposing the patch to excessive heat sources, such as hot water bottles, electric blankets, heat lamps, sunbeds, saunas or hot spa baths, as heat can increase the absorption of the active ingredient into the body, resulting in a greater risk of side effects.
5. The patient should tell his doctor once he got a fever while wearing the patch, as this might also increase the absorption of medicine through the skin.
6. Each patch should be worn for 7 days and then removed. New patches should be applied to a different area of skin, and one should avoid using the same area for the next 3–4 weeks. If a patch falls off before it needs changing, one should use a new one immediately, remembering that this patch should be replaced after 7 days.
7. Removed patches should be folded in half, sticky side innermost, and placed inside the open pouch or a piece of tin foil, for careful disposal away from children or animals. This is because used patches may still contain some active ingredient that may be harmful to children or animals.
8. The active ingredient of the patch, buprenoprhine, may cause drowsiness. One should not drive or operate machinery while wearing a patch, or for at least 24 h after removing the last patch. Alcohol should be avoided, as this may increase drowsiness.
9. The effect of buprenoprhine (including any side effects) can last for up to 30 h after removal of the last patch. If the physician is changing from this analgesic to another opioid painkiller, the new opioid, as a general rule, should not be administered within 24 h after removing the BuTran®s patch.
10. With prolonged use, the body may become dependent on this medicine. As a result, withdrawal symptoms such as feeling agitated, anxious, nervous or shaky, or having difficulty sleeping, may occur after the patient stops using the

medicine. This is rare, and if they occur, these effects usually disappear after a couple of weeks.

11. BuTrans® patches are not recommended for children and adolescents under 18 years of age, as they have not been studied in this age group.

Oral Transmucosal Fentanyl Citrate (OTFC) Stick for Treatment of Breakthrough Pain

The problem of breakthrough pain, lasting for 30 min to 2 h is often observed in patients with cancer pain (Fig. IV-16), which may present a major problem in chronic pain therapy. Breakthrough pain may appear at different instances such as

- Weight bearing/movement
- Walking/sitting

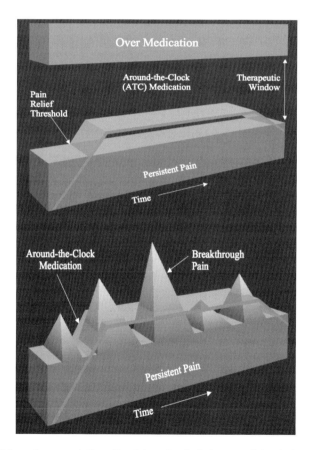

Figure IV-16. Schematic representation of breakthrough pain during around-the-clock medication where in spite of a stable and constant plasma blood level, peak nociceptive afferents break through the opioid barrier

- Defecation/urination
- Coughing/breathing
- Eating
- Spontaneously, or
- without a known cause.

Breakthrough pain is characterised by the following features. They present a

- Moderate to severe intensity
- Rapid onset (< 3 min in 43% of patients)
- Relatively short duration, and have a
- Frequency of 1–4 episodes per day

With a prevalence of 50%–89% the pathology usually is identical to persistent pain (Table IV-9):

Until recently it was advocated to alleviate breakthrough pain by the simultaneous oral intake of a fast acting morphine preparation. Presently, the oral transmucosal fentanyl citrate (OTFC) stick is available, where the active compound, due to its high lipophylicity is rapidly absorbed via the mucous membranes of the oral cavity.

The new galenic preparation of the potent opioid fentanyl is available as oral transmucosal fentanyl citrate (OTFC), also termed "the fentanyl lollypop". It enables rapid and sufficient high absorption through the mucous membrane with sufficient plasma levels within 5 min. Because of the high lipophilicity of fentanyl the opioid is rapidly absorbed through mucous membranes of the oral cavity thus bypassing reabsorption in the intestinal gut, avoiding the degradation through the first liver passage. The fentanyl lollypop (Actiq™, Cephalon company, Pennsylvania/USA) is available in six different concentrations (200, 400, 600, 800, 1200 and 1600 μg), which enables the patients to use the appropriate dose for treatment individual breakthrough pain intensity (Fig. IV-17). Because of the fast onset of action with a maximum of 5 min and a duration of 30 min to 2 h [31] (depending on the concentration being used), the patients starts with the lowest concentration and then increases the dose if breakthrough pain is not sufficiently relieved (Fig. IV-18). Compared to oral morphine sulfate instant release (MSIR), oral transmucosal fentanyl citrate results in a faster relief of pain, similar side effects

Table IV-9. Pathophysiology of breakthrough pain

Classification	Tissue damaged	Descriptors	Typical treatment
Somatic, nociceptive pain	General body tissues	Aching Throbbing Stabbing	Opioids
Visceral, nociceptive pain	Organs	Deep Dull Aching	Opioids
Neuropathic pain	Nervous system	Burning Tingling Lancinating	Adjuvant analgesics

Adapted from [29, 30]

Properties of mucuous membranes	Sublingual/transmucosal technology
Large surface area	
Uniform temperature	
High permeability	
Very well vascularized	
Rapid absorption	
Sufficient high amounts	
No resistance to highly lipophilic compounds	

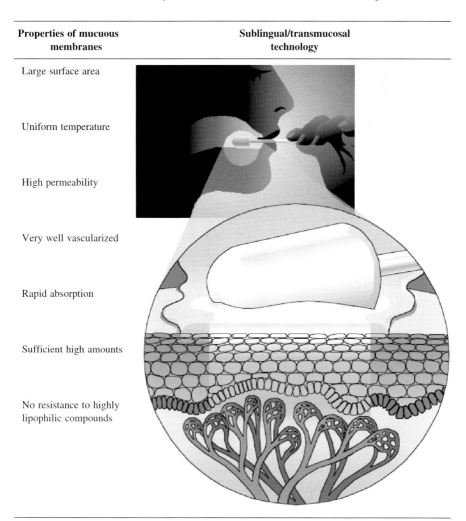

Figure IV-17. Summary of the potential advantages of the mucosal application of opioids, the oral transmucosal fentanyl citrate (OTFC) or sublingual buprenorphine for rapid relief of breakthrough pain

(sedation, nausea, constipation, disorientation) but a longer lasting and significantly better relief of breakthrough pain. Overall acceptance by patients is highly significant when compared to the usual oral morphine sulfate immediate release (MSIR) preparation [32].

While for the sake of practical use oral transmucosal fentanyl citrate is the appropriate compound when the transdermal fentanyl patch is used as this results in a 50% total bioavailability (Fig. IV-19). Also there is an equivalent when the buprenorphine patch is the preferred preparation for the long-term use of chronic

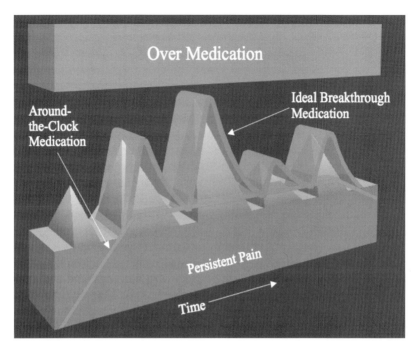

Figure IV-18. Schematic presentation of breakthrough pain and its treatment using the oral transmucosal fentanyl citrate (OTFC) lozenge

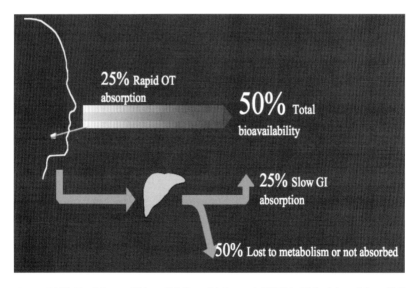

Figure IV-19. Total fentanyl bioavailability with fentanyl OTFC is 50%. Adapted from [33]

pain. The buccal formulation of buprenorphine in dosages of 0.4–08 mg/tablet represents another possibility to treat breakthrough pain when the patient uses transdermal buprenorphine treatment.

DIFFERENCES IN TRANSDERMAL TECHNOLOGY AND PHARMACOLOGY OF FENTANYL AND BUPRENORPHINE

Because of the difference in construction between both transdermal systems, the reservoir and the matrix composition, one has to be aware of possible side effects of the former. When using the old reservoir system, an additional rate limiting control membrane guarantees a steady stream of the active compound fentanyl into the skin. Contrary, in the matrix composition the active compound is incorporated in a polymer layer (Fig. IV-14). Because of this difference the reservoir system should never be cut in order to reduce the dose or use a damaged system for pain relief. By cutting the fentanyl reservoir patch in half the control membrane will no longer act as a rate limiting lining, which results in leaching of fentanyl and a dose dumping with an increase of opioid being taken up by the skin, with higher plasma level than necessary, resulting in respiratory depression, sedation and/or nausea [34]. In the matrix system, no such dose dumping is initiated whenever the transdermal patch is cut in half. In addition, dose dumping may also be induced by the use of a heating pad [35], a hot shower or heater when being applied over the site of the transdermal patch [36], all of which may result in toxicity with respiratory depression. In addition there have been reports where due to an allergic reaction, a local reactive hyperemia resulted in an increase in reabsorption of fentanyl, which is followed by severe side effects [37, 38]. But most of all there have been a number of reports dealing with the illicit use of fentanyl TTS by drug addicts, since the opioid can be extracted from the reservoir but not from the matrix system. For instance, illicit abuse of fentanyl from the reservoir patch was observed in cases with fatal overdose and with respiratory depression where the resultant dose of 5 mg of fentanyl was scraped from the patch and later injected [39] or heated and inhaled [40]. Overdose with respiratory depression from a transdermal fentanyl (reservoir) patch was also observed in a funeral employee who illicitly removed a patch from a dead body [41], or in a person who misused the patch by placing it into his mouth, which resulted in an increased reabsorption through the mucous membrane of the buccal cavity [42] or by chewing on the transdermal system [43, 44]. In addition, increased reabsorption with respiratory arrest was observed after topical administration of two (reservoir) patches on the well perfused scrotal area [45].

Aside from such scenarios of abuse, care deliverers assisting in the application of fentanyl patches in a nursing home are prone to absorb toxic levels of the drug. This has to be recognized when high doses and a frequent change of patches in elderly patients is necessary and/or the concurrent use of a steroidal spray and cream to decrease skin irritations in patients. This may result in an increase of opioid absorption, predisposing the caregiver to opioid intoxication [46]. The attractiveness of the fentanyl (reservoir) patch for illicit use is not too surprising since a 2.5 mg patch after being used therapeutically for 3 days, still has 0.7–1.22 mg of fentanyl remaining and a 10 mg patch has 4.46–8.44 mg of fentanyl remaining in the disposed patch [47]. Using the pharmacokinetic values of fentanyl with a volume of distribution of 4 L/kg and a potential lethal plasma concentration of $3.7 \mu g/L$ one can calculate the potential lethal dose for a 70 kg person to be $1.036 \mu g$, a concentration that is well within residual amount of the patch.

The use of this compound is not without problems since fentanyl's potency, as a narcotic has become an abuse challenge among health professionals, including anesthesiologists, physician pharmacists and nurses. By using a transdermal patch, recreational abuse of fentanyl is extremely dangerous due to the low concentration necessary to induce respiratory depression. As the use of transdermal patches within the management of chronic pain increases, therapeutic mis-adventures may be observed. Because of the ease of administration patients may apply more than one patch if they experience a sudden increase in pain. As the patch is capable of delivering higher than necessary doses of fentanyl multiple patches would result in overdose including death [48].

Presently, the new matrix technology, however, results in a much lower incidence of misuse in drug addicts. In fact there is no report in the literature involving the accidental overuse or the misuse of the buprenorphine patch by addicts. This is because the compound is a partial agonist with high receptor affinity, which first results in an antagonist affect at the binding site and only thereafter induces agonist effects at the same site [13, 49]. When taken by an opiate addict such antagonistic capabilities eventually may result in the precipitation or the increase in abstinence symptoms. In addition, buprenorphine is not a drug of choice for addicts, as it does not induce euphoric effects similar to heroin. Compared to morphine and fentanyl the much lower abuse potential of buprenorphine has been demonstrated conclusively by Jasinski and coworkers where the long-term pretreatment with morphine was followed by increasing doses of naloxone. This resulted in increase of abstinence symptoms, while similar intensities were not observed in individuals pretreated with buprenorphine [50, 51]. Last but not least, buprenorphine is fixed in the polymer matrix which practically makes it impossible to set free sufficient amounts of the drug for illicit use. Also, the development of tolerance, often observed after long-term use of pure μ-type ligands like fentanyl, purportedly is not observed with a partial agonist like buprenorphine. The most likely explanation for this difference is the diffrence in intracellular G-protein activation once buprenorphine binds to the receptor. Such a difference protects the binding site from desensitization (i.e. reduction in pharmacodynamic response to the same dose) and there is no need for an increase in doses in order to achieve a similar analgesic level. Since desensitization is due to an uncoupling of the binding site from the secondary mediator within the cell, the G-protein, the opioid related message can no longer be transmitted which results in a reduction of clinical efficacy (i.e. analgesia). In contrast, high affinity fentanyl-like ligands result in such an uncoupling, a characteristic trait of μ-type ligands, which is followed by the development of tolerance [52, 53].

Both transdermal patches are indicated for intense cancer pain and other non-malignant related chronic pain with a steady pain level, i.e. phantom pain, post herpetic neuralgia, severe osteoarthritis (OA), rheumatoid arthritis (RA), peripheral neuropathy and/or chronic degenerative back pain.

Recently three low-dose patches of buprenoprhine have been launched (BuTrans® 5, 10, 20 μg/h; Napp Pharmaceuticals-UK, and Purdue Pharma USA; Fig. IV-20), which specifically are designed for non-malignant pain such as osteoarthritis or chronic low-back pain, when non-opioid analgesics demonstrate insufficient relief.

While age does not affect the extent of absorption from *BuTrans®* patches, no dose adjustment is needed for the elderly. As with all other transdermal patches the following considerations should be observed when using one of the low-dose opioid patches. BuTrans® is contra-indicated in:
- patients with known hypersensitivity to the active substance buprenorphine or to any of the excipients,
- the treatment of opioid dependence and narcotic withdrawal,
- conditions in which the respiratory center and function are severely impaired or may become so,
- patients who are receiving MAO inhibitors or have taken them within the last 2 weeks,
- patients suffering from myasthenia gravis,
- patients suffering from delirium tremens,
- during pregnancy and lactation.

The following guidelines for approximate dose equivalents are given when converting from a less potent opioid to BuTrans®. However, due to the large inter-individual differences between patients they should be used as a guide to estimate a safe starting dose of the new opioid (Table IV-10).

One major prerequisite for the use of a transdermal system is that of a chronic but stable pain level. It is also important to keep in mind that the potential misuse either

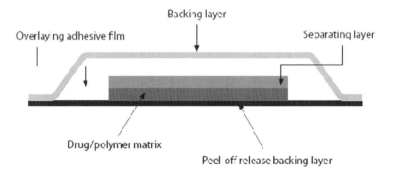

Figure IV-20. Structure of the low-dose buprenorphine patch BuTrans®

Table IV-10. Approximate dose equivalents when rotating from a less potent oral opioid to the low-dose patch BuTrans®

Oral daily dose	5 µg/h BuTrans®	10 µg/h BuTrans®	20 µg/h BuTrans®
Tramadol	< 30 mg/day	50–100 mg/day	100–150 mg/day
Codeine	30–60 mg/day	100–120 mg/day	150–180 mg/day
Dihydrocodeine	> 60 mg/day	> 120 mg/day	> 180 mg/day

by foul play, therapeutic misadventure or even assisted suicide may be considered when toxicity associated with the use of transdermal fentanyl or buprenophine is observed.

> **Both the fentanyl transdermal therapeutic (fentanyl TTS) and the buprenorphine transdermal system (buprenorphine TDS) are the only two non-invasive agents indicated in patients with gastro-intestinal malabsorption or who are unable to swallow**

CHANGE FROM ORAL MORPHINE TO A TRANSDERMAL OPIOID

The prior intake of oral opioids is no contraindication to switch to a transdermal patch because conversion from the oral to the transdermal opioid can be easily achieved by the use of a conversion table, always keeping in mind to adapt to the individual reaction by means of up- or down dosing. Therefore, careful and adequate titration of the dosage is the most relevant factor for a successful transition. Dose titration is determined by the need of the patient when switching from oral morphine to transdermal fentanyl:

1. Calculate the usual oral dose of morphine per 24 h.
2. By using a conversion scale for rough calculation of oral morphine to transdermal fentanyl.
3. Calculate the equianalgesic dosage of fentanyl TTS using the necessary dose of oral morphine per 24 h (Table IV-11).
4. Realize that short-term dose adaptation of the opioid dose is not possible when using the transdermal route of application. Therefore only patients with a stable pain level should be considered as possible candidates for a transdermal medication.
5. The lowest dose of the transdermal patch should be used as the initial dose. Consideration should be given to the previous opioid history of the patient as well as to the current general condition and medical status of the patient. The dose should not be increased before 3 days, when the maximum effect of a given dose is established. Subsequent dosage increases may then be titrated based on the need for supplemental pain relief and the patient's analgesic response to the patch.

Table IV-11. Conversion scale switching from oral morphine to transdermal fentanyl

Oral morphine (mg/day)	Fentanyl TTS ($\mu g/h$)	Size of patch $(cm)^2$
< 90	25	10
91–150	50	20
151–210	75	30
210–270	100	40
Each 60 mg/day	Each 25 μg/h	Each 10 cm^2

6. To increase the dose, a larger patch should replace the patch that is currently being worn, or a combination of patches should be applied in different places to achieve the desired dose. It is recommended that no more than two patches are applied at the same time, regardless of the patch strength. A new patch should not be applied to the same skin site for *the subsequent* 3–4 weeks. Patients should be carefully and regularly monitored to assess the optimum dose and duration of treatment.

7. Similar as in oral opioid therapy with slow release morphine, consider the possibility of breakthrough pain, and have a rescue medication available [30, 54].

8. For rescue medication of breakthrough pain, either morphine immediate release (MIR), the effervescent morphine tablet (Painbreak®), or the oral transmucosal fentanyl stick (OTFS) Actiq® is advocated.

9. While tumor pain patients should be given an opioid for rescue medication, patients with non-malignant pain should be given an NSAID.

ROTATION FROM ORAL MORPHINE TO TRANSDERMAL BUPRENORPHINE

Transition from morphine to buprenorphine is easily accomplished because of the number of spare binding sites, which act as a receptor reserve (see Fig. IV-7). When wanting to switch high dose morphine to buprenorphine the following conversion scale is only used as a rough estimate at start, which is followed by a titration period up to the desired effect (Fig. IV-21).

Successful conversion from high dose morphine to transdermal buprenorphine in chronic pain patients was demonstrated in 47 patients with chronic pain. Only a 5% of all patients were satisified with their current medication and after successfully switching to transdermal buprenorphine 77% reported a good to very good pain relief (Fig. IV-22).

In summary a transdermal opioid patch is indicated in the following category of patients with chronic pain:

1. in whom peak plasma levels of the opioid should be avoided,
2. who object to the daily intake of their medication,

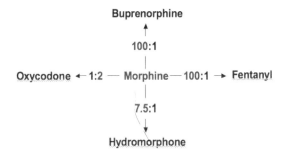

Figure IV-21. Chart for equivalent dosages when rotating from morphine to either fentanyl, hydromorphine or buprenorphine. Patients using very high daily dosages of morphine of < 240 mg/day and experience significant side effects, a 30% reduction of the buprenorphine dose at start of the titration period is advocated

3. who are unable to take a tablet orally,
4. who present malabsorption within the gastro-intestinal tract,
5. who repetitively experience emesis, nausea or hallucinations,
6. who ask for a long duration of action of up to 3 days,
7. where the first-pass effect through the liver is to be avoided,
8. where compliance of drug intake needs to be increased,
9. where administration by the clock is too cumbersome,
10. where due to progression of the underlying disease, a potent analgesic is indicated,
11. where breakthrough pain was effectively treated with an agent of the same molecular structure (i.e. fentanyl OTFC).

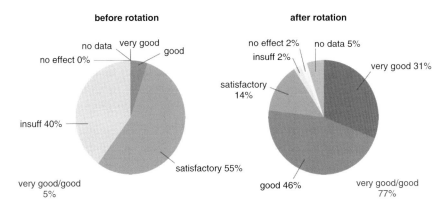

Figure IV-22. Pain relief before and after transition from oral morphine to transdermal buprenorphine in patients with chronic pain of various origin needing high (240 mg) to very high (> 500 mg) doses of daily oral morphine. Adapted from [55]

However, at the same time, the following contraindication should be considered when wanting to use a transdermal patch:
1. Painful conditions, which can be treated with another class of analgesics.
2. Dermatological conditions with an allergic reaction to the patch.
3. During pregnancy and during breast feeding.
4. Patients who do not present a stable painful condition.

Commonly Observed Side-Effects in Long-Term Pain Treatment with Opioids

According to a recent inquiry, treatment of tumor pain with opioids in patients is accompanied by a high degree of ignorance. This may be one of the reasons for an insufficient handling of the tumor patient. Thus, among other things, 51% of all general practitioners assumed tolerance to be a major obstacle in opioid therapy, 29% did not think that adjuvant use of co-analgesics to be justified, 27% considered it necessary to give opioids only parenterally and up to 29% believed the development of dependency a potential risk factor in long-term opioid therapy [56].

RESPIRATORY DEPRESSION

During medication with an oral opioid the possibility of a centrally induced respiratory depression occasionally may be considered and in a major review article the overall incidence was found to be 0.7% for all opioids used in long-term pain therapy (Table IV-12).

However, since pain is the physiological antagonist of a centrally mediated development of respiratory depression it becomes clear that under the presumption of a titrated opioid medication against individual pain, a clinically relevant respiratory depression does not develop. A respiratory depression, however, has to be expected if, in addition to the opioid the patient receives an additional neurolytic therapy to achieve freedom from pain, resulting in the development of a relative

Table IV-12. Incidence of respiratory depression following use of different opioids

	Total number of patients	Patients with respiratory depression	Incidence %
Morphine	3745	19	0.5
Buprenorphine	418	0	0
Hydromorphone	183	1	0.5
Methadone	150	6	4.0
Fentanyl TTS	388	9	2.3
Other opioids	814	5	0.6
Total	5698	40	0.7

overdose. In such cases the previous opioid dose has to be readjusted or completely omitted following each additional therapeutic intervention for pain attenuation. Therefore, each additional medication to opioids, such as sedatives (phenothiazines) or anxiolytics (diazepam) result in an increase of the centrally mediated analgesic effect. It, however, also results in an increase of pitfalls of potential side effects, in particular that of respiratory depression. It therefore is mandatory to reduce the present opioid dose by at least 25% before adding a sedative. By using additional techniques like nerve blocks, the opioid dose has to be reconsidered and possibly totally omitted.

Although the development of relevant hypoxia is possible after an opioid-based anesthesia, patients receiving oral opioids present a fundamental different situation:

1. The majority of patients already took opioids for some time; they cannot be considered as being opioid naive.
2. Patients with chronic pain take the opioid by mouth. This is of significance, because in comparison to the intravenous injection, there is a slower rate of absorption with lower peak plasma levels.
3. In patients with chronic pain there is no non-standard dosing, since the dose of the opioid generally is titrated against pain intensity. Thus titration makes an overdose improbable.
4. According to a recent survey it was pointed out that over the past 30 years patients who ingested morphine orally developed an overall incidence of a respiratory depression of 0.7%. Following transdermal Fentanyl-TTS the rate amounted to 2.3% and following intravenous morphine, the incidence of respiratory impairment rose to 4.5%. Such data suggest that respiratory impairment after oral opioid ingestion is not a problem, as there is a wide margin of safety following oral opioids.

Respiratory depression is not to be expected when using oral opioids for chronic pain treatment, because the dose necessary to induce respiratory depression is higher than the analgesic dose

---

DEVELOPMENT OF DEPENDENCY IN CHRONIC OPIOID USE

The risk of becoming dependent when ingesting opioids is an often expressed fear, which may lead to a reduced dosage with an ensuing insufficient pain release. Although often sited as a potential risk by the media that pain patients become addicted using chronic opioid medication, the media exaggerates the problem. As proven in a large-scale study only one (1) dependency was observed in a total of 1200 patients [57]. In addition, re-examining a total of 11,882 patients, a psychological dependency could only be observed in four cases, which amounts to an incidence of 0.03% [58, 59]. Also, psychological dependency could not be demonstrated using an opioid in the long-term therapy for pain of nonmalignant origin [60, 61]. This is explainable because the controlled release formulation of opioids makes the development of psychological dependency impossible. A sudden increase in peak plasma levels is not seen, which is a prerequiste to induce an "opioid-high". Also, all research studies point out that opioid intake is not the only factor leading to the development of dependency. Other, more important factors, like social surroundings and the basic personality structure have a much more important impact on the development of dependency [62]. In addition, the incidence of tolerance development after intake of potent morphinomimetics has clearly shown, that abuse of of non-opioid analgesics or combination of a weak opioid with a peripheral analgesic is found more frequently in dependent than in non-dependent patients [63, 64]. On the other hand, contrary to psychological dependence, physical dependency will develop within any long lasting therapy with opioids. This, however, does not justify reducing of dose or completely abolish the use of an opioid.

Prescribing controlled substances for legitimate medical uses requires special caution because of the potential for abuse and dependence. It therefore is essential for the prescriber to identify the subject with signs of potential abuse problems (Fig. IV-23). The following characteristic behavioral pattern is seen in subjects involved in drug diversion:

1. Strange stories surrounding why they need prescription medication.
2. Subjects demonstrate a reluctance to cooperate.
3. There is an unusually high or low understanding of the prescription medication.
4. Subjects often present episodes of lost or stolen prescriptions.
5. There is an exaggeration or feigning in symptoms.
6. There is a specific request for drugs.
7. The patient visits multiple physicians and/or pharmacies.
8. The patient insists on an appointment towards the end of office hours.
9. The patient calls or arrives after office hours or when his/her primary physican is not available.
10. The patient insists on being seen immediately because he/she are late for another appointment.
11. There is no interest in having a physical examination, and reluctance in giving permission to obtain past records or undergoing diagnostic tests.
12. The patient is unwilling/unable to give the name of a regular physician while claiming to have no health coverage (insurance).
13. The patient recites textbook symptoms or gives vague medical history.
14. The patient is slovenly or over-dressed. Signs that point to potential abuse:
    a. marks caused by injections,
    b. skin lesions caused by injecting drugs under the skin,
    c. track marks or scars in the underarm resulting from repeated injections,
    d. healing ulcers in the lower/upper extremities,
    e. pin-point constricted or widely dilated pupils,
    f. lethargy, drowsiness,
    g. posession of paraphernalia like syringes, bent spoons, and/or needles,
    h. a perforated nasal septum (cocaine abuse).

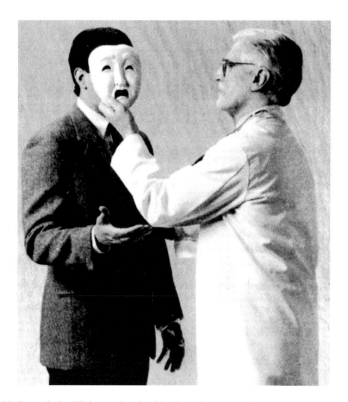

Figure IV-23. Demask the illicit user involved in drug diversion, who appears in the office faking a chronic pain syndrome

On the other hand, it is necessary to separate the subject with true dependency from the patient with pseudo-addiction. True physical dependency is considered a state of adaptation manifested by a specific class of drugs where withdrawal symptoms are produced by abrupt cessation, rapid drug reduction and/or administration of an antagonist. Pseudo-addiction wrongly accuses the patient of abusing the drug. The term pseudo-addiction describes the patient who demonstrates a behavior pattern that may occur when health care professionals undertreat pain resulting in a misinterpretation. Patients with unrelieved pain may
- become focused on obtaining medications,
- seem to present a pattern of drug seeking,
- display an agressive pattern to get access to the opioid,
- display doctor shopping, deception to obtain pain relief.
(for further information see Part V Detection of Illicit Use of Opioids in Primary Care, page 411 ff)

Pseudoaddiction can be distinguished from true addiction in that the behaviors resolve when pain is effectively treated

DEVELOPMENT OF TOLERANCE DURING LONG-TERM USE OF OPIOIDS

Tolerance development during opioid ingestion is characterized by the need to continuously increase the dose for sufficient pain relief. The underlying cause is that the organism has adapted to the drug and in order to achieve the same effect (analgesia), higher doses have to be given. The majority of investigations, where opioids were given for tumor pain however made clear, that proportional to the duration of an opioid therapy there is no necessity for dose adjustment [65] and occasionally the dose could be reduced or in some cases even be completely omitted [10, 66]. Therefore opioids, once they are used solely for the purpose of suppressing intense pain, result in fewer incidence of tolerance development. Moreoften, a necessary dose increase in tumor patients is not due to tolerance development, but rather is based on a progression of the underlying disease, which corresponds with an increase in pain intensity. Development of tolerance to the opioid-related inhibition of motility of the intestine and to miosis, in contrast to the development of tolerance to opioid-induced analgesia, never develops. If, in the process of pain therapy, genuine tolerance becomes evident, it is likely to be due to an adjustment of the organism to a foreign substance. This is accompanied with the necessity to escalating doses in order to achieve sufficient analgesia, and may be due to several possibilities:

1. Psychosocial and environmental factors, whereby the development of tolerance can be regarded as the beginning of a dependency development.
2. A pharmacokinetic dependent mechanism, whereby an insufficient absorption in the intestinal tract, or an interaction with other compounds results in an insufficient plasma level.
3. Metabolic causes, whereby an increase in activity of specific liver enzymes result in an increase of metabolic degradation with a reduced concentration of the pharmacologically active compound. Due to the habituation of the organism to the opioid, an increased metabolic rate results in major degradation, which is mirrored in a loss of efficacy. Then the dose must be sequentially increased in order to achieve a continuous and sufficient analgesic effect.
4. Tolerance development at the cellular and molecular level. Several adaptation processes at the cellular level have to be discussed all of which result in a reduction of the analgesic effect:
   - **Desensitization** of the receptor, which is due to a functional uncoupling of the receptor to its secondary intracellular mediator, the G-protein. Because phosphorilisation of the G-protein, a necessary step for mediation of effects is reduced, lesser amounts of protein kinases, especially the key-player PKC, are formed which results in lesser activation of ion-gated Ca^{++}- and K^+-channels. This process follows immediately within seconds after binding of a ligand to the specific μ-opioid receptor site.
   - **Internalization** of the receptor into the cell, also termed endocytosis. In such instances the receptor sequesters into the cell, thereby not being available any more for additional binding which results in a lesser binding rate and a

reduction in effects. Following internalization, the receptor again is recycled to the cell surface where it will be available for additional binding, a mechanism, which counteracts tolerance development. The process of internalization requires several minutes and it is important to note that internalization has been demonstrated for morphine and fentanyl while buprenorphine demonstrated rapid re-emergence at cell surface [21].

– **Downregulation** of the receptor is the key element in the cellular adaptation process to opioids resulting in long-term tolerance development. In this process the α-unit of the code G-protein in signal transmission is synthesized in lesser amounts by ß-Arrestin 2, resulting in a poorer transmission of all incoming signals. This process takes place within hours, and is most prominent during long-term application of potent opioids. Significance of ß-Arrestin 2 was documented by the fact that elimination of the appropriate gene resulted in a functional lack of ß-Arrestin 2 which was accompanied by a marked increase in analgesia and a significant extension in duration of action [67].

– **Inhibition of gene expresson** within the cell, the gene, which is responsible for the formation of new receptors (transcription) from protein molecules. This process is induced off within days during chronic intake of potent opioids.

– **Increase of protein kinase C (PKC) activity**. The key-player in intracellular phosphorylisation is PKC, which is activated via the second and intracellular mediator G-protein. PKC however in the long run also induces a compensatory activation of the excitatory N-methyl-D-aspartate (NMDA) receptor site. Due to activation of the NMDA-receptor there is an increase in transmembrane Ca^{2+}-Ion transfer (Fig. IV-24) with an ensuing overresponsiveness to all incoming nociceptive afferents (antiopioid effect). Because opioids by themselves do not have any effect on an overactive NMDA-receptor,

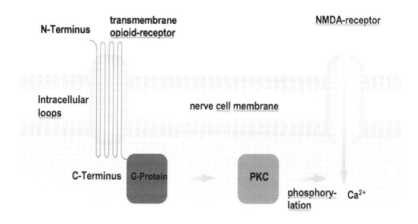

Figure IV-24. The N-methyl-D-aspartate receptor being activated by the long-term use of opioids

additional nonspecific NMDA antagonists such as ketamine, dextromethor-phane or memantine have to be given in order to attenuate this hyperactivity of the excitatory receptor system. Alternatively, methadone can be given, since the opioid by itself has a small but measurable NMDA-antagonistic property.

Tolerance development can be regarded as a self-regulating mechanism of the organism trying to adjust to the new situation in order to achieve homeostasis. Because of this opioid-induced imbalance in pro- and anti-nociceptive activity the organism responds by an increased activation of pro-nociceptive trans-mitters (Fig. IV-25) related to substance P, cholecystokinin (CCK) and NMDA activation.

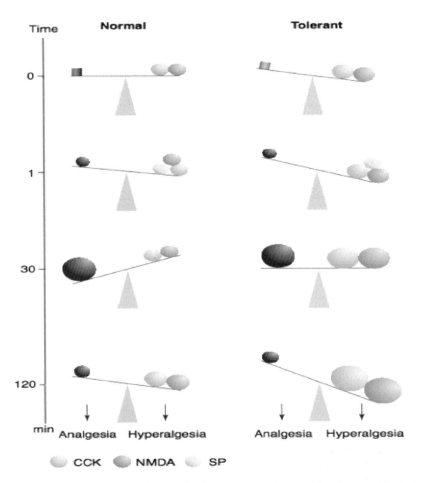

Figure IV-25. In order to balance the equation between pro- and anti-nociceptive transmission, the organism, during opioid ingestion, compensates this imbalance by activation of cholecystokinin (CCK), substance P (SP) and NMDA activation, resulting in tolerance development and the need for higher doses of an opioid. Adapted from [68]

Generally, tolerance development in the context of opioid therapy during chronic pain treatment:

- is more frequently observed in young than in elderly patients,
- is observed more often when short-acting opioids are used for pain therapy resulting in a so called. "roller coaster effect" with breakthrough pain. Therefore, once-a-day opioid intake is better than 4 times a day dosing,
- is particularly seen when opioids with a low intrinsic activity at the μ-receptor are used,
- is observed in individuals who take opioids when no pain is present,
- is likely to develop in patients who repeatedly and/or permanently need a rescue medication for sufficient pain attenuation,
- otherwise is a rare event, which however would be a desirable effect when it comes to respiratory depression, nausea, vomiting and hallucinations,
- more often is caused by a progression in the underlying disease and is not due to a reduced response of the receptor site to the ligand [69],
- usually is not to be expected when oral slow release opioid formulation is used to combat pain.

CONSTIPATION, A COMMON SIDE EFFECT OF OPIOIDS

A recent large US interview-based study ($n = 988$) of both cancer and non-cancer patients revealed that a significant proportion of terminally ill patients prefer not to increase opioid analgesic doses to levels which effectively control their pain, primarily as a result of side effects such as constipation and confusion [70]. Constipation is frequently seen in up to 90% of all patients, particularly when opioids are needed in large quantities. The incidence of constipation, in contrast to the oral opioids, is much smaller when a transdermal therapeutic system such as fentanyl TTS (Duragesic®) or buprenorphine TDS (Butrans®) is used. For instance, in a controlled metaanalysis oral morphine slow release demonstrated a constipation rate of 48% while equianalgesic doses of transdermal fentanyl resulted in an incidence of up to 17% [71]. However, constipation still may present a problem during long term application. This common side effect is related to opioid receptor sites in the intramural plexus of the intestine, the first barrier between the exterior and the interior milieu. There the majority of the immune system (Payer plaques) are located (Fig. IV-26) and binding of opioids results in the inhibition of propulsion.

In order to overcome constipation, a bulk producing laxative and/or a fecal softener is recommended and should be given parallel with the prescription medication. If a regular laxative such as lactulose (Dupholac®) is insufficient, a more aggressive therapy must be initiated using a stimulant laxative such as bisacodyl (Dulcolax®), which acts directly at sensory parasympathetic nerve endings of the colonic mucosa. Since constipation sometimes results in a more difficult task than actual pain therapy [72], with the beginning of any long-term opioid medication for pain therapy a bulk-producing fiber-supplement laxative

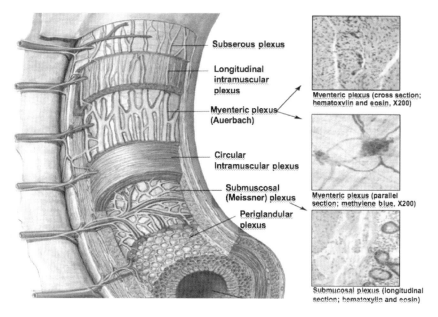

Subserous plexus

Longitudinal
intramuscular
plexus

Myenteric plexus (cross section;
hematoxylin and eosin, X200)

Myenteric plexus
(Auerbach)

Circular
Intramuscular plexus

Submuscosal
(Meissner) plexus

Myenteric plexus (parallel
section; methylene blue, X200)

Periglandular
plexus

Submucosal plexus (longitudinal
section; hematoxylin and eosin)

Figure IV-26. The intestinal mucosa and the different muscle layers where opioids bind to specific receptor sites found in Auerbachs plexus

such as (Metamucil®) should be prescribed, a necessary adjunct to overcome the inhibition of gastrointestinal transit. In addition, a fecal softener (Colace®), a hyperosmolar glycerin agent (MiraLax®, Fleet®Glycerin), a bisacodyl containing preparation (Fleet Biscodyl®) or a mineral oil enema (Fleet Enema ®) can be considered as laxatives. Certain cases of constipation need to be treated more agressively using monobasic sodium phosphate (Fleet®Prep Kit). Presently two peripheral selective opioid antagonists (i.e. methylnaltrexone, alvimopan) are under clinical phase 2 evaluation, which are able to reverse morphine-induced prolongation of gastrointestinal transit without however, antagonising centrally mediated analgesia [73, 74].

NAUSEA AND VOMITING

These side effects are experienced by approximately 40%–60% of all patients, who take potent opioids for pain relief. In the majority of cases these side effects are based on a stimulation of the chemoreceptors in the area postrema of the chemoreceptor trigger zone (CTZ), located within the medulla oblongata. To lesser extent they are due to a reduction in intestinal motility [10]. In general these side effects are only observed in the beginning of an opioid medication, they subside within the following days as there is the development of tolerance. Should nausea and emesis persist, neuroleptic agents such as metoclopramide (Reglan®), prochlorperazine

(Compazine®) or the more potent haloperidol (Haldol®) are agents of choice. The latter agent can be regarded as the most effective therapeutic intervention to overcome these phenomena. In addition, selective serotonin HT_3-inhibitors, which selectively act at the CTZ site, such as ondansetron (Zofran®), dolasetron (Anzemet®) or even a selective Δ^9-cannabinoid dronabinol (Marinol®) may be of benefit. Opioid-related nausea and emesis are seen mostly within the first 2–3 days with the start of medication, thereafter they subside as there is a development of tolerance and the additional medication can be stopped.

MARKED SEDATION

This is another opioid-related side effect, which has an incidence below 5%. It results in reduced vigilance and is a short-lived phenomenon, which subsides after the first days of medication. If, however, the opioid-related fatigue is pronounced, an additional central nervous stimulant such as methylphenidate extended release capsules (Ritalin® LA), dextroamphetamine extended release (Adderall® XR) or the wakefulness-promoting agent modafinil (Provigil®) should be prescribed.

PRURITUS

Although this side effcet is transient in nature, it can be managed with an antihistamine such as diphenhydramine (Benadryl®) or a sedative (prometazine) as needed.

Rotation from One Opioid to Another

Therapy of chronic pain, according to present recommendations, advocates the principle of the analgesic ladder. With this principle in mind, chronic pain first is treated by a peripheral analgesic. If this medication is not suffficient for relief, no time should be lost and a weak opioid, which later can be replaced by a more potent compound should be used. By doing so, one has to realize that different opioids interact with different receptors, and that a combination of a pure μ-ligand with a mixed agonist/antagonist, also in long-term pain therapy, is considered a major pharmacological mistake. This is because any simultaneous administration of a mixed class opioid with a pure agonist results in the displacement of the pure μ-ligand at the receptor site, resulting in a decrease of the analgesic effect. If the patient receives an agonist/antagonist for pain therapy (e.g. pentazocine, butorphanol), a more potent opioid with selective μ-characteristics (e.g. morphine), will not work accordingly and only after a wash-out phase, the new opioid is administered. During this time pain therapy is maintained by peripheral analgesics using derivatives from the class of non-steroidal antiinflammatory drugs (NSAIDs), which mediate their mode of action through inhibition of cyclooxygenase synthesis (COX-1, 2-inhibitors). Only after the elimination phase of the mixed agonist/antagonist, which may differ from one product to the other, slow titration with the new opioid

Table IV-13. Conversion from an oral opioid (24 mg/h) to the transdermal buprenorphine patch (μg/h)

TranstecPro® $\mu g/h$	33	52.5	70	87.5	105	122.5	140
Tramadol	150/300	450	600				
Morphine oral	30/60	90	120	150	180	210	240
Oxycodone oral	30		60		90		120
Hydromorphone oral	4/8	12	16	20	24	28	32
Fentanyl TTS (μg/h)	2.5		50		75		100
Buprenorphine sublingual	0.4/0.8	1.2	1.6	2.0	2.4	2.8	3.2

is initiated (Table IV-13). For such purposes a slow release medication such as Oxycontin® SR presents several advantages as it is as effective as immmediate release oxycodone. The agent has to be given only twice a day compared to 4 times daily. It presents a lesser incidence in side effects such as nausea, vomiting, somnolence and dizziness all of which result in a better compliance of patients [75].

OPIOID ROTATION FROM MORPHINE TO BUPRENORPHINE OR METHADONE

Contrary to mixed agonist/antagonists the partial μ-agonist and κ-antagonist buprenorphine due to its small number in receptors being occupied and the simultaneous high μ-affinity, still has significant receptor reserve. Pure μ-agonists such as morphine, fentanyl TTS or oxycodone can be added without any problems. The same holds true if the physician wants to convert from a pure μ-agonist morphine, hydromorphone or oxycodone to buprenorphine TTS (Transtec®), the transdermal form of the partial agonist which can be used for pain treatment. The following table can be applied for rotation, whereby certain patients need an individual lower dose than the calculated equivalent (Table IV-13).

On the other hand methadone represents a cost-effective alternative to oral morphine or transdermal fentanyl TTS, in particular when using its enantiomer levomethadone. This opioid especially is indicated, when tolerance development to the present opioid medication becomes obvious, a neuropathic pain component is present in the patient, and where high dosages of first-line opioids do not result in sufficient pain relief [76, 77, 78]. The rational for the use of methadone stems from the fact that this opioid also inhibits a NMDA-antagonistic profile and acts as a serotonin reuptake inhibitor [79, 80, 81]. Due to its special pharmacokinetic feature, characterized by a long elimation half-life, after a basic dose, the following doses are adjusted to effect. The following procedure is advocated when changing another opioid to methadone:

Day 1: The morphine dose is stopped and independent of the previous opioid dose, methadone 5.0–10.0 mg orally is given every 4 h.

Day 2: When pain is not sufficiently attenuated, the dose of methadone is increased by 30% every 4 h. When necessary, additional medication is given every hour until side effects of overdose become obvious.

Day 3: After 72 h the application interval is prolonged to 8 h. Any additional medication is similar to the single dose given every 3 h.

Day 4: In case of insufficient pain relief the dose of methadone is increased further by 30% given every 8 h. Requirement medication is similar to the single dose, every 3 h until sufficient pain relief or side effects become apparent.

OXYCODONE AND HYDROMORPHONE – ALTERNATIVE OPIOIDS FOR PAIN RELIEF

Although morphine is considered a reference agent for therapy with opioids, it does not denote that this is the drug of first choice when treating pain. Because of the metabolites of morphine, i.e. morphine-6-glucuronide, which is produced between 4.7% and 11%, and of morphine-3-glucuronide, which accumulates between 57% and 74%, there is a reduction in efficacy (Fig. IV-27). Such decrease in analgesic potency cannot be explained solely by the elimination half-life which is longer than the parent compound morphine.

Decrease in analgesia during long-term application of morphine is explained by the accumulation of the metabolites, which results in toxic excitatory effect (Fig. IV-28). This in particular applies to elderly patients, who typically show a reduction in kidney function with reduced elimination resulting in an accumulation of the two metabolites and an increase in side effects. Thus morphine-3-glucuronide can induce agitation, myoclonia, and hyperalgesia which may end up in somnolence and even seizures [81, 82], and after morphine-6-glucuronide miosis, sweating, nausea and vomiting as well as opioid intoxication may be observed as this metabolite has a higher affinity to the binding site [83, 84].

When using morphine for pain therapy and when marked side effects are observed in the patient, one should consider rotation to another opioid. In such instances it is rational rotating to a more potent compound such as oxycodone, which does not result in pharmacologically active metabolites or to an opioid with a higher receptor specificity like hydromorphone, fentanyl or buprenorphine. Due to this higher receptor specificity there is more selective binding of μ-ligands with lesser side-effect, findings which are corroborated by Pasternak and coworkers in genetically transmutagenic mice, who demonstrated the existance of at least a dozen different μ-receptor isoforms [85]. The change to a different opioid such as the controlled release form of oxycodone (OxyContin®SR), hydromorphone (Palladone®SR), or transdermal fentanyl and buprenorphine respectively is of practical importance, because these agents inherit the following favorable characteristics:

1. Oxycodone has a small first-pass effect through the liver; and after oral intake 84% of the actual dose is available for the mediation of effects (high bioavailability). This also holds true for hydromorphone, which contrary to morphine, after oral ingestion has a bioavailability of up to 36.4%.

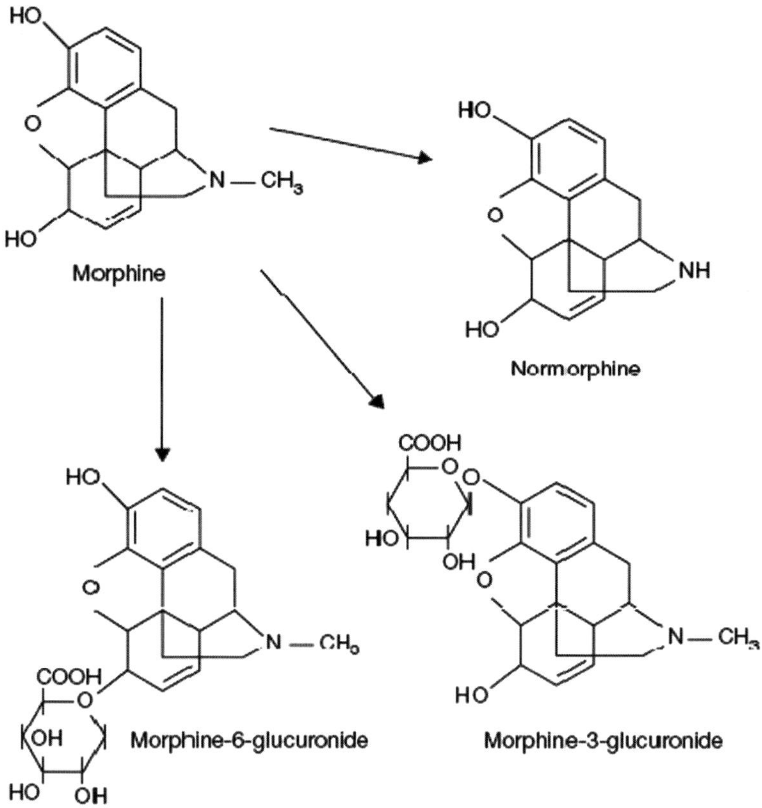

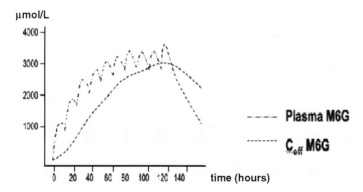

Figure IV-27. The major metabolites of morphine, which are the cause for often observed side-effects during long-term morphine treatment

Figure IV-28. Due to the active renal clearance of morphine metabolites, there is an accumulation in the elderly especially when morphine is given over a longer period of time, as they demonstrate an age-related reduction in renal clearance

2. Oxycodone in addition to hydromorphone, does not result in the formation of pharmacologically active metabolites. This is in sharp contrast to morphine where metabolites like morphine-3- and morphine-6-glucuronide are formed. Such difference is of particular importance in patients with limited liver and/or kidney function which otherwise would result in an accumulation of metabolites with an ensuing state of confusion (Fig. IV-28).

3. The metabolites of oxycodone are oxymorphone and noroxycodone, which are only formed by 10%. Such a low concentrations result in clinically lesser side-effects. During hydromorphone the majority of the compound is metabolised by 39% to the pharmacologically inactive hydromorphone-3-glucuronide, which primarily is eliminated via the kidneys.

4. For the metabolites of oxycodone, oxymorphone and noroxycodone, there is an elimination which parallels a decline in plasma levels of the mother compound; it therefore does not result in an accumulation of metabolites.

5. Oxycodone and hydromorphone, in regard to their analgesic potency, do not show a ceiling-effect. The dose of the opioid can be increased whenever necessary and as the dose is increased, in each case this is followed by an increase in effect.

6. Oxycodone and hydromorphone in regard to the central nervous system, are characterized by fewer side effects. This in particular applies when comparing both compounds with morphine, where hallucination, sedation and tiredness often can be observed.

7. Controlled release oxycodone achieves a maximal analgesic effect within 1 h; this is in complete contrast to controlled release morphine, where a time period of up to 3–4 h is necessary for maximum effect. When using controlled release hydromorphone, the maximum analgesic effect is to be expected after 2.5 h.

8. Unlike morphine, oxycodone and hydromorphone do not possess a negative stigma. Due to the association of morphine and dependency development many patients are still afraid to use opioids on a regular scale and in sufficient amounts.

9. Oxycodone and hydromorphone are pure μ-agonists with very little affinity to the κ-receptor. This is in contrast to buprenorphine, which is a partial μ-agonist and κ-antagonist, and specifically is in contrast to morphine which interacts with several μ-isoreceptors. This presumption could be demonstrated in receptor binding studies where the metabolite of morphine, morphine-6-glucuronide demonstrated selective interaction with its own distinct receptor, which is responsible in the mediation of excitatory effects [86].

10. Oxycodone similar to hydromorphone induces a lesser constipating effect when compared to morphine.

11. When using oxycodone there is a much faster equilibrium of dose and desirable effect. This is particularly true for the onset of a maximum effect, which takes much longer when controlled release morphine (MS Contin®) is used and is of substantial advantage in patients with pain.

12. Oxycodone, fentanyl and buprenorphine are also suitable for therapy of neuropathic pain, which usuallly is characterized by opioid resistancy.

13. The conversion factor of oral morphine to controlled release oral oxycodone shows a ratio of 2:1. If, however, the patient is first treated with oxycodone (opioid-naïve), it is advised to start with a lower dose in order to subsequently adapt to the next higher concentration. This course of action is only possible because the maximum effect of oxycodone can be judged within 1 h.

14. The conversion ratio of oral morphine to oral controlled release hydromorphone is 7.5:1. If however, the patient is first treated with hydromorphone (opioid-naïve), it is advisable to start with the lowest concentration of hydromorphone and adapt to the next higher dose only when necessary.

15. If opioid therapy should no longer be necessary, a patient on a daily dose of 20–60 mg of controlled release oxycodone can be withdrawn immediately. Tapering down of the dose however is necessary in patients with daily doses higher than 60 mg.

16. When performing opioid rotation it has to be emphasized that the usual conversion scales, which are available for computation, because of the large inter-individual variability should only be used as a rough estimate. When changing from morphine to hydromorphone or rotating from morphine to fentanyl TTS or buprenorphine TDS, it is conceivable that dose equivalency is only in one and not into both directions. Thus, when transferring oxycodone to morphine it does not correspond to the same dose relations when transferring from morphine to oxycodone. Therefore one should start with a low dose and quickly titrate up to the desired effect, which in the case with controlled release oxycodone can be achieved much faster as maximum receptor occupancy is reached within 1 h.

17. Because of pharmacologically inactive metabolites of hydromorphone, this agent particularly is indicated in pain therapy of the elderly patient.

18. Since elderly patients with chronic pain regularly demonstrate a reduction in kidney clearance, hydromorphone and buprenorphine offer several advantages as they are primarily metabolized by the liver and eliminated via the bile. Thus, serious side effects induced by the previous medication with morphine (i.e. dizziness, confusion, profound sedation, nausea) can be reduced by 80% [112] .

19. Because of functional impairment of liver activity in the elderly, one should start with half the usual recommended dose of oxycodone or hydromorphone.

20. In the elderly, multimorbid and cachectic patient with low plasma protein level, hydromorphone has attained special attention, because this compound demonstrates a low protein binding of only 8%. This is in marked contrast to fentanyl, which has a plasma protein binding of 90% and of buprenorphine with a binding capacity of 96% [38].

In summary, when changing from morphine to oxycodone, hydromorphone, or buprenorphine the following points have to be considered:

1. Start with the lowest dose of the opioid to switch to.
2. Rapidly titrate up to the desired effect for achieving a sufficient analgesia.

3. Generally, always switch to a more potent opioid with higher affinity for the opioid receptor. This particularly refers to morphine which is an opioid with little selectivity. Thus μ-opioid receptor mediated analgesia is less selective and specific than opioids with higher selectivity (e.g. oxycodone, hydromorphone, fentanyl buprenorphine) which are more suitable for rotation [115].
4. Do not rely on the equivalent doses derived from conversion scales.
5. When converting from morphine to oxycodone or hydromorphone, a stable analgesic effect only can be expected after 2 weeks. This is due to the time to excrete all active metabolites of morphine, such as morphine-6- and morphine-3-glucuronide. The higher potency of oxycodone in comparison to morphine seems to be based on the higher interaction of oxycodone at the κ-receptor with lower intrinsic activity at the μ-receptor [87]. Also hydromorphone, fentanyl and buprenorphine display a higher affinity to the μ- with lesser κ-receptor interaction than morphine, which results in a higher analgesic potency [115].

In the context of opioid therapy for chronic pain treatment, the following considrations have to be recognized:

- It is of no advantage to give 2 weak and two potent opioids at the same time.
- A weak opioid can only be added to a more potent opioid, once there are episodes of pain increase such as in breakthrough pain.
- Generally the patient should be instructed to add an additional fast release dose of the regular medication once there is breakthrough pain.
- Short-lasting opioids, such as pentazocine or pethidine (meperidine, USP) should be avoided, because the dosing interval is too short.
- Simultaneous and/or sequential ingestion of an agonist/antagonist (e.g., pentazocine, nalbuphine, dezocine) with a pure agonist (e.g., codeine, morphine) must be avoided. However, simultaneous administration of the partial μ-agonist, κ-antagonist buprenorphine (Buprenex®) with morphine, due to its special receptor kinetics, is possible since this compound does not replace the previous one.
- An opioid should be given in regular time-intervals; the latter depends on the duration of action of the specific opioid.
- If there is an insufficient analgesic effect, with a sufficient duration of action, an increase in the dose is required.
- If there is a sufficient effect in potency, but a reduced duration of action, a reduction in dosing interval is required. In order to avoid such a setting, controlled release opioids with longer dosing intervals of up to 12 and 24 h, or a transdermal opioid system (e.g. Duragesic®, TranstecPro®) should be prescribed. Both have a duration of up to 72 and 92 h/patch, respectively.
- Selection of the type of opioid depends on the intensity of pain. The latter is evaluated using pain rating scales such as the numeric pain intensity or the visual analogue scale (VAS) where $0 =$ no pain and $10 =$ worst possible pain. If VAS is between 1 and 4 one should start with a non-opioid. If pain intensity is higher, (VAS between 5 and 6) a contolled release opioid with medium

potency such as codeine, dihydrocodeine or tramadol is indicated. In such cases an active compound such as transdermal buprenorphine (TranstecPro®) may also be used because this substance in a reduced dose is sufficient for producing analgesia.

- A transdermal mode of administration should be considered if non-opioid analgesics are no longer effective. In cases with very intense pain (VAS 7–10), one should immediately start with an opioid of Level 3 in the WHO ladder (morphine, oxycodone, hydromorphone, fentanyl TTS or buprenorphine TTS).
- Rapidly titrate the dose of the opioids upwards to a point of sufficient pain relief.
- Together with the opioid, prescription of a laxative such as a fecal softener (Colace®), a hyperosmolar glycerin agent (MiraLax®, Fleet®Glycerin), a mineral oil enema (Fleet Enema ®) or a bisacodyl containing preparation (Fleet Biscodyl®) is mandatory.
- In the presence of neuropathic pain (pain due to chemotherapy, post radiotherapy pain, post surgical pain, plexopathy, paraneoplastic, radiculitis, post herpetic neuralgia, peripheral neuropathy of diabetic origin) additional medication which interacts at the NMDA-receptor (memantine, dextromethorphane, ketamine) or alternatively an antiepileptic of the second generation (gabapentin, lamotrigine, topiramate) and/or an antidepressive of the NASSA group (noradrenergic and specifically serotonergic antidepressant) like mirtazapine, and to a lesser degree a tricyclic antidepressant of the SSRI group (selective serotonin reuptake inhibitors) should be considered. Because of its simultaneous NMDA-antagonistic efficacy [116] the opioid methadone (Dolophine®) presents an alternative.
- When side-effects such as emesis are dominant, potent antiemetics such as low doses of a neuroleptic (Haldol® 0.5–1 mg) every 6–8 h or ondansetron (Zofran® 4 mg) are given.
- When marked sedation is troubling, the patient should receive an analeptic like dextroamphetamine, methylphenidate or modafinil.
- Additional corticosteroids are indicated in acute nerve compression, an increased intracranial pressure, anorexia, infiltration of soft tissue, distention of visceral organs and mood changes.
- When metastases of the bone are evident, biphosphonates are indicated.
- For break-through pain, the patient additionally receives fast release opioids, whereby the dose of the opioids is 5%–15% the entire daily opioid dose. The dosing interval should be long enough in order to take full effect. In case of controlled release morphine a liquid morphine solution, in case of trans-dermal fentanyl (Duragesic®) the oral transmucosal fentanyl citrate stick (OTFC; Actiq®), in case of transdermal buprenorphine (TranstecPro®) a buccal buprenor-phine tablet is administered.
- When oral therapy with opioids is insufficient or when side effects are dominant, change to another opioid (opioid rotation) is indicated. In certain cases change to methadone may be appropriate because the drug additionally blocks the NMDA-receptor and in addition results in a presynaptic inhibition of serotonine reuptake which results in potentiation of the analgesic effects [117].

- Once the patient is transferred to another opioid, in general the dose of the new opioids is reduced by 30%–50%. This is followed by titration of doses to the desired effect.
- As pure μ-ligands do not show a ceiling effect the dosage can be increased, titrating to a point of sufficient pain relief or side effects are not tolerated any more.

In extreme tumor-related pain, which cannot be controlled with the usual opioid medication, some authors (Bowlder, Mountain Seler, 1984, personnel communication) recommend a morphine-haloperidol-mixture given every 4 h. For preparation, use 5 ml of distilled water, and add 10–40 mg of morphine together with 0.25 mg of haloperidol.

As an ULTAMA RATIO epidural opioids via an external or internal pump, combined with a local anesthetic or an α_2-agonist like clonidine is possible. This is a final therapeutic option, whereby regional pain therapy is initiated by means of opioid receptor binding localized in the dorsal horn of the spinal cord (Fig. IV-29).

Compared to systemically applied opioids, peridural opioids result in lesser side effects since the dose can be reduced. Administered at an interval every 12–15 h, either morphine 3–5 mg or buprenorphine 0.15–0.3 mg diluted in 10–20 ml of 0.9% saline are injected as a "single shot" peridural injection. By a using a motor-driven pump, continuous peridural (0.2 mg/h of morphine or 0.018 mg/h of buprenorphine) opioid application, after a bolus application is possible. In neuropathic pain and in exercise-induced pain, the sole neuraxial application of an

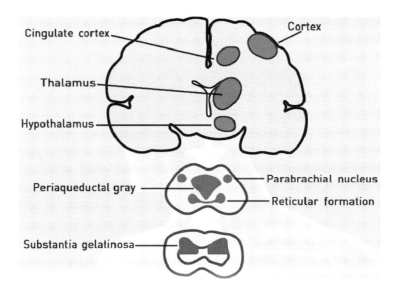

Figure IV-29. Parts of the central nervous system, which show an accumulation of opioid binding sites. Note, opioid receptors are also located in the substantia gelatinosa of the spinal cord where neuraxial opioids exert their analgesic action via blockade of nociceptive afferents. Adapted from [88]

opioid often is insufficient. In such cases, the combined application of an opioid together with a local anesthetic, with the α_2-agonist clonidine ($20\,\mu g/h$), or with the unspecific NMDA-antagonist like ketamine (0.1–0.5 mg/kg/day) significantly improves the attenuation of pain. For conversion from an oral to the intrathecal dose, on the first day of the neuroaxial application, 1/50 of the last daily oral opioid dose is administered while at the same time the oral dose is reduced by 50%. A neuroaxial dose (25%) is given initially, while the remaining quantity is infused over the whole day. Oral rescue medication should always be available where approximately 5% of the current total quantity of the opioid is given for breakthrough pain.

Preliminary clinical data suggest a pain-modulating effect of adenosine at the adenosine-A_1-receptor at the spinal cord. Also, neostigmine when given in combination with an neuraxial opioid, has demonstrated a significant opioid-sparing effect, which is due to an increase of intrathecal acetylcholine concentration. Larger clinical studies with both compounds are still pending.

Use of Opioids in Non-malignant Pain

Treatment with an opioid in nonmalignant pain of noncancer origin (i.e., pain due to rheumatic disorders, pain in chronic degenerative osteoarthritis) still is judged controversial [89–92]. While in acute pain states and in cancer pain, pathophysiology and assessment are better understood, and the use of opioids are a well-accepted standard of care. Presently there is no consensus regarding treatment modalities or the role of opioid analgesics for the treatment of patients who suffer from pain of nonmalignant origin. It generally is accepted however, that opioid therapy for nonmalignant pain is indicated if all other conventional, established pain-related interventions have failed. If this is the case, similar as in cancer-related pain therapy, opioid therapy in nonmalignant pain is characterized by the following:

- pain medication is given in a fixed time pattern (dosing by the clock);
- continuous surveillance in order to adjust the medication by either an increase or by a reduction of the dose;
- need for an opioid is derived from pain intensity and not the diagnosis;
- at start of the therapy, an opioid of low to medium potency is selected;
- opioid therapy is embedded into a parallel medication with other non-opioid analgesics;
- simultaneously with opioid therapy start the prophylactic medication for constipation;
- when considering opioids for chronic nonmalignant pain, rather than short-acting agents, long-acting formulations are recommended.

The latter is of major importance as short-acting opioids encourage a pattern of frequent dosing that increases the risk of both tolerance and abuse, while long-acting opioids are less likely to provide euphoric effects.

In chronic non-malignant pain it is necessary to evaluate whether a psychosomatic origin is not the crucial determinant for chronification. It therefore is necessary to exclude any type of psychosomatic pain from opioid therapy, since such patients are not appropriate candidates for opioid therapy since they demonstrate a potential development of tolerance, dependency, the illicit use and misadventure. Development of psychoreactive pain has to be assumed whenever the patient describes his/her pain syndrome while consulting family members, describing his/her complaints, and where a morphologic substrate is not or ever was present. The following points have to be recognized in chronic non-malignant pain in order to reason the use of opioid therapy:

1. Search for the cause of pain of non-malignant origin.
2. Previous unsuccessful conventional pain therapy using NSAIDs, COX-2 inhibitors or TCAs.
3. The otherwise therapy-resistant pain due to a benign disease.
4. Intense pain associated with degenerative joint disease.

Only when all prerequisites for opioid therapy in nonmalignant pain are fulfilled, then the risk for the development of abuse and dependency is practically non existent.

In summary, opioids in nonmalignant pain are only indicated when patients present a psychosocial stable environment and where previous treatment was ineffective. Just as pharmacological pain control will have limited benefits if it is not combined with a rehabilitation program, the opioid is likely to be ineffective, if pain interferes with compliance [93]. Pain-related non-malignant pathologies that possibly can result in the relief by an opioid are:

1. Severe osteoarthritis (OA) and cartilage distruction
2. Severe rheumatoid arthritis (RA)
3. Exessive generalized osteoporosis
4. Stenosis of the spinal canal
5. Degenerative disease of the vertebral column
6. Phantom limb pain
7. Central pain syndrome following stroke (thalamic mediated pain)
8. Postnucleotomy syndrome following failed back surgery
9. Postherpetic neuralgia (PHN)
10. Neuropathic pain when combined with co-analgesics

Opioids however, are contraindicated in patients with the following non-malignant pain-related conditions:

1. Trigeminal neuralgia
2. Migraine or chronic tension type headache
3. Functional intestinal pain
4. Functional urogenital pain
5. Crohn's disease
6. History of substances abuse
7. The patient with psychogenic or somatotopic pain
8. Absence of psychosocial stability of the patient
9. Insufficient control of effectiveness by the prescribing physician
10. The patient not signing an informed consent

Driving Ability While Taking an Opioid for Pain Relief

Opioids besides causing constipation also induce somnolence, hallucination and dizziness, side-effects which interfere with attention, vigilance and reaction time. In general therefore patients taking opioids for the relief of chronic pain should avoid driving a vehicle as there is a higher potential of driving accidents.

Since however, reaction of patients to an opioid shows a substantial individual variability, restriction of a driving permit really depends on the individual capability. It therefore is only reasonable to question the restriction of driving. Several studies have demonstrated that some patients taking opioids on a regular basis, in a driving simulator demonsterated an even better reaction time when compared to an opioid-free subject [118]. From such data it can be concluded that any opioid intake does not necessarily result in a reduction in the efficiency to perform complex sensomotoric tasks. Because of the large individual variability and the non-uniform data from previous studies, it can be concluded that the ability to drive in traffic must be judged individually in every patient taking an opioid for chronic pain treatment.

Since the ability to continue driving is very important to maintaining the quality of life of many patients with advanced cancer, and, although one may assume that they must stop driving while taking regular potent opioid analgesics, this is not necessarily so. The usual advice to patients is that they should not drive or engage in other skilled activities such as operating machinery when they first start on morphine or a similar opioid, or when they increase the dose. However, once the initial sedative effects have resolved and both the patient and physician are confident that cognitive and psychomotor performance are no longer impaired, driving and other similar activities may restart. This advice is based to a large extent on empirical experience and there have been few objective data to substantiate it. However, recent studies confirm, perhaps surprisingly, that morphine produces little measurable impairment of cognitive and psychomotor function [94], particularly in patients receiving continuous treatment with stable doses [95]. In one study, which used a battery of performance tests designed specifically to assess functions related to driving ability, chronic morphine use was associated with slower reaction times, more mistakes, and a slowing in ability to process visual information and perform motor sequences, but these changes were not statistically significant compared with a control group of cancer patients not taking morphine [96]. These data support the clinical impression that stable doses of morphine are unlikely to cause substantial impairment of the psychomotor skills required for driving, and allow us to continue to advise patients to this effect.

The following recommendations are given, whenever a patient taking an opioid for pain therapy wants to drive a vehicle [119]:

1. It is the duty of the physician who prescribes the analgesic to inform the patients on possible traffic-relevant side effects of an opioid therapy.

2. The patient should sign a written statement reflecting the type and the scope of the information with a counter signature of a witness.
3. The patient should undergo a critical self-evaluation.
4. The patient should receive a special opioid identity card, which shows the type of medication.

Apart from the documentation it is mandatory that the physician clarifies that driving is not indicated when the patient:

- is in the beginning or midst an adjustment phase of opioid therapy,
- is in need of dose correction (increase or reduction),
- presently is changing the type of the opioid medication,
- independent of opioid therapy, demonstrates signs of malnutrition,
- does not have a stable pain scale,
- does not show an effective reduction in pain intensity,
- in addition takes CNS active medication and/or alcohol.

If in doubt there is the possibility of a neutral check-up or test by the Department of Motor Vehicles or a similar independent institution. When using an opioid for non-malignant pain, control of progress with written documentation is mandatory. It should be pointed out that patients with chronic pain in addition should not be punished by revoking their driving license. And similarly in patients who regularly take an antihypertensive medication or are on an oral antidiabetic therapy but participate in the street traffic without restriction, it is only logical to increase quality of life in chronic pain patients being on a stable opioid medication.

In summary epidemiologic evidence indicates opioids are probably *not* associated with intoxicated driving, motor vehicle accidents fatalities, or motor vehicle accidents. This supports the contention that patients taking opioids may be allowed to drive. Determination should be individualized according to clinical factors, and stable opioid doses are *not* associated with impaired psychomotor/cognitive performance when evaluating driving performance.

New Options in Opioid Medication – The OROS® (Oral Osmotic Pump) System

OROS® technology employs osmosis to provide precise, controlled drug delivery for up to 24 h and can be used with a range of compounds, including poorly soluble or highly soluble drugs. OROS® technology can be used to deliver high drug doses meeting high drug loading requirements. ALZA's L-OROS™ technology, adapted for liquid formulations, can enhance the bioavailability of drugs with low solubility. This technique has several advantages:

1. Enhanced Bioavailablity: By targeting specific areas of the gastrointestinal tract, OROS® technology may provide more efficient drug absorption and enhanced bioavailability. L-OROS® technology can also enhance the bioavailability of drugs with low solubility.

2. Patterned Delivery: For many drugs, zero-order is not the optimal delivery profile. OROS® can be tailored to meet patterned delivery profiles to optimize a drug's therapeutic efficacy.
3. Reduced Variability: The osmotic driving force of OROS® and protection of the drug until the time of release eliminate the variability of drug absorption and metabolism often caused by gastric pH and motility. OROS® technology employs osmosis to provide precise, controlled drug delivery for up to 24 h and can be used with a range of compounds, including poorly soluble or highly soluble drugs. OROS® technology can be used to deliver high drug doses meeting high drug loading requirements. ALZA's OROS™ technology, adapted for liquid formulations, can enhance the bioavailability of drugs with low solubility.

The new Oros®-system combines both, a fast release of the agent hydromorphone from a tablet for dose-finding and the slow continuous liberation of the opioid for continuous plasma levels (Figure IV-30). Since hydromorphone shows little plasma binding, and is metabolized in only small amounts by the cytochrome-P450-system, clinically active metabolites are not present. Because of the continuous and steady release of the active agent within the gut, there is an effective 24 h duration of action resulting in the need of only one tablet per day. Due to such constant and reliable release, there is:

- a larger patient compliance,
- a natural 24 cycle for intake
- a steady and long duration of analgesia
- a stable plasma level for 24 h.

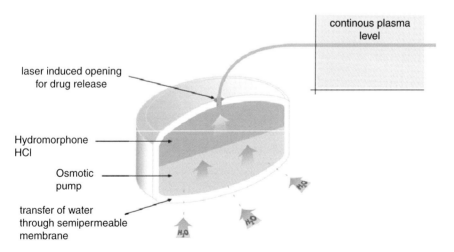

Figure IV-30. Schematic drawing of the mode of action of the osmotic active system Oros® where water migrates through a semipermeable membrane into the tablet resulting in the expansion of a osmotic pump. This leads to a continuous and steady ejection of hydromorphone through a microscopic hole within, out into the gut for reabsorption

The Oros® technology using the prolonged release tablets (Hydromorphone HCl), has has recently been marketed under the brand name Jurnista™. As a new prescription treatment for severe pain it has successfully completed the Mutual Recognition Procedure in Austria, Czech Republic, Estonia, Finland, Germany, Hungary, Italy, Latvia, Lithuania, Norway, Portugal, Slovak Republic, Slovenia and Spain. The countries mutually agreed to recognise the approval of Jurnista™ prolonged-release tablets (Hydromorphone HCl) by the Reference Member State, Denmark. The Hydromorphone HCl prolonged-release tablet was originally developed by ALZA Corporation and utilizes the OROS® Push-Pull delivery system to release the opioid hydromorphone at a consistent rate. It will be registered and marketed by Janssen-Cilag companies in Europe.

As with all opioid analgesics, hydromorphone exerts its pharmacological effects by binding to specific opioid receptors predominantly located on the Central Nervous System (CNS) and smooth muscle. Following oral dosing of Jurnista™ prolonged-release tablets, plasma concentrations reach a broad, relatively flat plateau region within 6–8 h post-dose and remain in this plateau region until approximately 24 h post-dose. This demonstrates that, as intended, hydromorphone is released in a consistent manner from the dosage form, with drug absorption continuing throughout the intestinal tract for approximately 24 h, consistent with once-daily dosing. Jurnista™ is available in four dosage strengths: 8 mg, 16 mg, 32 mg and 64 mg prolonged-released tablets.

When switching from another opioid medication to the Oros®-system, the following conversion guide can be used in order to facilitate the change (Figure IV-31).

In clinical trials with Jurnista™ prolonged-release tablets (Hydromorphone HCl), the most commonly reported adverse reactions are constipation, nausea and

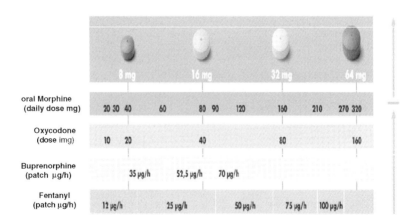

Figure IV-31. Conversion table for switching from an opioid to the Oros-technology based hydromorphone

vomiting. They can usually be managed by dose reduction, laxatives or antiemetics as appropriate.

Oxytrex™ Ultra-Low Dose Opioid Antagonist Combined with Oxycodone with Less Tolerance Development

Oxytrex™ contains a combination of oxycodone, an opioid agonist, and an ultra-low dose of naltrexone, an opioid antagonist. In the brain, opioid drugs usually inhibit the transmission of signals from neuron to neuron. However, with chronic use, the brain adapts to opioids, and the signals switch from being predominantly inhibitory to predominantly excitatory. This results in tolerance, or patients needing escalating doses of opioids to mask pain. Moreover, even when the pain stops, the brain continues to desire opioids, a process called physical dependence. Patients must endure unpleasant withdrawal symptoms to free themselves of the adverse effects of opiates.

Researchers at Albert Einstein College of Medicine discovered that combining an ultra-low dose of the opioid antagonist naltrexone with an opioid agonist prevents the physiological switch from the inhibitory to excitatory state. In general, opioid antagonists reverse the actions of opioid agonists. But it's all about the dose, at high doses, an antagonist and agonist do counteract each other, but at ultra-low doses an opioid antagonist actually turbo-charges the performance of the opioid agonist. This basic academic insight was translated by Pain Therapeutics Inc. into a novel opioid painkiller called Oxytrex™.

Opioid receptor excitatory signaling has long been associated with chronic opioid treatment [97]. Ultra-low-dose naloxone or naltrexone prevents this excitatory signaling and the associated opioid tolerance and dependence [97, 98]. It has been demonstrated that the excitatory signaling of opioid receptors underlying opioid tolerance and dependence is mediated by a G-protein coupling switch from Gi/o to Gs and that ultra-low-dose naloxone prevents this switch [98].

The research is based on the relatively new finding that mammals have two opioid receptor pathways. In addition to the inhibitory pathway that results in analgesia, there is also an excitatory pathway that, when stimulated, weakens analgesia, mediates side effects, and contributes to the development of tolerance and addiction. In vitro data have shown that chronic morphine exposure in Kreb's Ringer-incubated brain slices in morphine-treated slices results in a Go to Gs coupling switch that was blocked by co-treatment with ultra-low-dose naltrexone. Since a G-protein subunit Go is known to inhibit adenylyl cyclase and Gs is known to stimulate this enzyme, the chronic morphine-induced switch in morphine G-protein coupling switch from Go to Gs that was previously demonstrated in striatal tissue from chronic morphine-treated rats has been demonstrated in organotypic striatal slice cultures treated twice daily for 7 days. As seen in the in vivo treatment paradigm, ultra-low-dose naltrexone co-treatment attenuated the G-protein coupling switch that occurred following repeated morphine exposure to striatal slices. Measures of cAMP accumulation showed that the Gs protein, likely via both the α subunit and βγ dimer, is indeed stimulating adenylyl cyclase. These data suggested that the effect of ultra-low-dose naltrexone is a direct effect and not a consequence of altered morphine metabolism or of enhanced CNS access for morphine. Further, these data provided an additional system in which to probe the effects of ultra-low-dose opioid antagonists combined with an opioid agonist. Oxytrex™ (oxycodone + ultra-low-dose naltrexone) is one such example and has been shown to enhance opioid analgesia [99] and to decrease opioid dependence [100]. The mechanism of action of ultra-low-dose opioid antagonists in combination with opiates is thought to be a prevention of such excitatory signaling of opioid receptors. Specifically, ultra-low-dose opioid antagonists prevent a switch from Go- to Gs-protein coupling that has been shown to occur during chronic opiate administration and is thought to contribute to opioid tolerance [98, 101]. Especially, there are multiple signaling consequences of the switch to Gs coupling by MORs chronically exposed to opioids, and each may contribute differently to the various behavioral effects of long-term opioid administration such as analgesic tolerance, physical dependence, and the possibility of addiction [102]. Crain and Shen first demonstrated that opiates can produce excitatory as well as inhibitory effects by measuring action potential durations in electrophysiological recordings from mouse dorsal root ganglion neurons in vitro [97]. They observed that the excitatory effect (a prolongation instead of a shortening of the action potential) could be blocked by cholera toxin, an agent that blocks activation of the excitatory G-protein Gs. They therefore hypothesized that the excitatory effects of opiates were mediated by opioid receptors coupling to Gs instead of their usual inhibitory G-proteins, Gi and Go. The research of Crain and Shen also suggested that the excitatory signaling of opioid receptors underlies opioid tolerance and is regulated by GM1 ganglioside, since GM1 ganglioside administration essentially mimicks opioid tolerance [103]. The role of excitatory signaling of opioid receptors in tolerance was more explicitly demonstrated when Crain and Shen discovered that ultra-low-dose opioid antagonists prevented both the excitatory effects in vitro and opioid tolerance and dependence in vivo [101, 104]. Such paradoxical effects of opioid antagonists on pain sensitivity are thought to result from a bimodal G protein-coupled μ-opioid receptor. Its activity produces excitatory effects in response to ultra-low doses of agonist and inhibitory effects in response to high doses [97]. These excitatory and inhibitory effects are blocked (Fig. IV-32) by ultra-low (picomolar to nanomolar) and low (micromolar) doses of opioid antagonists, respectively [101].

Based on these preclinical data, Oxytrex™ a novel, next-generation painkiller is being developed exclusively by Pain Therapeutics Inc. for the treatment of severe chronic pain using oxycodone and naltrexone. Believing that Oxytrex™ provides strong pain relief and less physical dependence than currently marketed opioid painkillers, Oxytrex™ formulation combines an ultra-low-dose opioid antagonist naltrexone, with an opioid agonist, oxycodone, containing 0.001 mg of naltrexone and 10 mg of oxycodone.

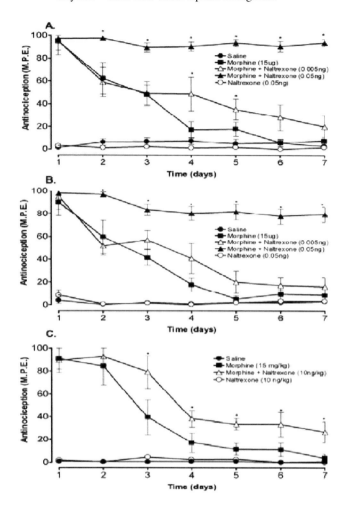

Figure IV-32. Time course of the effects of spinal (**A, B**) and systemic (**C**) naltrexone on the development of tolerance to chronic morphine in the tail-flick (**A, C**) and paw pressure (**B**) test. Morphine and naltrexone were administered as a single intrathecal (**A, B**) or intraperitoneal (**C**) injection once daily for 7 days. Nociceptive testing was performed 30 min following each injection. The data are presented as mean ± SEM for five to seven animals. * significant differences from the action of morphine alone ($P < 0.05$). MPE = Max. percent effect. Adapted from [104]

In previous clinical trials Oxytrex™ provided pain relief with minimal physical dependence, the drug really worked as intended. The patients had severe osteoarthritis pain, and many were waiting for knee or hip replacement surgery. In the 3 month study of 700 patients, Oxytrex™ reduced physical dependence by 55% and in the subset of patients older than age 50, physical dependence was reduced fivefold. Cases of severe physical dependence were reduced sixfold. Although the mechanism of action of ultra-low-dose opioid antagonists appears to be the specific prevention of G-protein signaling alterations of the mu opioid receptor that occur during opioid tolerance, multiple behavioral effects are seen with this co-treatment. First, the enhanced and prolonged analgesia provided by the addition of ultra-low-dose opioid antagonists increases the therapeutic index of the opiate. Since opiate analgesic efficacy is very often limited by side effects, this augmented analgesic efficacy may help to minimize the side effects of opiates, such as the problematic gastrointestinal and respiratory depressive effects. In addition, the reductions in constipation, somnolence and pruritis observed in the Phase II clinical trial were of a greater magnitude than would be expected from an opioid sparing effect [100]. A Phase III trial is on the way using the Oxytrex™ formulation in patients with severe chronic pain due to osteoarthritis.

Remoxy™ with ORADUR Technology, Opioid with an Abuse-Resistant Formulation

Abuse of controlled-release formulations of oxycodone and other prescription opioids is a large, fast-growing problem in the US. Simply crushing and dissolving these formulations can yield the full 12 h dose to produce an immediate, large spike in opiate blood levels and a powerful morphine-like high, as well as the potential for respiratory depression and death. In the US in 2002, oxycodone abuse resulted in over 22,000 Emergency Room visits (nearly 20% of ER visits due to abuse of narcotic analgesics), according to the Drug Abuse Warning Network (DAWN), a division of the Substance Abuse and Mental Health Services Administration (SAMHSA). This dramatic increase has coincided with the 1996 introduction and marketing of OxyContin® (Fig. IV-33). Between 2002 and 2003, the number of people over 12 years old reporting abuse of OxyContin® increased from 1.9 million

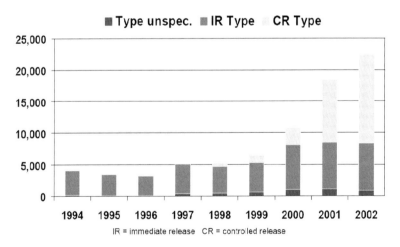

Figure IV-33. Emergency room visits involving oxycodone abuse. Adapted from DAWN

to 2.8 million, according to the National Survey on Drug Use and Health. Most alarmingly, in a 2005 survey conducted by the National Institute on Drug Abuse (NIDA), 5.5% of 12th-graders reported abusing OxyContin®.

Contrary to oxycodone slow release, the opioid is embedded in a sustained released oral gel-cap which provides unique characteristics. This is based on the ORADUR technology, which can take the form of an easy to swallow gelatin capsule that uses a high-viscosity base component, SABER™. This provides sustained release of active ingredients for a period of from 12 to 24 h (Durect Corporation Cupertino, Pain Therapeutics South San Francisco, and King Pharmaceuticals). Oral dosage forms based on the ORADUR gel-cap may also have the added benefit of being less prone to abuse than other controlled release dosage forms on the market today. Pain Therapeutics' Remoxy™ is an abuse-resistant version of long-acting oxycodone and has a sticky, high-viscosity capsule formulation (Fig. IV-34). This makes it difficult for drug abusers to inject or snort Remoxy™. Being a novel long-acting oxycodone formulation it is primarily designed to deter oxycodone abuse. In vitro tests show that Remoxy™ cannot be fragmented by forceful crushing, even after freezing at − 80 °C, and that its oxycodone content cannot be extracted by dissolution in alcohol or other common beverages. Ingesting OxyContin® after crushing and dissolving in water or alcohol produced plasma oxycodone levels even slightly higher than ingestion of an equivalent strength immediate release oxycodone tablet. In contrast, oxycodone plasma concentrations following similar treatment of Remoxy™ remained far below those of the comparable immediate release agent.

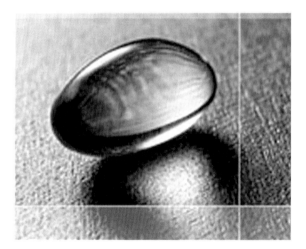

Figure IV-34. The soft-gel tablet Remoxy™ which has a sticky, high-viscosity mass that resists injection or snorting. Freezing, crushing or submerging Remoxy® in high-proof alcohol for hours at a time releases just a fraction of oxycodone compared to Oxycontin® at time points when abusers presumably expect to get high

The FDA has not yet evaluated the merits, safety or efficacy of Remoxy® and the company has just finished a large, pivotal Phase III registration study that can support a New Drug Application under an FDA filing strategy. However, Remoxy™ received a Special Protocol Assessment (SPA) from the FDA in February 2006, which specifies the Phase III trial objective, design, clinical endpoints, and analyses needed to support regulatory approval. Under the terms of the SPA, just one pivotal trial is required to file a New Drug Application. The randomized, double-blinded, placebo-controlled, multicenter trial will enroll 400 patients with moderate-to-severe osteoarthritic pain in the US. Patients will be randomized to either Remoxy™ (10 mg daily) or placebo for 12 weeks. After Remoxy™ receives marketing approval, the company Pain Therapeutics has a strategic alliance with King Pharmaceuticals to develop and market Remoxy™ and other abuse-resistant opioids.

Combining Oxycodone with the Opioid Antagonist Naloxone to Deter from Drug Abuse

OxyContin® is an opioid agonist and a Schedule II controlled substance with an abuse liability similar to morphine. Oxycodone can be abused in a manner similar to other opioid agonists, legal or illicit. This should be considered when prescribing or dispensing OxyContin® in situations where the physician or pharmacist is concerned about an increased risk of misuse, abuse, or diversion. OxyContin® Tablets are a controlled-release oral formulation of oxycodone hydrochloride indicated for the management of moderate to severe pain when a continuous, around-the-clock analgesic is needed for an extended period of time. OxyContin® tablets are NOT intended for use as a pro re nata (PRN) analgesic.

OxyContin® 80 mg and 160 mg tablets are for use in opioid-tolerant patients only. These tablet strengths may cause fatal respiratory depression when administered to patients not previously exposed to opioids. Oxycontin® tablets are to be swallowed whole and are not to be broken, chewed, or crushed. Taking broken, chewed, or crushed OxyContin® tablets leads to rapid release and absorption of a potentially fatal dose of oxycodone.

In order to overcome such disadvantages, Purdue Pharma investigational drug combined the opioid analgesic oxycodone with the opioid antagonist naloxone in the relation of 3.5:1. The company developed this formulation to reduce intravenous abuse, and potentially intranasal abuse, of OxyContin® (oxycodone HCl controlled release) tablets. This is an interim solution in response to reports of intravenous abuse in late 2000. It was assumed to be the most rapid, albeit partial, solution. The company had been pursuing other approaches prior to the naloxone project and is continuing to develop these other new drug candidates. These may have greater potential to deter not only intravenous abuse, but also the more common oral and intranasal abuse after first crushing the tablet. Developing new forms of pain relievers that are safe and effective for patients with pain while being more resistant to abuse is Purdue Pharma's research priority on developing abuse-resistant formulations.

Developing new medications that are safe and effective for patients in pain, and at the same time, resistant to abuse, is a very complex scientific and technical challenge. Prior data of the Worldwide Research and Development at Purdue Pharma recent Phase 1 studies have shown that the absorption or metabolism of naloxone is more variable than expected. Such variability has the potential to compromise pain relief in some patients. However, using lower doses of naloxone may not be sufficient to deter abuse. After reviewing the results of the Company's clinical data, company and FDA officials agreed that additional studies would be needed to fully assess the safety of this drug formulation in patients with pain as well as its potential to deter abuse. Furthermore, naloxone has significant limitations as an abuse deterrent. According to law enforcement sources, the majority of abuse of OxyContin® occurs orally or intranasally after crushing the tablets. The product's prescribing information therefore contains a warning clearly stating that OxyContin® Tablets are not to be swallowed whole and are not to be broken, chewed or crushed. While the oxycodone/naloxone formulation would deter abuse by intravenous injection, and possibly by the intranasal route ("snorting"), orally administered naloxone is, in most cases, rapidly metabolized and eliminated from the body. Therefore, naloxone is unlikely to be an effective deterrent to oral abuse of crushed OxyContin®.

Delivery of Opioids via the Lungs – The Aerosolized Liposome-Encapsulated Fentanyl (AeroLEF™)

AeroLEF™ is a proprietary formulation of free and liposome encapsulated fentanyl, a potent analgesic. It is intended for administration by pulmonary inhalation for the treatment of acute pain, including breakthrough cancer pain. AeroLEF™ is a product designed to meet the unique dosing needs of the individual, providing real-time patient directed pain relief. Using DELEX's proprietary Rapid Onset and Sustained Effect Delivery System (ROSE-DS) platform technology, AeroLEF™ provides rapid onset and extended pain relief to patients (Fig. IV-35). The development of AeroLEF™ as a pulmonary dosage form takes advantage of:

1. the lung's large absorptive surface and thin barrier to absorption, which permits rapid transport of the free fentanyl fraction into the blood stream.
2. the capacity of liposomes to function as reservoirs for the regulated release of encapsulated fentanyl over a period of time to extend the duration of action.

Currently, fentanyl is available in intravenous, transmucosal or transdermal formulations. The potential advantages of AeroLEF™ include:

1. simple, non-invasive administration,
2. rapid onset of relief that mimic intravenous,
3. extended duration of relief and
4. personalized patient-controlled dosing to match each patient's individual pain experience.

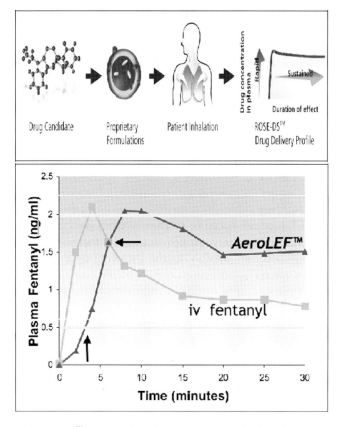

Figure IV-35. The AeroLEF™ system, mimicking intravenous application with fast onset and a long duration of action

AeroLEF™ has completed a Phase IIa trial for acute pain in post-surgical patients with positive results. In this study, 95% of patients successfully used AeroLEF™ to self administer fentanyl and achieve pain relief. AeroLEF™ demonstrated rapid onset (median time to first perceptible effect: 2.7 min) and sustained effect (average time to subsequent dosing: 3.7 h). A Phase IIb trial for acute pain and a Phase IIb trial for cancer pain are planned for the next years.

AERx® Pulmonary Delivery System for Morphine and Fentanyl

Another aerosol pulmonary delivery system with a built-in electro-mechanical liquid aerosol generator is shown in the following figure. The physical and mechanical details of the AERx® System is initated by an aerosol generated in about 1 s by means of mechanical extrusion of a piston of an aqueous formulation through an array of micron-sized laser micromachined holes. The extrusion causes the formation of aqueous jets that break up into droplets of sizes that relates to the sizes of the holes in the nozzle. The temperature controller warms up the dilution air to enhance stabilization of small, respirable droplets. The prototype system used for this study is a scaled-down version designed for inhalation delivery to dogs. For the majority of the studies described, the system was run at a flow rate of 15 L/min.

AERx® consists of a single-use, disposable drug container (the AERx Strip™) and a device that aerosolizes the drug formulation into the patient's inhalation air stream through a nozzle in the strip. The AERx® system has electronic components in the device in order to operate features related to dose titration, breath actuation and coordination, inhaled air temperature control, and electronic storage of dosing information (Fig. IV-36).

The AERx®Pulmonary Delivery System has unique features that guide the patient to breathe in an optimal manner each time a dose is taken, which enhances reproducibility and efficiency of delivery. The AERx® System delivers aerosolized medication from a dosage form comprising of a blister containing $50 \mu L$ of liquid drug formulation and a micromachined nozzle array. The aerosol is generated by extruding the formulation under pressure through an array of holes. The AERx® System also incorporates a temperature controller to minimize the effects of ambient air conditions and enhance the generation of aerosol droplets optimal for pulmonary targeting.

Nebulizers are relatively easy to use and no coordination is required, as the patient is instructed to breathe normally. However, a disadvantage of nebulizers is their low efficiency and poor reproducibility of delivery. The amount of aerosol reaching the lung from a jet or ultrasonic nebulizer has been estimated by several researchers at no more than about 10%, even when the nebulizer is operated to dryness. A significant contributor to this inefficiency is that nebulizers operate on the basis of continuous nebulization. Thus, a large proportion of the dose will never reach the patient. To improve delivery efficiency, it is important to deliver the aerosol only during the inhalation cycle. Aerosol delivered at the beginning of an inspiration can fill distal parts of the lung, while aerosol inhaled at the very end of the inspiration is likely to deposit predominantly in the oropharynx and central airways. The AERx® System is designed to sense the flow rate and volume and determine if it is optimum to deliver the targeted dose. The patient's inspiratory flow rate is measured and integrated. The actuation of the aerosol generation can occur only at the pre-programmed inspiratory flow rate and inspired volume to prevent delivery at suboptimal doses. Another critical issue for inhalation drug delivery is the potential for contamination with pathogenic microorganisms. Published reports on nebulizers show that contamination can be traced to multidose liquid packaging. Sterile unit-dose disposable systems such as the AERx® dosage form overcome this problem. The AERx® System thus has unique features that are highly desirable for delivering future therapies.

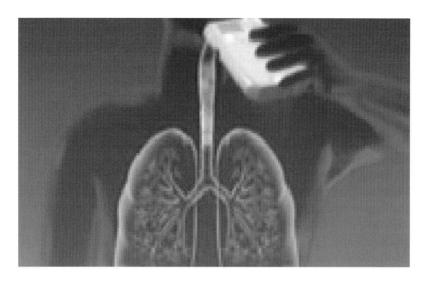

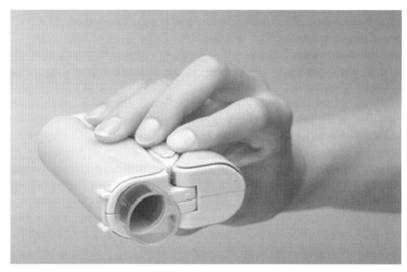

Figure IV-36. The AERx Essence® system offers a level of performance (efficiency and reproducibility) close to the existing AERx® system, but in a smaller and lower-cost package that does not have the dose titration, air temperature control, or dosing history features

The AERx® System has been previously used for the pulmonary delivery of both small molecules such as morphine [105, 106] and fentanyl [107]. It generally has been yielding emitted doses in the range of 60%–75%. The vast majority has been shown to deposit in the lung. Studies in normal fasting volunteers inhaling an aqueous solution of insulin from AERx® show that reduction in glucose levels is at least as reproducible as that achieved by subcutaneous injection, in both magnitude and time to maximum reduction in glucose levels. In a clinical study to evaluate pharmacokinetics of inhaled fentanyl delivered via the AERx® System, plasma concentration time courses for the AERx® System and intravenous route were comparable [107].

DUROS® Implant Technology for Chronic Pain Treatment

Just as ALZA Corporation's oral and transdermal technologies can improve therapy by controlling drug delivery over hours or days, the DUROS® was designed to bring the same benefits of continuous therapy for up to 1 year. DUROS® technology is the platform for an implantable drug-dispensing osmotic pump Chronogesic®. The system is shaped as a small rod with titanium housing, which can be as small as a matchstick, designed to release drugs (Fig. IV-37). The water drawn into the engine compartment expands the osmotic agent and slowly and continuously

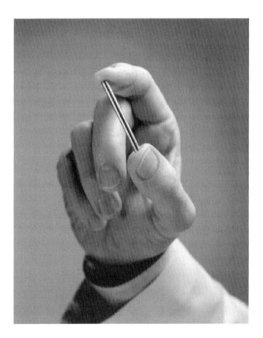

Figure IV-37. Size of the implantable DUROS® system for continuous opioid delivery. The DUROS® pump conceptually resembles a miniature syringe in which the drug is pushed out in highly controlled, minute dosages. Through osmosis, water from the body is slowly drawn through the semi-permeable membrane into the pump by salt (osmotic agent) residing in the engine compartment (Fig. IV-38).

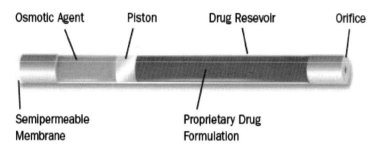

Duros Technology   Dimensions: 44mm L x 3.8mm D

Osmotic Agent   Piston   Drug Resevoir   Orifice

Semipermeable   Proprietary Drug
Membrane   Formulation

Figure IV-38. Cross section of the miniature cylinder implanted subcutaneouly via an applicator under local anesthesia. Salt in the cylinder attracks water that continuously drives a piston generating pressure to deliver an even viscous potent opioid using three different release rates of 2.5, 10, and $20\,\mu g/h$

displaces a piston to dispense small amounts of drug formulation from the drug reservoir through the orifice (Fig. IV-38). The osmotic engine does not require batteries, switches or other electromechanical parts to operate. The DUROS® system can be used for pain therapies requiring systemic or site-specific administration of a drug. To deliver drugs systemically, the DUROS® system is placed just under the skin, for example in the upper arm, in an outpatient procedure that is completed in just a few minutes using local anesthetic. Removal or replacement of the product is also a simple, quick procedure completed in the doctor's office (Fig. IV-39).

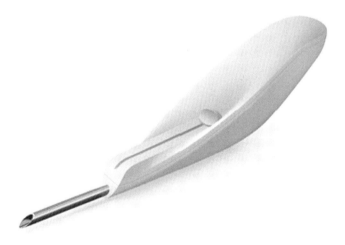

Figure IV-39. The Chronogesic® implanter for subcutaneous placement of the DUROS® system

The non-biodegradable, osmotically driven system is intended to enable delivery of small amount of the potent opioid sufentanil. The DUROS® implant is a miniature cylinder made from a titanium alloy, which protects and stabilizes the drug inside, using ALZA's proprietary formulation technology. Water enters into one end of the cylinder through a semipermeable membrane, and the drug is delivered from a port at the other end of the cylinder at a controlled rate appropriate to the specific therapeutic agent sufentanil.

The DUROS® pump operates like a miniature syringe loaded with a drug inside the drug reservoir (Fig. IV-38). Through osmosis, water from the body is slowly drawn through a semipermeable membrane into the pump by salt residing in the engine compartment. This water fills the pump, which slowly and continuously pushes a piston, dispensing the correct amount of drug out of the drug reservoir and into the body. The osmotic engine does not require batteries, switches or other electromechanical parts in order to operate. The amount of drug delivered by the system is regulated by the membrane's control over the amount of water entering the pump and by the concentration of the drug in the drug reservoir. The DUROS® system can be used for therapies requiring systemic or site-specific administration of a drug. To deliver drugs systemically, the DUROS® system is placed just under the skin, for example in the upper arm, in an outpatient procedure that is completed in just a few minutes using local anesthetic. Removal or replacement of the product is also a simple, quick procedure completed in the doctor's office.

Certain performance characteristics of the DUROS® system cannot be matched by drug delivery pumps on the market today. First, the pump can generate sufficient pressure to deliver highly concentrated and viscous formulations. Second, the system can be engineered to deliver a drug dosage at the desired dosing rate with a high degree of precision, to less than 1/100th of a drop per day on a continual basis. The titanium shell of the DUROS®system protects the drug formulation from degradation by enzymes and its passage through the body. As a result, the DUROS® system can store and release drugs in the body for up to 1 year.

DUROS® implant technology is specifically designed for the long-term delivery of the potent opioid sufentanil. Powered by osmosis, the technology incorporates a miniature titanium cylinder with the size of a match and can provide continuous drug delivery for up to 1 year.

The system incorporates several advantages for patients with chronic pain:

1. Continuous Delivery. Chronic conditions often require long-term treatment and multi-day dosing regimens. DUROS® can provide precise delivery with a single application of up to 1 year.
2. Improved Patient Compliance: Success in treatment of chronic pain is highly dependent on patient compliance. DUROS®, which can be applied and removed in an outpatient setting, helps promote compliance.
3. Enhanced Drug Stability: A common concern with long-term drug delivery is how the body's environment will affect stability. The design and non-aqueous formulation of DUROS® enhances drug stability until release (Fig. IV-40).

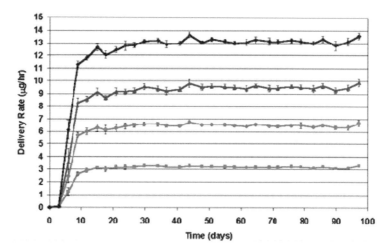

Figure IV-40. In vitro release rate from four different dosage strengths of the Chronogesic® system (mean ± SD)

Transdur™ Sufentanil Technology with 1 Week of Opioid Release

By avoiding the effects on the gastrointestinal tract and first-pass metabolism seen with some oral products, transdermal drug therapies can enhance therapeutic efficacy while decreasing side effects. Over the last few decades, numerous companies have introduced to the marketplace novel therapeutic products that utilize transdermal drug delivery technology. That tradition of innovation continues to be alive with DURECT company, which continues refining and improving various attributes of transdermal products with the development of the Transdur™ transdermal dosage form technologies. Developing small, non-irritating and user-friendly products with excellent skin-adhesion are the main objectives for the Transdur™ technology, which are major differentiating factors among patients and physicians. First generation transdermal products fall short of these objectives, in part, because of their use of a liquid drug-reservoir and skin-irritating additives such as alcohols.

Depending on the drug and its physicochemical properties, the Transdur™ technology provides compatible and functional transdermal formulations, resulting in thin solid state transdermal products that can deliver drugs, through intact skin, at a controlled rate up to 1 week. Transdur™ technology encompasses proprietary product components such as pressure sensitive adhesive formulations, skin permeation enhancers and carrier films depending on the application, which enable DURECT's scientists to expand the range of drugs that can be delivered transdermally (Fig. IV-41). Transdermal products based on Transdur™ technology improve convenience and compliance as well as cost-effectiveness, and provide highly reliable therapy to patients and health care provider.

The transdermal Transdur™-Sufentanil patch is a joint venture of Durect Corporation and Endo Pharmaceuticals Inc. It is intended to provide continuous delivery of sufentanil for up to 7 days from a single application, as compared to the 3 days of relief provided by currently available opioid patches. Sufentanil is an off-patent, highly potent opioid that is currently used in hospitals as an analgesic. The company anticipates that the small size of the sufentanil patch (Fig. IV-41), which is potentially as small as 1/5th the size of currently marketed transdermal fentanyl patches for a therapeutically equivalent dose and a longer duration of delivery, may offer improved convenience and compliance for patients.

In October 2004, a Phase I clinical trial for Transdur™-Sufentanil, consisting of a pharmacokinetic study in normal, healthy volunteers in Europe was initiated. The objectives of the clinical study were to determine the safety and tolerability of Transdur™-Sufentanil as well as to evaluate the pharmacokinetics of sufentanil following administration of Transdur™-Sufentanil. The study evaluated 24 subjects using Transdur™-Sufentanil. No clinically significant adverse events were reported. Some slight to moderate redness at patch site was observed by patients in the trial. Preliminary pharmacokinetics showed a rapid onset of the drug and the targeted plasma level over a 7 day period was achieved. A clinical trial of the Phase II program for Transdur™-Sufentanil was started in February 2005 at two clinical sites, one in the United States and the other in Europe. The clinical trial was an open-label study that was designed to evaluate the transition of chronic pain patients from Duragesic®, the commercial fentanyl patch, to the Transdur™-Sufentanil patch. The clinical study also evaluated the pharmacokinetics and safety of repetitive applications of Transdur™-Sufentanil in patients for a period of up to 4 weeks.

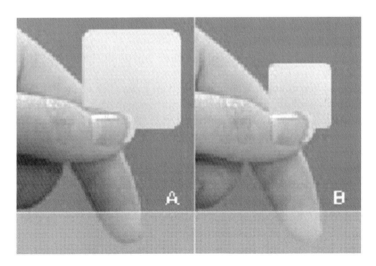

Figure IV-41. The Transdur™ patch equivalent to 100 μg/h (A) or 25 μg/h (B) of transdermal fentanyl where instead of 3 days the opioid is being released for 7 days

Evaluation of plasma level data indicate that Transdur™-Sufentanil performed as designed by achieving its target delivery profile of providing a rapid onset of drug and a delivery duration of over 7 days. Targeted plasma levels over the consecutive 4 week period (repetitive applications of Transdur™-Sufentanil) were achieved as intended. The product was tolerated well with no apparent safety issues over the 4 week treatment period. As this was an open label study, conclusions on efficacy cannot be drawn; on the average, pain levels remained stable after the transition to Transdur™-Sufentanil.

Endo Pharmaceuticals will have the exclusive rights to develop, market and commercialize Transdur™-Sufentanil in the US and Canada and full marketing rights in the rest of the world.

Effervescent Buccal Fentanyl Tablet for Treatment of Breakthrough Pain

Lipophilic opioids are more efficiently absorbed across the oral mucosa than hydrophilic opioids [108]. Fentanyl also enters the central nervous system (CNS) faster, rapidly crossing the blood-brain barrier once it is in the systemic circulation. The rate constant for the equilibrium of fentanyl between the blood and CNS is 6 min [109], whereas the rate constant for morphine is approximately 17 min [110].

The rapid onset of pain relief with oral mucosal delivery devices is attributable to the lipophilic nature of fentanyl. However, the lipophilic nature of fentanyl also makes it more difficult to dissolve in saliva, which is the first step in the buccal delivery of a solid dosage form. Fentanyl, which has a pKa of 8.4, is a weak base and, in its ionized form, is much more soluble in aqueous solutions. Therefore, dissolution is favored by a low pH, in which the ionized, less lipophilic form of fentanyl predominates. However, absorption across the buccal mucosa is favored by a high pH, in which the more lipophilic, nonionic form is more common [111].

OraVescent® technology (Cephalon Inc, Salt Lake City Utah, USA) utilizes the principles outlined above to enhance the oral transmucosal delivery of drugs such as fentanyl that are characterized as weak bases. The Fentora® buccal tablets take advantage of effervescence to bring about the pH changes necessary to optimize drug absorption.

Effervescence reactions involve the production of carbon dioxide from the combination of an acid and bicarbonate in an aqueous solution. Initially, when hydrogen ions from an acid in solution combine with bicarbonate, carbonic acid is formed. Carbonic acid rapidly dissociates into carbon dioxide and water. In open systems, carbon dioxide dissipates into the atmosphere and the equilibrium reactions favor the breakdown of the acid. The equilibrium reactions can be summarized as:

$$H + HCO_3 - > H_2CO_3 - > CO_2 \text{ and } H_2O.$$

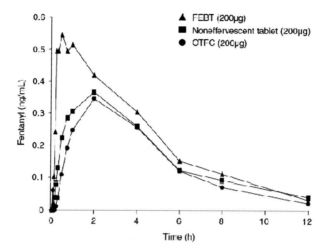

Figure IV-42. Serum fentanyl concentrations after administration of fentanyl effervescent buccal tablets (FEBT) 200 μg, fentanyl 200 μg tablets without effervescent agents, and oral transmucosal fentanyl citrate (OTFC) 200 μg. Adapted from [112]

Fentanyl effervescent buccal tablets (FEBT Fentora®) contain citric acid, sodium bicarbonate, sodium carbonate, and fentanyl citrate. As the tablets dissolve, citric acid lowers the pH. As the hydrogen ions combine with bicarbonate (and carbonate), carbon dioxide is formed. Dissipation of the carbon dioxide increases the pH. This process leaves sodium citrate and excess sodium bicarbonate in the solution.

Preliminary data suggest that use of fentanyl effervescent buccal tablets (FEBT) results in a faster onset and in plasma levels exceeding the non-effervescent tablet and those of oral transmucosal fentanyl citrate (Fig. IV-42). Due to the promising results the company is planning to market the product on a large scale.

Intrathecal DUROS® Opioid Delivery Using a Precision Miniature Catheter

To deliver drug to a specific target site, DURECT company developed a proprietary miniaturized catheter technology that can be attached to the DUROS® system to direct the flow of drug directly to the target organ within the spinal cord. Undergoing preclinical evaluation, this site-specific delivery enables a therapeutic concentration of a drug to be present at the desired target opioid receptor sites without exposing the entire body of the patient to a similar dose. The precision, miniature size, and performance characteristics of the DUROS® system allows continuous site-specific delivery, using DUROS® with a miniature catheter are presented (Fig. IV-43).

The precision DUROS® Intrathecal Opioid Delivery System is indicated for a number of chronic pain conditions, which include chronic back and leg pain, chronic cancer pain, complex regional pain syndromes (usually in the foot or

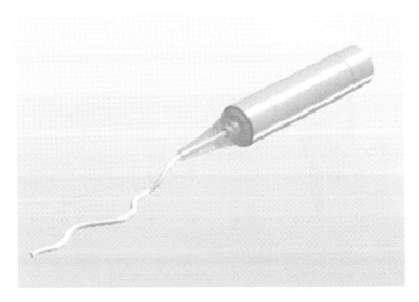

Figure IV-43. The DUROS® opioid intrathecal delivery system

hand), and painful neuropathy. By directly delivering opioids, such as morphine or hydromorphone, into the intrathecal space surrounding the spinal cord using the DUROS® system, significantly smaller doses of the drug are required to elicit pain relief. A DUROS® Intrathecal (opioid) delivery system presently is at the preclinical stage.

The figure illustrates the DUROS® intrathecal (opioid) delivery system with a catheter, which is surgically implanted subcutaneously near the target-site of drug administration. The proprietary miniature catheter is attached to the DUROS® system and tunneled under the skin to the site where opioid is to be delivered. The DUROS® system is designed to deliver the drug at a constant, preset rate through the catheter to the targeted intrathecal site for a prescribed duration of approximately 3 months. The proprietary catheter has a hold-up volume of about $20\,\mu l$.

DUROS® Intrathecal Opioid Delivery System has a nominal volume-pumping rate of $10\,\mu l/day$ ($0.42\,\mu l/h$). The following figure demonstrates a constant volume-pumping rate from a DUROS® system over 100 days. The in vitro pumping rate was determined by placing the systems in an aqueous buffer solution at $37\,°C$, and by measuring the effluent from the systems at preset time intervals. Both the initial start-up time and completion of systems pumping action are predictable and reproducible between different systems (Fig. IV-44). By varying the drug concentration in the reservoir, the opioid can be intrathecally administered at the rate from 10 to $100\,\mu g/h$.

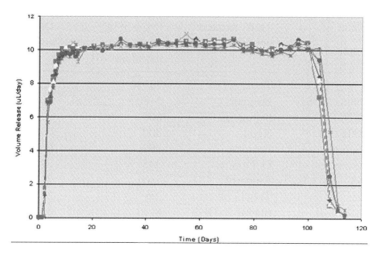

Figure IV-44. In vitro release rate from the DUROS® opioid intrathecal delivery system

Appendices: Duration of Action and Dosing of Opioid Analgesics

APPENDIX IV-1

Oral, transdermal, sublingual, buccal, and nasal preparations of different opioids; their analgesic potency and duration of action

Generic name of opioid	Trade name of opioid	Potency in relation to morphine = 1	Duration of action (h)
Morphine immediate release	Morphine sulfate MSIR	1	4
	Oxy IR	1	4
	OxyFast	1	4
	Roxanol	1	4
	Oramorph SR	1	8–12
Morphine sustained release	MS Contin	1	8–12
	Kadian	1	18–24
Propoxyphene	Darvon	1/50–1/25	4–6
Oxymorphone Sup	Numorphan	12–15	3–6
Oxymorphone extended - release	Opara	12–5	12
Buprenorphine subl.	Buprenex	20–30	8–10
Buprenorphine TDS	Transtec	20–30	72

Generic name of opioid	Trade name of opioid	Potency in relation to morphine = 1	Duration of action (h)
Buprenorphine TDS	TranstecPro	20–30	92
Buprenorphine TDS	Butrans	5–20	92
Fentanyl TTS	Duragesic	800	72
Fentanyl OTFC	Actiq	800	20–30 min
Fentanyl buccal	Fentora	800	60 min
Methadone	Dolophine	3–5	22–48
Meperidine	Demerol	1/10	2–4
Pentazocine	Talwin	1/6	3–4
Butorphanol nasal spray	Stadol	8–11	3–4
Codeine	Codeine Sulfate	1/10	4
Tramadol	Ultram	1/10–1/5	3–4
HydromorphoneTbl	Dilaudid	7	4–6
HydromorphoneCR	Palladone	7	8–12
Oxycodone Tbl	Roxicodone	2	4–6
Oxycodone SR	OxyContin	2	8–12
Morphine extended release	Avinza	1	24
Hydromorphone OROS technology	Jurnista	7	24

APPENDIX IV-2

Potent oral and sublingual opioid analgesics Step 3 of the analgesic ladder, their initial dose for pain therapy

Opioid	Initial daily dose
Morphine fast release	4–6 times 10 mg
Morphine extended release	2–3 times 30/60 mg
Methadone	3 times 10–20 mg
Hydromorphone sustained release	2–3 times 8/16 mg
Buprenorphine sublingual	3 times 0.2–0.4 mg
Oxycodone extended release	2 times 10/20 mg
Hydromorphone extended release	2 times 4/8 mg
Morphine sulfate extended release	Once 30/60/90/120 mg

APPENDIX IV-3

Equianalgesic doses of different opioids when compared to oral morphine

Opioid	Mean duration of action (h)	Dose per patient per day (mg)	Equianalgesic dose to morphine = 1
Buprenorphine subl. (Buprenex)	8–10	2–3 times 0.2 mg	40–50
		2–3 times 0.4 mg	60–120
Pentazocine (Talwin)	2–4	6–8 times 25 mg	25–35
		6–8 times 50 mg	50–70
Meperidine (Demerol)	2–4	6–8 times 50 mg	40–50
		6–8 times 100 mg	75–100
Methadone (Dolophine)	3–5	6 times 5 mg	60
		6 times 10 mg	120
Morphine (Oxy IR)	4–5	6 times 10–30 mg	60–180
Morphine (MS Contin)	8–12	2 times 10–200 mg	40–400
		once 30–60–100 mg	
Morphine (Kadian)	12–24	6–8 times 50 mg	60–120–200
		6–8 times 100 mg	
Tramadol (Ultram)	3–6	3–4 times 50 mg	30–40
			60–80
Propoxyphene (Darvon)	4–6	6–8 times 30 mg	40–50
Codeine (Codeine Sulfate, Phosphate)	3–4	6–8 times 60 mg	15–30
		2–3 times	30–60

Opioid	Mean duration of action (h)	Dose per patient per day (mg)	Equianalgesic dose to morphine = 1
Fentanyl TTS (Duragesic)	72	diff. patch sizes 25–50–100 μg/h	600–800
Fentanyl buccal (Fentora)	1	100–200–400– 600–800 μg	600-800
Buprenorphine TDS (TranstecPro)	96	diff. patch sizes 35–52.5–75 μg/h	200–400
(Butrans)	96	5–10–20 μg/h	5–20
Oxycodone CR (OxyContin)	8–12	2 times 10/20/40/80/160	15–30–60–120–240
Hydromorphone (Palladone)	8–12	2 times 4/8/16 mg	10–20–40
Morphine ER (Avinza)	24	once 30–60–90–120	60–90–120–200
Hydromorphone OROS (Jurnista)	24	once 8–16–32–64 mg	10–20–40–60

APPENDIX IV-4

Indications for use of opioids with and/or without adjuvants

Indication
- Chronic pain, not attenuated by other methods.
- Intolerable side effects of peripheral analgesics or NSAIDs.
- Insufficient pain relief by NSAIDs.
- Contraindications for use of NSAIDs (e.g., peptic ulcer formation).
- Progression of underlying disease with the necessity to increase the dose of peripheral analgesic.
- Temporary increase in pain intensity where NSAIDs are insufficient.
- Painful syndromes which only respond to opioids.

Examples for use of opioids in chronc pain therapy
- Intense pain in OA where pain results in immobilization.
- Intense pain in osteoporosis where pain results in immobilization.
- Intense back pain, failed back surgery, stenosis of spinal canal, and/or chronic arachnoiditis.

- Post herpetic neuralgia.
- Phantom limb pain.
- Thalamic pain.
- Tumor related pain.
- Peri-, post-operative pain for prevention of chronification.
- Acute pain in trauma.

Contraindications for use of opioids
Relative
- Simultaneous use of benzodiazepines unless otherwise indicated.
- History of dependency.
- Intolerable side effects.

Absolute
- Pain that can be treated sufficiently with other methods.
- Hypersensitivity to opioids.

References

1. Wood, P.L., *k Agonists analgesics: evidence for $\mu2$ and delta opioid receptor antagonism.* Drug Dev Res, 1984, **4**: pp. 429–435.
2. Mercadante, S. and F. Fulfaro, *World Health Organization guidelines for cancer pain: a reappraisal.* Ann Oncol 16, 2005, **16**: pp. IV132–IV135.
3. Mercadante, S., *World Health Organisation guidelines: problem areas in cancer pain management.* Cancer Control, 1999, **6**: pp. 191–197.
4. Foley, K.M., *Changing concepts of tolerance to opioids*, in *Current and Emerging Issues in Cancer Pain: Research and Practice*, C.R. Chapmann and K.M. Foly, Editors, 1993, Raven Press: New York. pp. 331–350.
5. Taeger, K., *Pharmakokinetik der Opiate Dolantin, Morphin und Fentanyl.* Anästh Intensivmed, 1981, **22**: pp. 28–37.
6. Nielsson, M.I., et al., *Pharmacokinetic of methadone maintenance treatment: characterization of therapeutic failures.* Eur J Clin Pharmacol, 1983, **25**: pp. 497–501.
7. Wörz, R. and J. Berlin, *Behandlung chronischer Schmerzsyndrome mit Antidepressiva.* Der Schmerz, 1989, **3**: pp. 1–7.
8. Yuan, C.S., et al., *Methylnaltrexone for reversal of constipation due to chronic methadone use: a randomisesd controlled trial.* JAMA, 2000, **283**: pp. 367–372.
9. Becker, G., Galandi, D., and H.E Blum. *Peripherally acting opioid antagonists in the treatment of opiate-related constipation: A systematic review.* J Pain Symptom Manage, 2007, **34**: 547–565.
10. Twycross, R.G., *Opioid analgesics in cancer pain: current practice and controversies.* Cancer Sur, 1988, **7**: pp. 29–53.
11. Budd, K., *Buprenorphine and the transdermal system: The ideal match in pain management.* Int J Clin Pract, 2002, **133**: pp. 9–14.
12. Gal, T.J. and C.A. DiFazio, *Prolonged antagonism of opioid action with intravenous nalmefene in man.* Anesthesiology, 1986, **64**: pp. 175–180.
13. Heel, R.C., et al., *Buprenorphine: a review of its pharmacological properties and therapeutic efficacy.* Drugs, 1979, **17**: pp. 81–100.

14. Tao, P.-L., P.-Y. Law, and H.H. Loh, *Decrease in delta und mu opioid receptor binding capacity on rat brain after chronic treatment*. J Pharmacol Expt Ther, 1986, **240**: pp. 809–816.

15. Atkinson, R.E., P. Schofield, and P. Mellor, *Opioids in the treatment of cancer pain*, in *London Int Congress and Symposium Series*, D. Doyle, Editor, 1990, Royal Society of Medicine: London. pp. 81–87.

16. Greenwald, S.K., *Buprenorphine's effects on brain opioid receptors and behavior of heroin abusers*. Neuropsychopharmacology, 2003, **28**: pp. 2000–2009.

17. Sadee, W., J.S. Rosenbaum, and A. Herz, *Buprenorphine: differential interaction with opiate receptors subtypes in vivo*. J Pharmacol Exp Ther, 1982, **223**: pp. 157–162.

18. Walsh, S.L., K.L. Preston, and M.L. Stitzer, *Clinical pharmacology of buprenorphine: ceiling effects at high doses*. Clin Pharmacol Ther, 1994, **55**: pp. 569–580.

19. Budd, K., *High dose buprenorphine for postoperative analgesia*. Anaesthesia, 1981, **36**: pp. 900–903.

20. Dahan, A., et al., *Comparison of the respiratory effects of intravenous buprenorphine and fentanyl in humans and rats*. Br J Anaesth, 2005, **94**: pp. 825–834.

21. Zaki, P.A., et al., *Ligand-induced changes in surface μ-opioid receptor number: relationship to G-protein activation*. J Pharmacol Expt Ther, 1999, **292**: pp. 1127–1135.

22. Engelberger, T., et al. *In vitro and ex vivo reversibility of the opioid receptor binding of buprenorphine*, in *Pain in Europe IV*, 2003, European Federation of the International Association for the Study of Pain Chapters: Prague, Czek Republik.

23. Ventafridda, V., et al., *A validation study of the WHO method of cancer pain relief*. Cancer, 1987, **59**: pp. 851–856.

24. Ahmedzai, S. and D. Brooks, *Transdermal fentanyl versus sustained-release oral morphine in cancer pain: preference, efficacy, and quality of life*. J Pain Symptom Manag, 1997, **13**: pp. 254–261.

25. Bach, V., et al., *Buprenorphine and sustained release morphine – effect and side effects in common use*. Pain Clin, 1991, **4**: pp. 78–93.

26. Hug, C.C.J., *Pharmacokinetics of new synthetic narcotic analgesics*, in *Opioids in Anesthesia*, F.G. Estafanous, Editor, 1984, Butterworth: Boston. pp. 50–60.

27. Bullingham, R.E., et al., *Buprenorphine kinetics*. Clin Pharmacol Ther, 1980, **28**: pp. 667–672.

28. Helmers, J.H., et al., *Sufentanil kinetics in the elderly*. Beitr Anästhesiol Intensivmed, 1987, **20**: pp. 376–377.

29. Patt, R.B. and N.M. Ellison, *Breakthrough pain in cancer patients: characteristics, prevalence and treatment*. Oncology, 1998, **12**: pp. 1035–1052.

30. Portenoy, R.K. and N.A. Hagen, *Breakthrough pain: definition, prevalance and characteristics*. Pain, 1990, **41**: pp. 273–281.

31. Lichtor, J.L., et al., *The relative potency of oral transmucosal fentanyl citrate compared with intravenous morphine in the treatment of moderate to severe postoperative pain*. Anseth Analg, 1999, **89**: pp. 732–738.

32. Coluzzi, P.H., et al., *Breakthrough cancer pain: a randaomized trial comparing oral transmucosal fentanyl citrate (OTFC®) and morphine sulfate immediate release (MSIR®)*. Pain, 2001, **91**: pp. 123–130.

33. Ashburn, M.A. and J.B. Streisand, *Oral transmucosal fentanyl – help or hindrance?* Drug Safety, 1994, **11**: pp. 295–300.

34. Klockgether-Radke, A.P., P. Gaus, and P. Neumann, *Opioidintoxikation durch transdermales Fentanyl*. Anaesthesist, 2002, **51**: pp. 269–271.

35. Fröhlich, M., A. Gianotti, and A.H. Modell, *Opioid overdose in a patient using a fentanyl patch during treatment with a warming blanket*. Anesth Analg, 2001, **93**: pp. 647–648.

36. Newsham, G., *Heat-related toxicity with fentanyl transdermal patch*. J Pain Symptom Manage, 1998, **16**: pp. 277–278.

37. Griesinger, M., *Fentanyl transdermal system: unsafe in unexperienced hands*. P & T, 2002, **27**: p. 132.

38. Farmer, S.E., *Hyperaemia of the skin results in increased absorption rate of fentanyl via a transdermal drug delivery system*. Br Med J, 2002, **324**: p. 286.

39. De Sio, J.M. and D.R. Bacon, *Intravenous abuse of transdermal fentanyl therapy in chronic pain patient*. Abesthesiology, 1993, **79**: pp. 1130–1141.

40. Marquardt, K.A. and R.S. Tharratt, *Inhalation abuse of fentanyl patch*. J Toxicol Clin Toxicol, 1994, **32**: pp. 75–78.

41. Fannagan, L.M., J.D. Butts, and W.H. Anderson, *Fentanyl patches left on dead bodies – potential source of drug for abusers*. J Forens Med, 1996, **41**: pp. 320–321.

42. Kramer, C. and M. Twaney, *A fatal overdose of transdermal administered fentanyl*. J Am Osteopath Assoc, 1998, **98**: pp. 385–386.

43. Parucker, M. and W. Swann, *Potential for duragesic® patch abuse*. Ann Emerg Med, 2000, **35**: p. 244.

44. Arvantis, M.L. and R.C. Sartonik, *Transdermal fentanyl abuse and misuse*. J Emerg Med, 2002, **20**: pp. 58–59.

45. Schneir, A.B., S.R. Offerman, and R.F. Clark, *Poisoning from the application of a scrotal transdermal fentanyl patch*. Foster North American College of Clinical Toxicology, Annual Meeting, 2001.

46. Gardner-Nix, J., *Caregiver toxicity from transdermal fentanyl*. J Pain Symptom Manage, 2001, **21**: pp. 447–448.

47. Marquardt, K.A., R.S. Tharratt, and N.A. Mussalam, *Fentanyl remainuing in a transdermal system following three days of continuous use*. Ann Pharmacother, 1995, **29**: pp. 969–971.

48. Edinboro, L.E. and A. Poklis, *Fatal ferntanyl intoxication following excessive transdermal application*. J Forensic Sci, 1997, **42**: pp. 741–743.

49. Dum, J.E. and A. Herz, *In vivo receptor binding of the opiate partial agonist, buprenorphine, correlated with its agonistic and antagonistic actions*. Br J Pharmacol, 1981, **74**: pp. 627–633.

50. Jasinski, D.R., J.S. Pevnik, and J.D. Griffith, *Human pharmacology and the abuse potential of the analgesic buprenorphine*. Arch Gen Psychiatry, 1978, **35**: pp. 501–516.

51. Bickel, W.K., et al., *Buprenorphine: dose-related blockade of opioid challenge effects in opioid dependent humans*. J Pharmacol Exp Ther, 1988, **247**(1): pp. 47–53.

52. Chakrabarti, S., et al., *The mu-opioid receptor down-regulates differently from the delta-opioid receptor: requirement of a high affinity receptor/G protein complex formation*. Mol Pharmacol, 1997, **52**: pp. 105–113.

53. Cvejic, S., et al., *Thr353, located within the COOH-terminal tail of the delta opiate receptor, is involved in receptor down-regulation*. J Biol Chem, 1996, **271**: pp. 4073–4076.

54. Twycross, R.G., *Relief of pain*, in *The Mangemement of Termninal Malignant Disease*, C. Saunders, Editor, 1984, Edward Arnold: London. pp. 64–90.

55. Freye, E., et al., *Opioid rotation from high dose morphine to transdermal buprenorphine (Transtec®) in chronic pain patients*. Pain Practice, 2007, **7**: pp.121–137.

56. Elliott, T.E. and B.A. Elliott, *Physicians attitudes and beliefs about use of morphine for cancer pain.* J Pain Sympt Manag, 1992, **3**(7): pp. 141–148.

57. Porter, J. and H. Hick, *Addiction rare in patients treated with narcotics.* New Engl J Med, 1980, **302**: pp. 123–126.

58. Jick, H., et al., *Comprehensive drug surveillance.* JAMA, 1970, **213**: pp. 1455–1460.

59. Babayan, E.A., V.K. Lepakhin, and G.M. Rudenko, *Opioid analgesics and narcotic antagonists*, in *Meyers's Side Effects of Drugs*, M.N.G. Dukes, Editor, 1980, Exerpta Medica: Amsterdam. p. 105.

60. Taub, A., *Opioid analgesics in the treatment of chronic intractable pain of non-neoplastic origin*, in *Narcotic Analgesics in Anesthesiology*, L.M. Kitahata and J.G. Collins, Editors, 1982, Williams and Wilkins: Baltimore. pp. 199–208.

61. Portenoy, R.K. and K.M. Foley, *Chronic use of opioid analgesics in non-malignant pain. Report of 38 cases.* Pain, 1986, **25**: pp. 171–186.

62. Robbins, L.N., D.H. Davis, and D.M. Nurco, *How permament was Vietnam drug addiction.* Am J Public Health, 1974, **64**: pp. 38–43.

63. Maruto, T., D.W. Swanson, and R.E. Finlayson, *Drug abuse and dependency in patients with chronic pain.* Mayo Clin Proc, 1979, **54**: pp. 241–244.

64. Tennant, F.S. and G.F. Kelman, *Narcotic maintenance for chronc pain: medical and legal guidelines.* Postgrad Med, 1983, **73**: pp. 81–94.

65. Schultheiss, R., J. Schramm, and J. Neidhardt, *Dose changes in long- and medium-term intrathecal morphine therapy of cancer pain.* Neurosurgery, 1992, **31**(4): pp. 664–670.

66. Twycross, R.G. and S.A. Lack, *Symptom control in far-advanced cancer pain relief*, 1983, Pittman: London.

67. Bohn, L.M., et al., *Enhanced morphine analgesia in mice lacking β-arrestin 2.* Science, 1999, **286**: pp. 2495–2498.

68. Colpaert, F.C., et al., *Large-amplitude 5-HT1A receptor activation: a new mechanism of profound central analgesia.* Neuropharmacology, 2002, **43**: pp. 945–958.

69. Kanner, R.M. and K.M. Foley, *Pattern of narcotic drug use in cancer pain clinic.* Ann NY Acad Sci, 1981, **362**: pp. 162–172.

70. Weiss, S., et al., *Understanding the experience of pain in terminally ill patients.* Lancet, 2001, **357**: pp. 1311–1315.

71. Clark, A.J., et al., *Efficacy and safety of transdermal fentanyl and sustained-release oral morphine in patients with cancer and chronic non-cancer pain.* Curr Med Res Opin, 2004, **20**: pp. 1419–1428.

72. Fallon, M.T. and G.W. Hanks, *Morphine, constipation and performance status in advanced cancer patients.* Palliat Med, 1999, **13**: pp. 159–160.

73. Liu, S.S., et al., *ADL 8-2698, a trans-3,4-dimethyl-4-(3-hydroxyphenyl) piperidine, prevents gastrointestinal effects of intravenous morphine without affecting analgesia.* Clin Pharmacol Ther, 2001, **69**: pp. 66–71.

74. Yuan, C.S., et al., *The safety and efficacy of oral methalnaltrexone in preventing morphine-induced delay in oral cecal transit time.* Clin Pharmacol Ther, 1997, **61**: pp. 1–9.

75. Hale, M.E., R. Fleischmann, and R. Salzmann, *Efficacy and safety of controlled-release versus immediate release oxycodone: randomized, double-blind evaluation in patients wiith chronic back pain.* Clin J Pain, 1999, **15**: pp. 179–183.

76. Clark, K.J. and K. Turner, *The rediscovery of methadone for cancer pain management.* Med J Aust, 2001, **174**: pp. 547–548.

77. Davis, M.P. and D. Walsh, *Methadone for relief of cancer*. Supp Care Med, 2001, **9**: pp. 73–83.
78. Ripamonti, C. and E.D. Dickerson, *Strategies for the treatment of cancer pain in the new millenium*. Drugs-Aging, 2001, **61**: pp. 955–977.
79. Ebert, B., S. Andersen, and P. Krogsgrad-Karsen, *Ketobemidone, methadone and pethidine are non-competitve N-methyl-D-aspartate (NMDA) antagonists in the rat cortex and spinal cord*. Neurosci Lett, 1995, **187**: pp. 165–168.
80. Gorman, A.L., K.J. Elliott, and C.E. Inturrisi, *The D- and the L-isomers of methadone bind to the non-competitive site on the NMDA receptor in the rat forebrain and spinal cord*. Neurosci Lett, 1997, **223**: pp. 5–8.
81. Morley, J.S. and K.J. Makin, *The use of methadone in cancer pain poorly responsive to other opioids*. Pain Rev, 1998, **5**: pp. 51–58.
82. Smith, G.D. and M.T. Smith, *Morphine-3-glucuronide: evidence to support its putative role in the development of tolerance to the antinociceptive effects of morphine in the rat*. Pain, 1995, **62**: pp. 51–60.
83. Rossi, G.C., et al., *Antisense mapping of MOR-1 in rats: distinguishing between morphine and morphine-6β-glucoronide antinociception*. J Parmacol Expt Ther, 1997, **281**: pp. 109–114.
84. Osborne, R.J., S.P. Joel, and M.L. Slevin, *Morphine intoxication in renal failure: The role of morphine-6-glucuronide*. Br Med J, 1986, **292**: pp. 1548–1549.
85. Pan, Y.X., et al., *Identification and characterization of three new alternative spliced mu-opioid receptors*. Mol Pharmacol, 1999, **56**: pp. 396–403.
86. Rossi, G.C., et al., *Novel receptor mechanisms for heroin and morphine-6β-glucuronide analgesia*. Neurosci Lett, 1996, **216**: pp. 1–4.
87. Ross, F.B. and M.T. Smith, *The intrinsic antinociceptive effects of oxycodone appear to be k-opioid receptor mediated*. Pain, 1997, **73**: pp. 151–157.
88. De Castro, J., J. Meynadier, and M. Zenz, *Regional opioid analgesia. Physiopharmacological basis, drugs, and clinical application*, 1991, Kluwer Academic Publishers: Dordrecht.
89. Large, R.G. and S.A. Schug, *Opioids for chronic pain of non-malignant origin-caring or crippling*. Health Care Anal, 1995, **3**: pp. 5–11.
90. Portenoy, R.K., *Opioid therapy for chronic non-malignant pain: clinician's perspective*. J Law Med Ethics, 1996, **24**: pp. 269–309.
91. Thomsen, A.B., N. Becker, and J. Eriksen, *Opioid rotation in chronic non-malignant pain patients. A retrospective study*. Acta Anaesthesiol Scand, 1999, **43**: pp. 918–923.
92. Kumar, K. and D. Demeria, *Review: the role of opioids in the treatment of chronic nonmalignant pain in the elderly*. Ann Long-Term Care, 2003, **11**: pp. 34–40.
93. Marcus, D.A., *Treatment of nonmalignant chronic pain*. Am Fam Physician, 2000, **61**: pp. 1331–1338.
94. O'Neill, W.M., et al., *The cognitive and psychomotor effects of morphine in healthy subjects: a randomised controlled trial of repeated (four) oral doses of dextropropoxyphene, morphine, lorazepam and placebo*. Pain, 2000, **85**: pp. 209–215.
95. Zacny, J.P., *Should people taking opioids for medical reasons be allowed to work and drive?* Addiction, 1996, **91**: pp. 1581–1584.
96. Vainio, A., *Driving ability in cancer patients receiving long-term morphine analgesia*. Lancet, 1995, **346**: pp. 667–670.

 97. Crain, S.M. and K.F. Shen, *Opioids can evoke direct receptor mediated excitatory effects on sensory neurons.* TIPS, 1990, **11**: pp. 77–81.
 98. Wang, H.-Y., et al., *Ultra-low-dose naloxone suppresses opioid tolerance, dependence and associated changes in Mu opioid, receptor-G protein coupling and Gβγ signaling.* Neuroscience, 2005, **135**: pp. 247–261.
 99. Chindalore, V.L., et al., *Adding ultra-low-dose naltrexone to oxycodone enhances and prolongs analgesia.* J Pain, 2005, **6**: pp. 392–399.
100. Burns, L.H., *Ultra-low-dose opioid antagonists enhance opioid analgesia while reducing tolerance, dependence and addictive properties,* in *Recent Devevelopment of Pain Research,* 2005, Kerala/India: Research Signpost. pp. 115–136.
101. Crain, S.M. and K.F. Shen, *Ultra-low concentrations of naloxone selectively antagonize excitatory effects of morphine on sensory neurons, thereby increasing its antinociceptive potency and attenuating tolerance/dependence during chronic cotreatment.* Proc Natl Acad Sci, 1995, **92**: pp. 10540–10544.
102. Wang, H.Y. and L.H. Burns, *Gβj that interacts with adenylyl cyclase in opioid tolerance originates from a Gs protein.* J Neurobiol, 2006, **66**: pp. 1302–1310.
103. Crain, S.M. and K.F. Shen, *GM1 ganglioside-induced modulation of opioid receptor-mediated functions.* Ann NY Acad Sci, 1998, **845**: pp. 106–125.
104. Powell, K.J., et al., *Paradoxical effects of the opioid antagonist naltrexone on morphine analgesia, tolerance, and reward in rats.* Pharmacology, 2002, **300**: pp. 588–596.
105. Ward, M.E., A. Woodhouse, and L.E. Mather, *Morphine pharmacokinetics after pulmonary administration from a novel aerosol delivery system.* Clin Pharmakokinet Ther, 1997, **62**: pp. 596–609.
106. Dershwitz, M., et al., *Pharmacokinetics and pharmacodynamics of inhaled versus intravenous morphine in healthy volunteers.* Anesthesiology, 2000, **93**: pp. 619–628.
107. Boyle, F., L.E. Mather, and J. Lam. *Inhaled fentanyl via the AERx system for the treatment of breakthrough cancer pain.* In *19th Annual Scientific Meeting, American Pain Society,* 2000, Atlanta, GA.
108. Weinberg, D.S., C.E. Inturrisi, and B. Reidenberg, *Sublingual absorption of selected opioid analgesics.* Clin Pharmacol Ther, 1988, **44**: pp. 335–342.
109. Scott, J.C., K.V. Ponganis, and D.R. Stanski, *EEG quantification of narcotic effect: the comparative pharmacodynamics of fentanyl and alfentanil.* Anesthesiology, 1985, **62**: pp. 234–241.
110. Kramer, T.H., R.H. d'Amours, and C. Buettner, *Pharmacodynamic model of the effects of morphine-6-glucuronide during patient controlled analgesia.* Clin Pharmacol Ther, 1996, **59**.
111. Streisand, J.B., J. Zhang, and S. Niu, *Buccal absorption of fentanyl is pH-dependent in dogs.* Anesthesiology, 1995, **82**: pp. 759–764.
112. Pather, S.I., J.M. Siebert, and J. Hontz, *Enhanced buccal deleicvery of fentanyl usingthe oravescent drug delivery system.* Drug Delivery Tech, 2001, **1**: pp. 54–57.
113. Lee, M.A., M.E. Leng, and E.J. Tiernau. *Retrospective study of the use of hydromorphone in palliative care patients with normal and abnormal urea creatinine.* Pall Med, 2001, **15**: pp. 26–34.
114. Bruera, E., et al. *Opioid rotation in patients with cancer pain.* Cancer, 1996, **78**: pp. 852–857.
115. Chen, Z.R., et al. *Mu receptor binding of some commonly used opioids and their metabolites.* Life sci, 1991, **48**: pp. 2165–2171.

116. Morley, J.S. and K.J. Makin. *The use of methadone in cancer pain poorly responsive to other opioids.* Pain Rev, 1998, **5**: pp. 51–58.
117. Ripamonti, V., et al. *Switching from morphine to oral methadone in treating cancer pain: what is the equianalgesic dose ratio?* J Clin Onkol, 1998, **16**: pp. 3216–3221.
118. Sabatowski, R., et al. *Driving ability under long-term treatment with transdermal Fentanyl.* J Pain Symp Manag, 2003, **25**: pp. 38–47.
119. Vainio, A., *Driving ability in cancer patients receiving long-term morphine analgesia.* Lancet, 1995, **346**: pp. 667–670.

Part V

Detection of Illicit Use of Opioids in Primary Care

Contents

Introduction

The CASA National Survey of Primary Care Physicians and Patients on Substance Abuse is the most comprehensive nationally representative survey of how primary care physicians deal with substance-abusing patients [1]. This survey carried out in 1999 found that 94% of primary care physicians failed to diagnose substance abuse when they were presented with a description of early symptoms of alcohol abuse in an adult patient. In addition, 41% of pediatricians failed to diagnose illegal drug use when presented with a classic description of a drug-abusing teenage patient [1].

Only a small percentage of physicians considered themselves "very prepared" to diagnose illegal drug use (16.9%), alcoholism (19.9%), and prescription drug abuse (30.2%). In contrast, 82.8% felt "very prepared" to identify hypertension, 82.3% diabetes, and 44.1% depression [1]. According to the survey, physicians are missing or misdiagnosing patients' substance abuse for several reasons, including: lack of adequate training in medical school, residency programs, or continuing medical education courses; skepticism about treatment effectiveness; discomfort discussing substance abuse; time constraints; patient resistance; and concern that they will not be reimbursed for the time required to screen and treat a substance-abusing patient [1].

The CASA (Center on Addiction and Substance Abuse) report made a number of recommendations, including increasing substance abuse training in medical school, residency programs, and continuing medical education courses; expanding coverage by Medicare, Medicaid, private insurers, and managed care for substance abuse treatment services; and holding primary care physicians liable for negligent failure to diagnose substance abuse and addiction and encouraging their patients to seek help [1].

Many medical students are taught that if opioids are prescribed in high doses or for a prolonged time, the patient will invariably become an addict. Therefore, the common wisdom is to prescribe the lowest possible dose at the longest possible dosing interval. As a result, opioids are frequently prescribed in doses that are inadequate and at time intervals beyond the duration of action of the drug, resulting in poor analgesia [2].

Weissman and Haddox first introduced the term pseudoaddiction in 1989 to describe the iatrogenic syndrome of abnormal behavior developing in direct consequence of inadequate pain management [3]. They described the natural history of pseudoaddiction as a progression through three characteristic phases including:
(1) Inadequate prescription of analgesics to meet the primary pain stimulus;
(2) Escalation of analgesic demands by the patient associated with behavioral changes to convince others of the pain's severity; and
(3) A crisis of mistrust between the patient and the healthcare team.

Treatment strategies include establishing trust between the patient and the healthcare team and providing appropriate and timely analgesics to control the patient's level of pain [3]. The behavior ceases when adequate pain relief is provided [4]. Pseudoaddiction is not a diagnosis, but rather is a description of a clinical interaction.

The need for higher doses of an analgesic, however, may be due to the development of tolerance. By definition, tolerance is a state of adaptation in which exposure to a drug induces changes that result in a diminution of one or more of the drug's effects over time [4]. Tolerance develops to some drug effects much more rapidly than other effects of the same drug. For example, tolerance rapidly develops to the euphoria produced by opioids, but tolerance to their gastrointestinal effects develops more slowly [5, 6, 7]. Tolerance is variable over time and between patients. Doses plateau for long periods of time in most patients in the absence of progressions of the underlying pathology [7]. Because tolerance develops rapidly to euphoria-producing effects of opioids [7], addicts tend to increase their daily dose, depending on their financial resources and availability of the drug [6].

The development of tolerance is rarely treatment limiting, and tolerance alone is rarely the sole reason for increasing doses [5].

Tolerance is only one of several potential contributors to increasing dosage requirements. Pharmacodynamic tolerance refers to adaptive changes that have taken place within systems affected by the drug, so that response to a given concentration of the drug is reduced (e.g. drug-induced changes in receptor density or efficiency of receptor coupling to signal transduction pathways) [6, 7].

Pharmacokinetic (or dispositional) tolerance refers to changes in the distribution or metabolism of the drug after repeated drug administration, such that reduced concentrations are present in the blood and subsequently at the sites of drug action. Many variables can influence the absorption of drugs, which can have profound effects on the clinical efficacy of a drug [6, 7]. For example, rapid weight gain, such as during pregnancy, creates a new volume of distribution, and more medication may be needed to achieve the desired effect [7]. Furthermore, dietary intake, other medications, or illness can affect the absorption of opioids.

There is a distinction between the patient who is physically dependent, but not out of control with medication, and the addict who is. The physically dependent patient's quality of life is improved through use of the medication, whereas the addict's quality of life is severely impaired (Table V-1). Use of medication continues

Table V-1. Addiction is a disease; medication compliance is not addiction Adapted from [2]

	Physical dependence	Addiction
Out of control with medications		✓
Medications improve quality of life	✓	
Use continues in spite of problem		✓
Denial about any problems		✓

or increases despite adverse consequences to the addict; however, the physically dependent patient will complain or seek to deal with negative consequences, such as side effects, by trying to cut down on the medication. The addict is unaware or in denial about the problems caused by the medication; the physically dependent patient is concerned about these problems [2].

Physical Dependency

Physical dependence is commonly seen with addiction, but it is important to distinguish them [8, 9, 10, 11]. Physical dependence – the capacity for withdrawal syndrome to ensue – can occur following adaptive changes from repeated exposure to the drug, by either stopping or rapid reduction of the drug, or upon the administration of an antagonist [10]. The universe of addiction is much smaller than the universe of physical dependence to drugs, yet most of the universe of addiction is included in the universe of physical dependence. Physical dependence is certainly a focus of treatment in addiction, but that is not why someone is an addict [9].

Some people may experience an addictive pattern, but not be physically dependent; for example, some binge alcohol drinkers or "chippers" who use heroin periodically.

Physical dependence is not a clinical problem if patients have an adequate supply of the medication, are warned to avoid abrupt discontinuation, use a tapering regimen if treatment cessation is indicated, and opioid antagonists (including agonist-antagonist agents) are avoided [10]. Knowledge of equianalgesic doses of opioids is essential when changing drugs or routes of administration.

Physical dependence may be evident in subgroups such as the patient with angina who obtains relief from nitroglycerin or a steroid-dependent asthma patient [9]. A hypertensive patient receiving clonidine may have a good therapeutic response, but if the drug is stopped abruptly there may be a withdrawal syndrome consisting of rebound increased blood pressure, temporarily higher than that prior to beginning the medication [6]. Studies have shown that approximately 50%–70% of adult patients with hypertension or asthma experience recurrence of symptoms each year, due to noncompliance with treatment, to the point where they require additional medical care to reestablish symptom remission [11].

Other examples include rebound insomnia, which commonly occurs when hypnotics are rapidly withdrawn from a patient who regularly takes higher doses; withdrawal symptoms when some SSRIs are discontinued abruptly; rebound acid hypersecretion after long-term use of acid inhibitors to inhibit gastric acid secretion; rebound psychosis after discontinuation of antipsychotics; and seizures when antianxiety agents (benzodiazepines) are abruptly withdrawn following their use for long periods of time [6, 12, 13].

Addiction and diversion are also possible reasons for requesting dose escalation [7]. Disease progression, a new disease entity, or increased functional activity, may also result in the need for dose escalation [7]. Psychologic or emotional factors, such as stress, anxiety, and/or depression, may also underlie an apparent decrease in analgesia by heightening a patient's sensitivity to pain [5, 7].

A drug-to-drug interaction can result in a clinically significant increase or decrease in the effects of one or both drugs. For example, inhibition of CYP450 2D6 by selective serotonin reuptake inhibitors or quinidine prevents the production of morphine from codeine, a prodrug dependent on the activity of CYP450 2D6 [14]. Rifampin and phenytoin accelerate the metabolism of methadone and can precipitate withdrawal symptoms [6]. A number of antihistamines (e.g. hydroxyzine) enhance the analgesic effects of low doses of opioids.

Differences in bioavailability among formulations of a given drug can have clinical significance. For example, morphine has significant first-pass metabolism in the liver, which results in 2- to 6-fold decreased availability of orally administered morphine compared with parenteral delivery [2, 6]. Failure to recognize this when switching patients from parenteral to oral doses will result in significant undermedication of the patient, which can cause him or her to seek additional medication for treatment of pain [2]. And finally, unrealistic expectations of efficacy can also lead the patient to request dose escalation.

Advances in the neurobiology of drug addiction have provided increasing evidence that prolonged exposure to drugs of abuse produces long-lasting effects in cognitive and drug-rewarding circuits – for this reason, addiction should be considered a chronic medical illness [8]. Therefore, the appropriate standards for treatment and outcome expectations would be found among other chronic illnesses [11].

A literature review was performed to compare addiction with three chronic illnesses: type 2 diabetes mellitus, hypertension, and asthma. These disorders are widely believed to have effective treatments that must continue throughout a patient's life [11]. Genetic heritability, personal choice, and environmental factors were found to be comparably involved in the etiology and course of all four disorders. The natural history of and treatment strategies for addiction strongly resemble those of diabetes, hypertension, and asthma; for example, similar to the pancreas deteriorating in diabetes, the brain changes during addiction [15]. Drugs of abuse activate the dopamine reward circuit, which is connected to areas of the brain that control memory, emotion, and motivation. Eventually, the dopamine circuit becomes blunted and drugs simply push the circuit back to normal, no longer propelling the person toward euphoria; some of these brain changes appear to be long-lasting. Addiction parallels diabetes, asthma, and hypertension in other ways as well. All worsen if left untreated; susceptibility can be inherited; medications ease symptoms but do not affect a cure; recurrence is routine; and each can be triggered or exacerbated by voluntary behavior – overeating, smoking, not exercising, having a drink, or using a drug.

It is estimated that 40%–60% of patients treated for alcohol or other drug addiction return to active substance abuse within a year following treatment discharge. Likewise, treatment for the three chronic disorders also has major problems of medication adherence, early drop-out, and relapse [11].

Across all of these chronic medical illnesses, adherence and outcome were poorest among patients with low socioeconomic status, lack of family and social supports, or significant psychiatric co-morbidity [11].

Definitions and Concepts in Physical Dependency

Most exposures to drugs that are considered to have addiction potential do not result in the disease of addiction [11]. Each person has a particular underlying genetic risk for developing addiction if exposed to a certain type of drug in a certain environment [16, 17, 18]. Environmental factors play a critical role, and exposure to the drug(s) of abuse plays an essential role. Although the choice to try a drug may be voluntary, the drug effects can be influenced profoundly by genetic factors [11, 18]. In addition, enduring and possibly permanent neuroadaptive responses to long-term drug use may contribute to persistency of drug intake, relapse, and craving [11, 19].

The interaction of the drug with a person's biology involves reinforcement pathways – the reinforcing effects of certain drugs contribute largely to their abuse liability [20, 21]. These reinforcing properties are associated with their ability to increase neurotransmitters such as dopamine and serotonin levels of in the brain. The neuronal pathways of drug addiction are components of the mesocortico-limbic dopaminergic systems [20]. Cocaine, amphetamines, ethanol, and opioids all increase extracellular fluid dopamine levels in the nucleus accumbens, although through different mechanisms [11, 8, 6, 22]. The mesolimbic circuit has been implicated in acute reinforcing effects, memory, and conditioned responses linked to craving and the emotional and motivational changes of the withdrawal syndrome [19, 8]. The mesocortical dopamine circuit is involved in the conscious experience of the effects of drugs, drug craving, and the compulsion to take drugs [19]. Generally, addictive drugs act as positive reinforcers (producing euphoria) or negative reinforcers (alleviating symptoms of withdrawal or dysphoria) [8]. Drug characteristics such as rapid onset and intensity of effect increase the potential for abuse [8].

Personality and personal choice is clearly involved in the initiation of drug use – some individuals are inherent risk takers and have novelty-seeking traits, while others are more risk averse [8]. The interaction of the environment with biology creates an individual's psychologic make up (Figure V-1), influencing their learning and how they will respond to environmental stimuli [8, 11].

Addiction is not merely a disorder of drug abuse, and the widely held view of drug addiction as a moral or behavioral problem rather than a medical disease undermines treatment efforts [15]. To devise effective treatment strategies for addiction, it is necessary to understand the interactions of pharmacologic, biochemical, psychiatric, genetic, behavioral, social, and spiritual realms.

Twin studies have established substantial genetic influences on substance abuse disorders [23, 16, 24, 25, 17]. Alcoholism is the best-studied addiction: about 40%

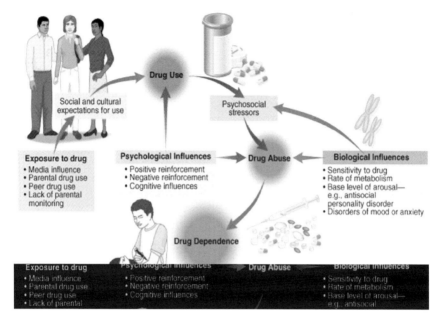

Figure V-1. An integrative model of substance related disorders

of the risk for the disease appears inherited [15, 26]. In addition, the environment and social influences play a role in the development of substance disorders [23, 16, 18]. There is considerable psychiatric co-morbidity among substance abusers, and these patients may have more serious substance abuse histories, poorer outcomes, and increased relapse [27, 28, 29, 8]. Spirituality has long been emphasized as an important factor in recovery from addiction. People with strong spiritual beliefs are healthier, heal faster, and live longer than those without them. A report by the National Center on Addiction and Substance Abuse concluded that clinicians should understand better the importance of spirituality and religion to the prevention and treatment of addiction, and of the spiritual and religious resources available in their communities [30].

In summary, addiction therefore can be considered

- A primary, chronic, neurobiological disease, with genetic, psychosocial, and environmental factors influencing its development and manifestations (Figure V-2)
- Characterized by behaviors that include one of more of the following:
  1. Impaired control over drug use
  2. Compulsive use
  3. Continued use despite harm
  4. Craving

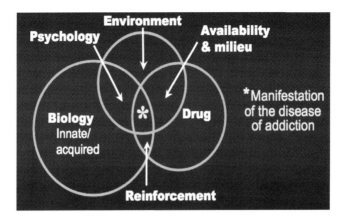

Figure V-2. Addiction: A multi-factor disease state

Terminology in Illicit Use of Opioids

Reward is a stimulus that the brain interprets as intrinsically positive or as something to be attained [8].

Craving is an intense desire to re-experience the effects of a psychoactive substance; it is the cause of relapse after long periods of abstinence [8].

Relapse is a resumption of drug-seeking or drug-taking behavior after a period of abstinence. Priming (new exposure to a formerly abused substance), environmental cues (people, places, or things associated with past drug use), and stress can trigger intense craving and cause a relapse [8].

Addiction is a primary, chronic, neurobiologic disease, with genetic, psychosocial, and environmental factors influencing its development and manifestations. It is characterized by behaviors that include one or more of the following: impaired control over drug use, compulsive use, continued use despite harm, and craving.

Contrary, **physical dependence** is a state of adaptation that is manifested by a drug-class-specific withdrawal syndrome that can be produced by abrupt cessation, rapid dose reduction, decreasing blood level of the drug, and/or administration of an antagonist.

Lastly, **tolerance** is a state of adaptation in which exposure to a drug induces changes that result in a diminution of one or more of the drug's effects over time.

There are several misconceptions of chronic opioid therapy that routinely can cause later addiction:

1. Opioids lead to significant cognitive impairment
2. Absolutely contraindicated in persons with addictive disorders
3. Opioid doses will require continual escalation
4. Adequate pain control with opioids now will lead to poor response later.

Physicians can help minimize the potential for abuse of opioid pain medications by considering the agents' delivery route, bioavailability, and pharmacokinetics. In this respect, a little caution is able to minimize opioid abuse.

Bioavailability of Pain Medicine Related to Abuse

The one thing that inhibits good pain therapies is that the prescriber is afraid of abuse and diversion. It is recommended to match opioid half-life with the indication. In this sense short-acting drugs are for short-acting problems and long-acting drugs for long-acting problems. The same goes for route of delivery. One should match the route with the indication. For example, transdermal patches may be less than ideal for acute situations but work well in a chronic setting.

When choosing the optimal route, one should avoid options with poor bioavailability. Low bioavailability means that higher doses are needed to get the required effect, because there is lesser amount of the active dose being absorbed resulting in low plasma levels with less effect (Table V-2). If one tries to compensate this by a higher loading dose, the excess loading contributes to the amount of drug available for abuse and diversion. For example, the bioavailability of oral oxymorphone is 10%. Ten times the intravenous dose would be required to achieve the same response orally.

Many medical students are taught that if opioids are prescribed in high doses or for a prolonged time, the patient will invariably become an addict. Therefore, the common wisdom is to prescribe the lowest possible dose at the longest possible dosing interval. As a result, opioids are frequently prescribed in doses that are inadequate and at time intervals beyond the duration of action of the drug, resulting in poor analgesia [31]. A recent study of 130 cancer patients evaluated the possible influence of oral opioids, pain, and performance status on cognition. The investigators found that use of long-term oral opioid treatment in cancer patients per se did not affect any of the neuropsychological tests used in the study, and that unrelieved pain itself may deteriorate performance more than oral opioid treatment [32].

In addition, data indicate that chronic opioid analgesic therapy should not be unilaterally contraindicated in patients with addictive disorders [31]. A survey of

Table V-2. Differences in bioavailability of opioid agents commonly used in pain medicine

Opioid	Bioavailability
Fentanyl patch	30%–70%
Fentanyl transmucosal	50%–65%
Oral hydromorphone	30%–35%
Oral morphine	30%
Oral oxycodone	60%–80%
Oral oxymorphone	10%

38 patients suggests that chronic opioid analgesic therapy initiated for chronic non-malignant pain can be safely and often effectively continued for long periods of time. Escalation of dose and tolerance to the analgesic effects were not encountered [33].

Evidence is accumulating of considerable psychiatric co-morbidity among substance abusers. Patients with Axis II (personality) disorders often have more serious substance abuse histories, alcohol-related consequences, and longer treatment histories [27]. A more structured approach may be valuable in helping to organize and coordinate the timing of addiction, pain, and psychiatric interventions [34].

Impulsivity and failed attempts at controlling pain or addiction may also indicate need for a more structured setting. In such cases, consultation with a specialist in pain medicine, a psychologist, or psychiatrist, may be warranted depending on the expertise of the practitioner and the complexity of the presenting problem. The management of pain in patients with a history of addiction or co-morbid psychiatric disorder requires special consideration, but does not necessarily contraindicate the use of opioids [35]. Consultation should also be considered when the treating physician becomes aware of behaviors that may indicate medication misuse, such as unanticipated positive urine drug tests or inflexibility about treatment options [9]. In addition, when patients are unresponsive to therapy, with unimproved function, unmanageable side effects, or impending surgery, a consult should be considered.

Physicians should know when and how to make an appropriate referral. If a chronic pain patient is found to be suffering from an addiction, it is incumbent upon the physician to initiate and support drug treatment interventions. Addiction treatment for patients with chronic pain includes referral to and involvement with formal drug treatment [36, 2]. There is accumulating evidence of considerable psychiatric co-morbidity among substance abusers. Persistent non-compliance, suicidal ideation, and failed attempts at pain management are also reasons for considering referral.

Avoiding Abuse Liability When Prescribing Opioids

Rationally prescribing opioid analgesics will minimize the chances for abuse. When prescribing a controlled substance, the physician should inform the patient of the conditions under which the medication will be prescribed, provide written instructions about appropriate use of the medication, ensure that the patient can understand these rules, and have them sign an agreement [2]. It is important to set the dose of the medication at an effective level – not at the lowest possible level. Get feedback from the patient – if the dose of medication is inadequate, titrate the dose until it is effective [2].

Give sufficient medication to the patient to last until the next appointment. This should also include rescue doses for a sudden increase in a patient's pain level [2]. Ask the patient to bring any remaining medications in the original bottles when he or she returns for their next visit. Examine these bottles to ensure that other physicians are not also prescribing for the patient, the prescription has not been altered, and to determine if the patient is consistently using one pharmacy. Also count any remaining medication to determine use patterns [2]. It is necessary to monitor for lost or stolen prescriptions. The patient should be responsible for prescriptions. One approach is to give the patient a refill on the first lost prescription. The patient is then informed that further lost or stolen prescriptions will result in periods without medication.

Another way of monitoring a patient is to obtain random urine drug screens to determine whether the patient is taking other drugs with the prescribed medication. Such screens may also determine whether the patient is taking the prescribed medication. However, it is essential to know what drugs at what levels will be identified – contact the laboratory to determine whether the specific drugs you are testing for will be identified. Use standard cut-off levels to monitor for presence or absence of drug [2].

Adjunctive medication to treat all aspects of the patient's pain should be employed as necessary [2]. To reduce problems with regulatory agencies, physicians should provide good documentation for everything that occurs during the treatment of the patient. If a medication change occurs, the decision-making process should be noted on the patient's chart. If concerns arise about addictive problems, the plan to assess them should be documented in the chart. The patient should be evaluated as often as necessary. On subsequent visits, outcome measures of opioid therapy including pain relief, use or reduction of pain medications, sleep, functional and social activities, and treatment satisfaction should be recorded [2]. It may be necessary to work with significant others in the patient's life, such as spouse, close friend, employer, or another family member. These individuals sometimes will control the medication, dispensing it appropriately [2].

When the patient no longer needs the medication, it is important to know how to safely discontinue the treatment. This means maintaining this dosing interval and decreasing the total daily dose by about 10% every 2–3 days. Physicians should know the pharmacology of all the drugs that they prescribe. This includes an understanding of the pharmacokinetics and phamacodynamics. Because there is a range of opioids currently available, including full agonists, mixed agonist-antagonists, and partial agonists, it is important to understand the difference between these agents and the relationship they have to each other [2]. Since most opioids have significant first-pass effect, so higher oral doses are needed than parenteral doses.

Although a lesser problem, however, it was observed that physicians who contribute to the problem of prescription drug abuse have been described by the American Medical Association as dishonest-willfully misprescribing for purposes of abuse, usually for profit; disabled by personal problems with drugs or alcohol; dated in their knowledge of current pharmacology or therapeutics; or duped by various patient-initiated fraudulent approaches. Even physicians who do not meet any of these 4D descriptions (dishonest prescription, disabled personal problems, dated in knowledge, duped by patients) must guard against contributing to prescription drug abuse through injudicious prescribing, inadequate safeguarding of prescription

Part V

forms or drug supplies, or acquiescing to the demands or ruses used to obtain drugs for other than medicinal purposes [37].

Avoiding Illicit Use by Ongoing Assessment and Documentation

Review of treatment efficacy should occur periodically to assess the continued analgesia, functional status of the patient and quality of life, adverse effects, and indications of aberrant drug-related behavior [35]. Certain "drug-seeking" behaviors that are either more or less predictive of addiction have been outlined. However, none of these behaviors are absolutely predictive of an addictive disorder or diversion [38].

What are some signs of drug-seeking behavior for illicit purposes? A classic one that law enforcement investigators relate is that drug seekers want an appointment toward the end-of-office hours or they telephone or arrive after office hours when staff are anxious to leave after a long day.

Secondly, drug seekers may insist on being seen immediately or demand immediate action because they're in a hurry to catch a plane or they're late for a meeting. They don't want the physician to do a thorough assessment. There is a need to reschedule those people – if they come back, the physician probably got a patient with a legitimate pain management issue; if they don't, that's one less thing for you to worry about.

Another indicator of drug-seeking behavior is that the individual is not interested in having a physical examination or undergoing diagnostic tests. These individuals are unwilling to give permission to obtain past medical records: "I had a bad time with the doctor, and I don't want that to prejudice your viewpoint," or "I was in a malpractice suit against the doctor and those records are unavailable." That is not true – they should be available.

Drug seekers will often be unable to recall the hospital or clinic where their past records are kept or claim that it went out of business or burned down. They may also be unwilling or unable to supply you with the names of past healthcare practitioners.

They claim to be from out of town and to have lost their prescription or forgotten to pack their medication or they say it was stolen from or left in their bag on the plane.

They may exaggerate or feign medical problems, for example, complain of renal colic and prick a finger to add blood to the urine specimen, so you might believe a renal stone was not visible on x-ray. Their complaints may be hard to determine objectively, such as a migraine, tic, or toothache.

Another indicator of drug-seeking behavior is reciting textbook symptoms or giving an extremely vague, disorganized medical history in which nothing seems to fit.

Drug seekers will often have no interest in a referral or good medical care – they want a prescription and they want it now. They may show an unusual knowledge of controlled substances, but this must be taken in context. Patients who have attended pain clinics may have been taught what is appropriate for them, what works, and know the names of these medicines. But be cautious about someone who claims to have never seen a specialist, but is familiar with many drug names.

Requesting a specific drug and unwillingness to try any other treatment with no medical justification is another suspicious behavior, as is claiming allergy to non-opioid analgesics or to all but one opioid.

TYPICAL DRUG SCAMS TO OBTAIN A PRESCRIPTION OPIOID

Scams to watch out for include hospital employees who have access to the surgery schedule posing as a family member of a patient – they call the surgeon to claim the pain medication is not working: "Can you prescribe something else and call it in, and I'll go and pick it up for them?"

Another scam is reading the obituaries and contacting prescribers for a prescription, posing as an out-of-town relative of the deceased. This could be for a prescription for themselves because they have a grief problem, or they might risk that the prescriber has not yet been informed of the death. When the prescribers are out of town, a drug seeker may read the nursing home obituaries and call them on their return or call the prescribers' partners for a prescription while they are away.

Another example of a drug scam is a practitioner who calls in a prescription for deceased patients and picks up the medication for personal abuse or diversion, claiming to deliver the medication to the patient's home.

The final example here is of an abuser posing as a pharmacist or regulator calling a practice to request DEA numbers of all the prescribers because there is a local issue with diversion and stolen scripts. The DEA does not need to call to ask for your DEA number, because they gave it to you. However, this scam has worked very successfully – an 18-year-old working after school thinks it is the right thing to do and provides the information to the scammer.

Scams are limited only by the imagination of the drug seeker.

Prescribing Opioids – The Controlled Substances Act from 1979

The controlled substances Act from 1979, where the legal definition of a narcotic drug does not necessarily relate to its pharmacology, is defined by law enforcement needs. For medical use, the term "opioid" is preferable and changed to "narcotic."

"Narcotic drugs" defined, not by known pharmacology, but by law enforcement needs, for example are:

1. Opium derivatives
2. Cocaine
3. Marijuana
4. Hallucinogens
5. Amphetamines
6. CNS depressants

Title 21 Code of Federal Regulations (CFR), part 1306.05, paragraph (a) is the citation style used for federal regulations. This citation says that all prescriptions for controlled substances shall be dated as of, and signed on, the date when issued and shall bear the full name and address of the patient ... and the name, address, and registration number of the practitioner. The key element here is that post-dating a prescription cannot be in compliance with federal law, and state law echoes this. It should be remembered, state law can be more restrictive than or equally restrictive to federal law, but it cannot be more lax.

What do you do if you want to give a patient more than one month's supply of a Schedule II medication, which is not refillable, but his or her insurance company will only pay for one month at a time? Write two prescriptions today, date them today, sign them today, and put a note to the pharmacist on one of them – "please do not fill before" – and put in the date a month from today. Nothing in federal law prohibits that, although automatic expiration dates for prescriptions may prohibit that in some states.

The second tenet of the Controlled Substances Act is that for a prescription for a controlled substance to be effective, an individual practitioner acting in the usual course of his or her professional practice must issue it for a legitimate medical purpose. This, again, is a direct quote from federal regulations reiterating the point made earlier that it must be for a legitimate medical purpose in the usual course of practice and be documented.

This section also states that pharmacists, by federal and state law, have what is referred to as a "corresponding responsibility" to ensure that the drugs they dispense are being dispensed for a legitimate medical purpose. This means that if a pharmacist calls to the physician with a question about a prescription, one should not consider this a nuisance; the physician should not consider this as someone trying to second guess. It should be considered that an intelligent, dedicated, law-abiding pharmacist is trying to make certain that he or she is complying with the federal and state regulations. The physician should welcome those calls and work in collaboration with your local pharmacist to provide optimal care for your patients and prevent diversion of controlled substances.

Many practitioners think that emergency telephone prescriptions for Schedule II controlled substances are for their convenience. However, under federal law, it must be a bona fide emergency and the quantity must be limited to that amount necessary to adequately treat the patient for the emergency period [3]. One cannot use an emergency prescription for a month's supply to save the patient a trip. The law also requires that the pharmacist immediately reduces the order to writing. Pharmacists therefore, should make a reasonable effort to determine that the oral authorization came from a registered practitioner [3]. They may call back after a few minutes, getting your office number from the telephone directory, to ensure that you did authorize that emergency prescription.

The law requires that the physician authorizing the prescription delivers the original written prescription, matching what the pharmacist took down by telephone, to the pharmacist within 7 calendar days. On this must be written: "Authorization for Emergency Dispensing." Therefore, if the DEA or pharmacy board inspects their controlled substance records, for every emergency prescription that was dispensed more than 7 days previously, a matching prescription will close the loop and demonstrate that the pharmacist is practicing lawfully.

What are the conditions of an emergency? This again is a three-pronged test. The immediate administration of the substance is necessary for proper treatment; no appropriate alternatives are available, including a non-controlled drug – for example, the patient cannot tolerate ibuprofen or it is ineffective; and it is not reasonably possible for the practitioner to provide the patient with a written prescription prior to dispensing – not because the physician is teeing up on the fourth hole.

What does federal law say about treating chronic pain with opioids? The Controlled Substances Act of 1970 says that any registrant – a practitioner who has a DEA number – can administer or dispense narcotic drugs to persons with intractable pain in which no relief or cure is possible or none has been found after reasonable efforts [39]. It clearly states that it is appropriate to give this type of medication for chronic pain.

What is the position of the DEA on prescribing controlled substances for someone with pain due to cancer and prescribing opioids for someone with chronic pain not due to cancer?

The positions by the DEAs are directly quoted from the Physician's Manual: An informational outline of the Controlled Substances Act [40]. It says: "Controlled substances and, in particular, narcotic analgesics, may be used in the treatment of pain experienced by a patient with a terminal illness or a chronic disorder." The first sentence specifies that controlled substances can be used not only for terminal illness, but also for any chronic disorder [41].

These drugs have a legitimate clinical use – that is why they are legally on the market – and the physician should not hesitate to prescribe, dispense, or administer them when they are indicated for a legitimate medical purpose [40]. Again it has to be pointed out that "legitimate medical purpose" is important. It is the position of the DEA that these controlled substances should be prescribed, dispensed, or administered when there is a legitimate medical need" [41].

This is a very straightforward statement; the DEA does not want to be the entity that is responsible for a patient not receiving pain medication or other controlled substance treatment when it is legitimately needed.

In summary, federal law does not preclude the use of opioids as analgesics for legitimate medical purposes, including treating chronic pain and treating pain in addicted patients. However, federal law does prohibit the use of opioids to treat addiction without a separate DEA registration in a Narcotic Treatment Program (NTP) [39]. So any registrant can treat *pain* with opioids in an addicted patient; they can detox or maintain addiction in a hospital if the addict is admitted for reasons other than addiction, such as a motor vehicle accident, but once the addicted patient is an outpatient, a physician cannot maintain their addicted state outside of a Narcotic Treatment Program.

Lastly, federal law is not static; things are changing. For example new laws are in place that will allow the office-based treatment of addiction with particular opioids that are indicated for that purpose. This is a radical change that reverses many years of federal law and the prevailing custom.

Typical Patterns as Predictive Signs of Aberrant Drug-Related Behavior

1. Selling prescription drugs
2. Prescription forgery
3. Stealing or "borrowing" drugs
4. Injecting oral formulations
5. Obtaining prescription drugs from non-medical sources
6. Concurrent abuse of alcohol and illicit drugs
7. Multiple unsanctioned dose escalations
8. Repeated episodes of prescription "loss"

Contrary, aberrant drug-related behaviors are probably less predictive of addiction and could represent pseudo-addictive behavior [38].

1. Aggressive complaining about the need for higher doses
2. Drug hoarding during periods of reduced symptoms
3. Requesting specific drugs
4. Prescriptions from other physicians
5. Unsanctioned dose escalation
6. Unapproved use of the drug
7. Reporting psychic effects not intended by the physician
8. Use of multiple pharmacies.

It is important to note, that extended-release formulations with low bioavailability pose a particular risk for diversion and abuse. For example, a drug that is 10% bioavailable would require 10 times the intravenous amount to achieve the same response; to use a short-acting compound for long-acting pain with twice-daily dosing, the amount of drug needed goes up again, meaning that a lot of drug is now available for diversion and abuse. In contrast, methadone is rarely abused for practical reasons. The drug has a 100% bioavailability. The same amount of drug is available regardless of how it's administered. In addition, methadone is long lasting, based on the nature of the molecule resulting in a large volume of distribution (Vd), a lesser clearance (Cl) and a long elimination half-life (t1/2ß), so an extended-release formulation isn't necessary. One should get suspicious about a patient possibly diverting or abusing opioids, if he claims, "this is a great drug to start with".

Transdermal delivery of opioids involves a delay in onset of action for about 4–8 h. It is for this reason, that these drugs are not an option for breakthrough pain. In the setting of outpatient cancer breakthrough pain, it's important to have a fast-, and short-acting compound readily available. This avoids layering on excess opioids when breakthrough pain resolves after a short time.

Avoiding Drug Diversion from Medical to Illicit Use

There are a number of new and upcoming ways to avoid the potential for abuse. One problem is that sustained release opioid drugs can be crushed or rapidly extracted with alcohol. The sucrose acetate isobutyrate extended release (SABER) technology overcomes this problem because the viscous gel locks the drug into the matrix (i.e. Remoxy^{RM}), despite attempts to crush, melt, or extract it with alcohol.

Another option is to add antagonists, such as naloxone and naltrexone. Naloxone has a bioavailability of 3% when taken orally, so when a patient takes a drug like buprenorphine and naloxone in a 4:1 ratio sublingually (i.e. Suboxone^{TM}), they're not having any inhibition of the μ-opioid receptor due to the naloxone. But if they attempted to crush and inject the drug, there would be 100% bioavailability of naloxone, and it would inhibit the action of buprenorphine. A similar drug containing oxycodone and naltrexone is being developed by Pain Therapeutics Inc. and currently is in phase III trials. What they're finding in their studies is that there may be less euphoria and less physical withdrawal related to this compound, compared with just the native oxycodone. Also, in 2006, the U.S. Food and Drug Administration approved Ionsys^{TM} (fentanyl iontophoretic transdermal system). This patient-activated analgesic system is indicated for the short-term management of acute postoperative pain in adult patients requiring opioid analgesia during hospitalization. The system made by Alza Corp. and marketed by Janssen Pharmaceutical delivers a preprogrammed, 40-μg dose of fentanyl through the skin over a 10-min period, and the drug has 100% bioavailability. In addition, AcelRx is developing a sublingual sufentanil "nanotab", which is six times smaller than a nitroglycerin pill, having a 90% bioavailability. Abusers could crush this if they wanted to, but it's along the order of methadone – they're not going to get any advantage by crushing and injecting it.

Another problem is the tracking of opioids. While it is easy to track a pair of socks through FedEx or UPS from New Jersey to California, yet when the physician writes an OxyContin® prescription, he has absolutely no idea how it's used. With the technology that's available to track mail, there should also be a better way to track the use of prescription opioids. Currently, Purdue Pharma uses radio-frequency identification (RFID) tags on their bottles of OxyContin®. However, this technology tracks the drugs from the manufacturer to the pharmacy only while it does not help a physician to monitor patient use.

AcelRx is planning to use computerized dispensers for nanotab products that will allow physicians to download a patient's dosing history. Such technology also could be helpful in assuring that dosing regimens do not confuse patients.

Avoiding Illicit Use by Combining Opioids with Antidepressants/Antiepileptics

Antidepressants and antiepileptics are both effective in treating neuropathic pain, but a combination performs best. Nearly 80% of patients who took a combination of antiepileptics and antidepressant medications had a greater than 50% Visual Analogue Scale (VAS) improvement, a statistically significant finding. Whereas clinical trials have shown clear evidence in favor of using antidepressants and antiepileptic medications alone in treating chronic pain, no studies have been designed to focus on the effect of combining antidepressants and antiepileptics for the treatment of neuropathic pain. Over a 2-year period Dr. Robinson and collegues of Beth Israel Deaconess School, Harward Medical at Boston reviewed 6,129 charts with an initial encounter and a diagnosis of neuropathic pain. They also analyzed VAS, medical procedures, and antidepressant and antiepileptic use and dosage at each visit. Patients who had a 50% or greater improvement in their VAS score were considered to have a favorable response. Of the charts reviewed, 3,370 patients had at least one antidepressant or antiepileptic prescribed. All of the antidepressant and antiepileptic drugs analyzed had favorable responses in more than 70% of patients. There was a statistically significant level of improvement among patients who were prescribed tertiary amines and among patients who were prescribed a combination of antiepileptic and antidepressant medication. A total of 939 patients received the combination, with 79.4% reporting a VAS score improvement of 50% or greater. About 19.4% of patients who received combination therapy had no response, and 1.2% had an unknown response.

The investigators stressed that addiction should be insured, treated, and evaluated like other chronic illnesses [11]. No single treatment is appropriate for everyone, and addicted individuals with co-morbid mental illness need to receive integrated treatment for both disorders. Recovery from addiction is a long-term process that often requires multiple treatment episodes. Unfortunately, many physicians that do see addiction as a medical problem tend to treat it as an acute, rather than chronic disorder. The concept of addiction as a medical disease has yet to gain acceptance with a large proportion of physicians. They, like many others in society, often regard abuse or alcohol as moral or behavioral problems.

The best addiction treatments teach patients the biologic origins of their disease while helping them understand how their behavior affects the individuals around them. Calling addiction a disease does not absolve personal responsibility [15] and it is noted that the different drugs also demonstrate a difference in addiction liability

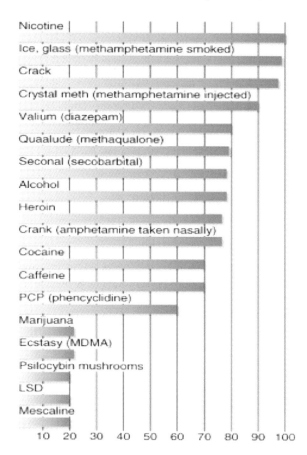

Figure V-3. Relative ranking of the addictive potential inherent in different drugs

(Figure V-3). Experts were asked in regard to todays commonly used drugs and their addictiveness. Rating was done according to
– how easy it is to get hooked on the substance,
– how hard it is to stop using it,
– how much does the drug effect the persons health.

Demask the Patient Prone to Develop Illicit Use

When the physician has the suspicion of a possible abuse of prescription analgesics, he should gather information from multiple sources to validate patient responses or concerns of others. An unanticipated positive urine drug screen or worsening results are often indications that drug abuse is occurring [42]. However, contrary to belief, no behavior is absolutely predictive of aberrant drug use or addictive disease, so a differential diagnosis must be made. These behaviors may be appropriate responses to either under-relieved or well-relieved pain [36]. In the former, drug-seeking behaviors arise when a patient cannot obtain tolerable relief with the prescribed dose of analgesic and seeks alternate sources or increased doses of analgesic – pseudoaddiction [36, 3]. Alternatively, a patient receiving good pain relief may take steps to ensure adequate medication supply, as they fear not only reemergence of pain, but also the emergence of withdrawal symptoms [36]. Psychiatric factors, such as anxiety or depression, a personality disorder, or changes in cognitive state, such as mild encephalopathy due to the treatment regimen or their underlying psychiatric problems, may be responsible for the behaviors identified. Responses of family members and others in the patient's environment may also affect a patient's perception of their pain [5]. These behaviors may be the result of increasing pain due to disease progression, or development of a new medical condition. Non-restorative sleep has also been associated with worsening pain [43]. Criminal activity – diverting the medications to the "street" – may also be an explanation for these behaviors. Although none is pathognomonic, the following behavior patterns could indicate an addiction:

1. Pseudoaddiction
2. Psychiatric diagnosis with
   a. Depression
   b. Personality disorder, and/or
   c. Anxiety

On the other hand there are other traits, which might mislead the supposition of an addiction:

1. Mild encephalopathy
2. Social stressors
3. Other medical diagnosis
4. Inadequate instruction by healthcare provider
5. Non-restorative sleep
6. Criminal activity

Further Stigma of Persons with a Potential Drug Addictive Behavior Pattern

Principles of good medical practice should guide the prescribing of opioids. Initial evaluation of the patient should include a review of previous diagnostic studies to determine if the patient has previously been treated for a pain syndrome [35, 44]. The American Pain Society recommends that patient management include complete history and physical examination, an initial comprehensive pain assessment, including an evaluation of biologic, psychological, or social factors that may be contributing to pain, as well as an assessment of the overall impact of pain on function. Pain assessment should focus on the type of pain, intensity, location, duration/time course, and effects on lifestyle [44].

The role nicotine plays in the patient's life should be established, including a question about the time of day he or she has the first cigarette. The severity of tobacco addiction correlates with the time to first cigarette of the day, the most important cigarette of the day, and the number of cigarettes smoked daily. Patients who smoke within minutes of arising, or even before getting out of bed, and whose first cigarette of the day is the most important are often severely addicted [45].

A positive family history of substance use, whether for alcohol or prescribed or illicit drugs, mental health and emotional problems, are risk factors for addictive disease in all clinical populations [9, 46]. Therefore, it is necessary to ask the patient about both alcohol and illicit drug abuse among immediate family members (i.e., parents, siblings, children) and second-degree relatives (i.e., grandparents, uncles, aunts, cousins) [46].

Participation or recommended participation in drug abuse treatment programs should be determined. Patients who have undergone an opioid detoxification in the past may be at higher risk for addictive disease [36].

Nearly all drugs of abuse alter sexual function [7]. Although the perception exists that drugs enhance sexual performance, drug use typically decreases performance and may cause impotence or other sexual dysfunction.

The Alcohol Addictive Patient

An alcohol and drug history should be included in the initial assessment, for example using the CAGE questionnaire or Trauma questions, to assess potential for substance abuse problems [47, 42, 48].

The Trauma Test is another screening tool used to assess the potential for substance abuse. It is a noninvasive method of obtaining information that can provide an important adjunct to diagnosis, and its brief structure provides a cost-effective screening procedure in clinical practice. The Trauma Test is composed of the following five questions:

Since your 18th birthday, have you:

1. Had any fractures or dislocations to your bones or joints (excluding sports injuries)?
2. Been injured in a traffic accident?
3. Injured your head (excluding sports injuries)?
4. Been in a fight or assaulted while intoxicated?
5. Been injured while intoxicated?

A positive response to two or more questions indicates a strong potential for alcohol abuse. Clinicians should use this tool in conjunction with laboratory tests and a brief questionnaire that directly inquires about problems related to alcohol use [42, 48].

Collateral information can be obtained from family, employers, and previous medical records [42]. Sudden loss of a job or frequent job changes for no apparent reason is often a consequence of substance abuse [42]. Unexplained financial or family problems can also result from substance abuse. Patients with a history of driving under the influence or a history of two or more non-sport-related traumatic events (after age 18 years) are considered at high risk for substance abuse [42]. Therefore, the prescribing physician should be alert to the eating disorder, addiction, and sexual abuse triad – if two are present, look for the third [49]. It is because of this triad that researchers have recommended that all women entering substance abuse treatment should be screened for eating disorders [50].

During the initial assessment ask for the following:

1. Has drug/alcohol use ever contributed to a problem for them or those close to them?
   - Incorporate CAGE and Trauma questions into patient interview
2. Gather collateral information from
   a. Family
   b. Work
   c. Legal medical records
3. Be alert to the eating disorders, addiction, and sexual abuse triad. If two are present, look for the third.

The National Institute of Alcohol Addiction and Abuse recommend use of the CAGE questionnaire for possible alcohol problems. Clinicians should then ask the quantity and frequency questions of all patients who drink alcohol [51, 52]. If two of four questions are positive, diagnosis of a history of alcohol abuse or dependency has a sensitivity of 74% and a specificity of 91%:

1. Have you felt the need to cut (C) down on your drinking (or drug use)?
2. Have people annoyed (A) you by criticizing your drinking (or drug use)?
3. Have you ever felt bad or guilty (G) about your drinking (or drug use)?
4. Have you ever needed an eye-opener (E) the first thing in the morning to steady your nerves or get rid of a hangover?

Another test is the CRAFT, a screening instrument for problematic adolescent substance use. It is a six-question, "yes" or "no" type questionnaire. Like the CAGE, the CRAFT takes about one minute to complete, and can be incorporated into any type of evaluation [53]. While items 1, 2, and 5 pertain to personal drinking or drugging, and are heavily endorsed by adolescents with substance use disorders, only item 6 relates directly to the criteria for abuse [53]. A CRAFT score of two or higher is optimal for identifying problem use, abuse, or dependence having a sensitivity 76% and a specificity 94%. Positive screens should be followed by a more complete substance use history [54].

CRAFT is a developmentally appropriate screening tool for adolescents [54]. It is verbally administered, simple to score, and easy to remember. CRAFT is composed of the following six questions:

1. Have you ever ridden in a car (C) driven by someone (including yourself) who was "high" or had been using alcohol or drugs?
2. Do you ever use alcohol or drugs to relax (R), feel better about yourself, or fit in?
3. Do you ever use alcohol or drugs while you are alone (A)?
4. Do you ever forget (F) things you did while using alcohol or drugs?

5. Do your family or friends (F) ever tell you that you should cut down on your drinking or drug use?
6. Have you ever gotten into trouble (T) while you were using alcohol or drugs?

This tool offers clinicians a practical means of identifying adolescent patients who need more comprehensive assessment or referral to substance abuse treatment specialists [54].

An optimal marker of excessive alcohol consumption has not been found. Although γGT is the most widely used test as a marker, however, elevated levels are also caused by nonalcoholic liver disease, most hepatobiliary disorders, obesity, diabetes mellitus, hypertriglyceridemia, and the use of liver microsome-inducing drugs [55]. Also, elevated Mean Corpuscular Volume (MCV) is another frequently used marker for alcohol abuse. Combinations of more than one marker give better sensitivity. Determining both MCV and γGT levels greatly improves the estimate of daily consumption. In particular, it permits tracking of false-negative subjects who exhibit low γGT levels despite high alcohol consumption [56].

In alcoholic hepatitis, the activity of serum alanine aminotransferase (ALT) is depressed relative to that of aspartate aminotransferase (AST). An AST: ALT ratio greater than 2 may indicate alcoholic hepatitis [45].

There are initial laboratory assessments directing to a potential addiction liability:

1. Elevated
   a. γGT (or other liver function tests)
   b. MCV (mean corpuscular volume)
2. Detectable blood alcohol concentration
3. Elevated γGT + MCV highly suggestive of alcoholism
4. AST: ALT ratio > 2 may indicate alcoholic liver disease
   γGT = gamma-glutamyltranspeptidase;
   MCV = mean corpuscular volume;
   AST = aspartate aminotransferase;
   ALT = alanine aminotransferase

The Most Common Signs of Alcohol Addiction

Alcohol consumption and abuse can have a variety of cutaneous manifestations, including palmar erythema and spider angioma (also known as spider telangiectasis, arterial spider, spider nevus, or nevus araneus) [57]. Alcohol can also induce diseases/disease states with dermatologic manifestations [57]. Many endocrine changes are seen in patients with chronic alcoholism. Signs of hypogonadism and hyperestrogenism are seen in male patients. Hypogonadism is manifested by loss of libido and potency, testicular atrophy, reduced fertility, and reduced facial hair growth [57]. Gynecomastia, vascular spiders, changes in fat distribution, loss of body hair, and change of pubic hair to a female distribution [57] manifest hyperestrogenism. In contrast, female patients with alcoholism rarely manifest signs of masculinization. They may demonstrate breast atrophy or menstrual irregularities [57].

In 30% of patients with alcoholic hepatitis, the liver is enlarged, smooth, and occasionally tender [45].

In summary the following signs are significant for alcohol abuse:
1. Alcohol on breath during exam
2. Cutaneous manifestations
   a. Palmar erythema
   b. Spider angiomata
3. Endocrine changes (in males)
   a. Gynecomastia
   b. Testicular atrophy
4. Enlarged or tender liver

Concomitant Sequelae of Alcoholism

Chronic pancreatitis often develops in alcoholic patients, and is frequently associated with diabetes [45]. Also, secondary hypertension may be associated with the use of excess alcohol [45], while gastritis is common, and may be related to alcohol's effect on gastric secretions, which increase in volume and acidity while the pepsin content remains low [45].

Both the direct toxic action of alcohol and the accompanying nutritional deficiency, particularly of thiamine, are considered responsible for the frequent peripheral neuropathy [45], while alcohol-induced sexual dysfunction may occur only or predominantly during intoxication [45]. Following excessive alcohol consumption, diarrhea and tremulousness are common symptoms [58].

Common Comprehensions on Prescription Drug Abuse

The street value of a prescription drug is dependent on whether it is a brand or generic. Even abusers know that they get what they pay for when buying a brand-name drug. Drugs that have a quick onset – immediate-release or injectable drugs – are more sought after, as well as those that have a greater intensity. The demand for drugs with a short duration of action is consistent with the rate hypothesis of reinforcement – the faster the drug enters the system, the quicker it causes the dopamine surge in the nucleus accumbens, which is associated with euphoria. Street value also depends on whether the product can be injected or snorted successfully.

Prescription drug abuse occurs because the controlled substances that work effectively for patients with legitimate need are commonly prescribed. As controlled substances are prescribed more often, their availability increases. As a result, opportunities for diversion increase because more people have access to the drug for abuse or diversion, either directly or indirectly because a family member is receiving it legitimately. An example was a woman who admitted under oath to giving M

& Ms® candy in place of pain medication to her grandmother who was dying of cancer, so that she could divert and abuse the pain medication.

There is a perception that abusing pharmaceutical drugs is safer than abusing street drugs. A pharmaceutical drug is easily identified (determined by the indicia on the pill), it is pure, and there is less risk of contracting HIV or hepatitis if not injecting and sharing needles. However, the risk of sexually transmitted disease may remain unchanged if a drug abuser with impaired judgment has sex with other abusers who are sharing needles.

There is often a correlation between the currently popular illicit drugs of abuse and the type of prescription drugs sought by diverters. Heroin is often interchanged with prescription opioids; benzodiazepines are used to soften the crash from cocaine withdrawal; methamphetamines are substituted with amphetamines; and cariso-prodol is reported to enhance the "high" of hydrocodone. In addition, there is a population that abuses only prescription drugs, as well as a population that primarily abuses illicit drugs, and a population that migrates from one to the other.

Another perception, particularly among the young, is that a prescription drug is safer because "it's just a prescription drug": "If my 80-year-old grandmother takes them, how bad can they be?" They don't realize that the grandmother, who has pain, has built up tolerance to the respiratory depressant effects of the medication over time. Healthy 18-year-olds who abuse their grandmother's pain medication are taking a big risk – they do not have the same pain condition and their bodies are not adapted to the presence of that drug.

There is also the issue of low or no acquisition cost for prescription drugs. For example, Workers' Compensation, the VA Health System, and Indian Health Services usually have zero acquisition costs; Medicaid has a small co-pay; and private insurance companies may have a small or no co-pay. This may motivate some individuals to profitably sell all or part of their medication.

PHYSICAL SIGNS AND SYMPTOMS OF HARD DRUG ABUSE

Drug abusing individuals frequently develop medical sequelae of that behavior. Smoking or snorting cocaine and other drugs can cause respiratory problems, atrophy of the nasal mucosa, and perforation of the nasal septum [42]. On the other hand, needle marks may be present on the skin from recent injections, or "tracks" may be present over veins from repeated injections. Injection is not always confined to the obvious sites. Many users will inject into the axilla, under the tongue, under the breast, in the legs, and even into the dorsal vein of the penis [42]. Many heroin addicts begin with subcutaneous injections ("skin popping") and may return to this mode when extensive scarring makes their veins inaccessible (Figure V-4). As addicts become more desperate, cutaneous ulcers may be found in unlikely sites [45].

How can the medical practitioner protect himself from diversion? By being a good practitioner. Protecting yourself from diversion boils down to two basic tenets: be a

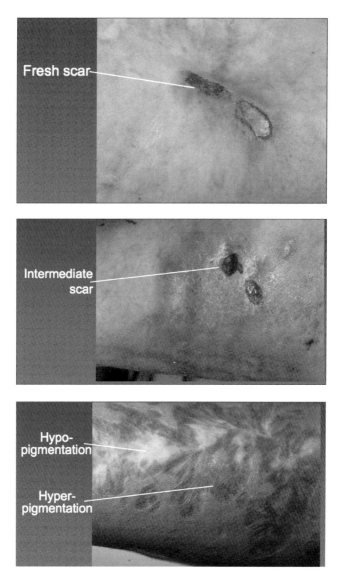

Figure V-4. Fresh, intermediate and old skin-popping scars resulting from subcutaneous injection of drugs

careful, thoughtful practitioner, and document, document, document! Investigators accept that even the best practitioners are going to be fooled once in a while, but you don't want to be fooled routinely. You do want to be cautious because you want to protect your ability to serve your community and those patients in need.

Obtain a history and perform a physical examination that is appropriate to the complaint and do document all findings !!! Look for signs of drug abuse because some diverters are also abusers. They resort to diversion in order to feed their habit. Signs of drug abuse include inflamed nares and a perforated septum in individuals without a history of significant facial trauma. Tracks – multiple, linear, and often hyperpigmented scars – can be found over the arms, wrists, axillae, neck, groin, between the toes, on the breasts, and the dorsal vein of the penis.

When abusers run out of veins, they will resort to "skin popping," which is the subcutaneous injection of drugs. Skin-popping scars are irregular or round and look like small-pox vaccination scars, except they are multiple and not found where expected over the deltoid muscle. Skin-popping scars can be found all over the body and are a common cause of abscesses. In 1999, skin abscesses due to skin-popping heroin were the number one admitting diagnosis at San Francisco General Hospital's emergency department, for which the hospital provided more than $18 million in un-reimbursed medical care. The typical progress of drug abuse is from snorting or smoking, to intravenous injection, followed by skin-popping when no access to veins remains.

Signs and symptoms to look for in order to detect a past or a present abusive behavior.
1. Inflamed, ulcerated, or perforated nasal septum (Figure V-5).
2. Continual sniffing
3. Needle tracks along venous access sites (Figure V-6)
4. Poor venous access
5. Multiple small skin ulcerations
6. Subcutaneous use – "skin popping" (Figure V-4)
7. The typical "pin-point" pupil (Figure V-7)

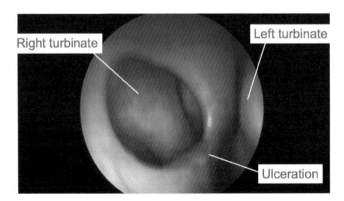

Figure V-5. Looking into the left nares one can see the left turbinate, as expected, and also the right turbinate, which you should not be able to see because a wall – the septum – should be present. Instead there is a healed hole. One can also see some ulceration present

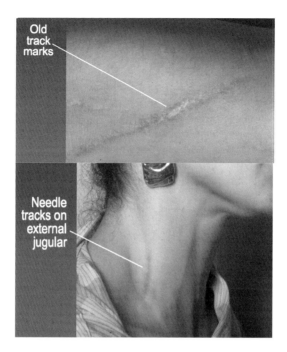

Figure V-6. Needle tracks at accessible veins are typical for the injection of illicit drugs

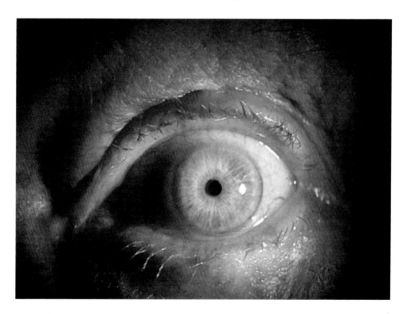

Figure V-7. A jaundiced eye with a small pupil is suggestive of hepatitis C resulting from intravenous drug abuse. Constricted pupils are a characteristic of opioid use. The photograph was taken in normal light, so the small pupil is not an artifact of flash photography

Such a perforated septum may be the result of piercing, trauma, or repeated snorting of cocaine, which is both vasoconstrictive and locally irritating to the nasal mucosa.

In addition, injecting drug users are at risk for infective endocarditis and valvular murmurs [45].

Alcohol or drug addiction problems often lead to a disturbance of lifestyle in which adequate nourishment is neglected. Absorption and metabolism of nutrients are also impaired. Drug addicts are often emaciated [45]. Cocaine causes intense coronary arterial spasm and users may present with cocaine-induced angina or MI [45].

THE RED FLAGS DURING INITIAL ASSESSMENT

Inconsistent information provided by the patient, a history of substance abuse, past or present participation in detoxification or other treatment programs (AA, NA), history of adverse consequences related to substance abuse, including legal issues, and a family history of substance abuse are all red flags for problematic substance abuse [42, 9, 36].

The physician should be sensitized in case of:
1. Inconsistent information provided
2. History of substance abuse
3. Past or present participation in treatment programs (AA, NA)
4. History of adverse consequences related to substance abuse, including legal issues
5. Family history of substance abuse

A history of problems with employers, family, or school, such as frequent change of jobs for no apparent reason or unexplained financial problems, may be indicative of impulsivity, and can be the result of substance abuse [42]. Some patients' manipulativeness can be detected by observation. For example, when a physician has the impression that his or her responses are being intensely studied by the patients. Patients with pseudologica fantastica or Münchhausen's syndrome, or those who are adept at deceit, can be persuasive to a degree that is unusual in comparison to ordinary clinical encounters. When the interaction with the patient creates unease or discomfort for the physician, suspicion that a manipulator may be present is justified [37].

In summation, aberrant drug related features characterize behaviors, which are more likely to be predictive. Adapted from [38]:
- Prescription forgery
- Concurrent abuse of related illicit drugs
- Repeated prescription losses
- Selling prescription drugs
- Multiple unsanctioned dose escalations
- Stealing or borrowing another patient's drugs
- Injecting oral formulations

- Obtaining prescription drugs from non-medical sources
- Concurrent abuse of alcohol and illicit drugs
- Repeated episodes of prescription "loss"

However, there are aberrant drug related behaviors, which are less predictive. Adapted from [38]:

- Drug hoarding during periods of reduced symptoms
- Acquisition of similar drugs from other medical sources
- Aggressive complaining about the need for higher doses
- Unapproved use of the drug to treat another symptom
- Unsanctioned dose escalation one or two times
- Reporting psychic effects not intended by the clinician
- Requesting specific drugs

Also, when prescribing drugs with abuse liability, for his own safety the physician should observe the following:

1. Set clear rules and expectations for the patient; have them sign an agreement.
2. Begin the dose of medication at the appropriate level to treat the condition and titrate as necessary; get feedback from the patient.
4. Give sufficient medication to last between appointments, plus rescue doses.
5. Ask the patient to bring any remaining drugs to the next meeting in original bottles – provides information on pharmacies used, alterations of prescription, other prescribing physicians, and patterns of use.
6. Monitor for lost or stolen prescriptions.
7. Obtain random UDS (urine drug screens); know what drugs laboratory screens actually identify.
8. Use adjunctive medications as necessary.
9. Document your decision-making process.
10. Evaluate the patient at appropriate intervals.
11. Involve significant others in treatment plan.
12. Know how to safely discontinue medications.
13. Know the pharmacology of the drugs used.

When interpretating aberrant drug-related behavior, realize that none are pathognomonic, and could indicate

1. Addiction
2. Pseudoaddiction
3. Psychiatric diagnosis, with
   a. Depression
   b. Personality disorder
   c. Anxiety
   d. Mild encephalopathy
   e. Social stressors
4. Other medical diagnosis
5. Inadequate instruction by healthcare provider
6. Non-restorative sleep
7. Criminal activity

Use of Urine Drug Screening (UDS)

Physicians must understand the process of any kind of urine drug screening that will have the implication of discharging a patient or altering their treatment plan. Urine drug screening was designed to detect illicit and/or licit non-prescribed drug abuse, not to monitor adherence to treatment regimens.

Physicians must be sure that they are getting a high-quality laboratory process. The Department of Health and Human Services (DHHS) Substance Abuse and Mental Health Services Administration (SAMSHA) has a certification program for analytical laboratories [59]. It is important to understand how the specimen is collected, what is being prescribed, and the retention times. Many prescribed opioids are not part of a standard UDS; for example, you must specifically ask for oxycodone and hydrocodone. With a formalized quality-controlled collection procedure, UDS can be a valuable tool – for example, an unexpected result can support decision to refer to a specialist. Interpretation requires information – physicians should get to know their laboratory director and consider a medical review officer consultation.

Urine drug screening is typically a two-step procedure. The first step uses proprietary immunoassays to detect the presence of a drug or metabolite in the urine. Specimens identified as positive on the initial immunoassay test are confirmed using gas chromatography/mass spectrometry [59]. There can be multiple reasons for a negative urine drug screen, including the cutoff points used by the testing laboratory. The specificity and sensitivity of immunoassays vary depending on the assay type and specific test performed. Antibodies are seldom specific to a single drug or drug metabolite; therefore cross-reactions cause false positive results. Positive results based on immunoassay tests alone are referred to as "presumptive positives" and must be confirmed using a different assay technique. Be aware that a positive opiates screen cannot distinguish between morphine, codeine, or heroin [59]. Even confirmation by gas chromatography/mass spectrometry (GC/MS) has variables in the assay procedure that affect its sensitivity, specificity, and reliability [59]. Although GC/MS can quantitate the level of drug in the urine, no inference can be made about how much was taken because the levels of drugs or drug metabolites in urine are affected by numerous factors.

Summary of reasons for false negative/positive UDS
1. High cut-off points of the test being used
2. "Presumed, false positive" results may be due to the tremendous variability in specificity and sensitivity of assay type and the specific test performed
   a. Assay methods being used
   b. Laboratories being involved
   c. Technicians being a human source of error

N.B. Urine drug levels are not related to blood levels either detected or not detected

An example of a common error of interpretation is when the UDS of a patient taking a hydrocodone preparation is reported as "positive" for opiates, which may occur because there is some cross reactivity. The GC/MS, however, confirms the presence of hydrocodone and hydromorphone. Therefore, the patient is accused of abusing street drugs or doctor shopping. The solution is to understand the metabolism of hydrocodone and, therefore, know that a fraction of hydrocodone is metabolized to hydromorphone. Also, in order to eliminate the identification of most individuals who have ingested poppy seeds, the DHHS raised the testing levels for opiates from 300 to 2,000 ng/mL. They also established a new requirement to test for 6-MAM, a metabolite that comes only from heroin, for specimens that test positive for morphine [60].

Cases have been documented of cocaine ingestion by drinking tea made from coca leaves. Although such tea may be available for purchase by (apparently) unknowing consumers, the product-containing active cocaine and/or related metabolites-is illegal under US DEA and FDA regulations, and does not constitute an "alternative valid medical explanation" [59].

Cocaine is a local, vasoconstrictive anesthetic, not resembling other local anesthetics that are more commonly employed in ENT procedures. A positive urine test through medical use can be checked through documented medical records, prescription forms, or contact with the prescribing practitioner [59]. Immunoassay screening tests cross-react with various amphetamine-related drugs that are not abused, for example, dopamine, isoxsuprine (a vasodilator), and ephedrine (an asthma medication). GC/MS confirmation distinguishes the cross-reacting compounds, assuring that results are not false positive. The Vicks® Vapor Inhaler contains desoxyephedrine, which is the *l*-form of methamphetamine. A separation of *d*- and *l*-methamphetamine isomers should reveal 100% *l*-methamphetamine following Vicks® Vapor Inhaler use; more than 20% of *d*-methamphetamine suggests a source of *d*-methamphetamine other than the inhaler [59].

Summary of Considerations When Using Urine Drug Screening (UDS)

1. Ingestion of poppy seeds in cakes or cookies results in opiate positive screening. This has been addressed by a higher cut-off change on 12/01/98
2. Cocaine positive reaction. Illicit under CSA, where use of herbal teas are not a valid explanation. Even in ENT, cocaine does not resemble other local anesthetics in the analysis.
3. Methamphetamine/amphetamine positive may be due to either prescription use or demonstrate a cross reactivity (e.g. Vicks® Vapor Inhaler containing desoxyephedrine, the *l*-form of methamphetamine).
   CSA = controlled substance act;
   ENT = ear, nose, and throat;
   CSA = controlled substance act.

> **Note, most semisynthetic and synthetic opioids (Table V-3) are *not* reliably detected by commonly used screens**

INDICATIONS FOR RANDOM URINE DRUG TESTING

1. For presence of illicit drugs or controlled substances not prescribed
2. Verify patient is taking prescribed medication
3. Verify unexpected results with a more definitive test (e.g. GC/MS) GC/MS = gas chromatography/mass spectrometry

The term urine drug "screening" actually is a misnomer since it implies screening for all drugs [60]. In reality, it is not possible to prove the presence or absence of all drugs, and the testing procedure is open-ended and evolving [61].

All urine drug testing is not equal. No "standard" Urine Drug Test (UDT) is suitable for all purposes and settings – rather, a multitude of options exist that healthcare professionals should adapt to their clinical needs. Standard tests exist only for federally regulated industries, such as those under the purview of the Department of Transportation [59]. Therefore, healthcare professionals must indicate to the testing laboratory whether the presence of any particular substance or group of substances is suspected or expected [61]. Strong lines of communication with laboratory personnel or technical support staff of the manufacturer of point-of-care testing devices are necessary to learn what can and cannot be reasonably expected of a particular test and/or laboratory.

Controversies exist regarding the clinical value of UDTs, partly because most current methods are designed for, or adapted from, forensic or workplace deterrent-based testing for illicit drug use. These are not necessarily optimized for widespread clinical applications [60]. However, when used with an appropriate level of understanding, systematically, and with follow-up documentation, UDTs can improve healthcare professionals' ability to manage therapy with prescribed drugs (including controlled substances), to diagnose substance misuse, abuse, or addiction, when present, to guide treatment, and to advocate for patients.

Table V-3. Summary of commonly used derivatives from the opium poppy, and their semisynthetic and totally synthetic opioid agents

Opiates – natural from opium poppy plant	Semisynthetic – derived from the opium poppy plant	Total synthetic opioids
Codeine	Hydrocodone	Meperidine
Morphine	Oxycodone	Fentanyl
Thebaine	Hydromorphone	Sufentanil
	Oxymorphone	Propoxyphene
	Buprenorphine	Methadone
		Heroin

Federally regulated testing is the most established use of UDTs. The "Federal Five" drugs or drug classes that are tested for in federal employees and federally regulated industries (e.g., the Department of Transportation) are marijuana (active ingredient: tetrahydrocannabinol (THC), cocaine metabolites (e.g. benzoylecgonine), opiates, phencyclidine (PCP), and amphetamine/methamphetamine [59]. The immunoassay screening and confirmatory cut-off concentrations for the Federal Five are federally mandated [59]. However, these levels are likely to be too high to be of value in clinical practice [62]. Federally regulated testing has split-sample* and chain-of-custody† requirements [59], but these are not always applicable to clinical practice [62].

Non-regulated testing is used for an increasing range of purposes. It is particularly important in settings outside the federally regulated system that testing laboratory personnel be aware of the purpose of testing so that they can customize their methodology and interpretation of results, if necessary, to meet these needs [60]. Many forensic uses of UDTs have possible legal implications; for example, candidates for employment; testing parents involved in child custody cases; applicants for driver's license renewal after drug-related revocation/suspension; persons within the criminal justice system; and claimants for insurance or workers' compensation [20, 21]. The scope of non-regulated workplace testing often involves immunoassays for drugs in addition to the Federal Five; for example, methadone, propoxyphene, benzodiazepines, and barbiturates [59].

Urine drug testing is also used for clinical purposes. In contrast to forensic testing, which assumes that the majority of donors will be negative for substances that may have misuse liability, in therapeutic testing the vast majority of donors are expected to be positive for the drug(s) of interest to demonstrate adherence to therapy [62].

The UDT can be an important tool at the healthcare professional's disposal, together with history and physical examination, to evaluate patients (e.g., pregnant women at risk for substance misuse; prior to a medical procedure), to support assessment and diagnosis (e.g., treatment decisions made in emergency departments; to assist in the diagnosis of drug misuse or addiction prior to starting or during treatment with controlled substances), and to monitor adherence to and help manage therapy with controlled substances [60, 61, 21, 20, 63, 64, 65].

A UDT can aid the healthcare professional to diagnose, or rule out, misuse of illicit or non-prescribed licit drugs [62]. UDT tests that corroborate the clinical history of self-reported use should be used to assist the patient in discontinuing illicit drug use; UDT results that are in conflict with the patient's self-report should be further investigated, with significant tightening of barriers. However, UDTs assess only the presence of a particular drug and/or its metabolite(s) in a specific concentration at a specific moment in time and do not generally provide definitive

---

* split-sample: splitting a single urine void into two separate bottles labeled A and B; bottle A is tested; bottle B remains sealed and available for testing at the discretion of the donor

† chain-of-custody: a legal term that refers to the ability to guarantee the identity and integrity of the specimen from collection through to reporting of the test results

information regarding addiction or impairment. It is important to remember that drug misuse or a concurrent addictive disorder does not rule out another medical problem, such as pain, but does require careful evaluation and use of a treatment plan, and referral to a pain specialist or program experienced in the treatment of substance misuse, when indicated.

With accurate record-keeping and due care, healthcare professionals can use UDTs to advocate for patients in family, workplace, and contested situations as documentation of adherence to the agreed-upon treatment plan and absence of undisclosed substances [62]. Diversion or trafficking of controlled substances occurs when patients, who may or may not be drug misusers, attempt to obtain a prescription for abusable drugs for illicit distribution or sale [62, 66]. To determine whether the patient is taking the medications prescribed or to decrease the risk of diversion, it is essential to know the characteristics of the testing procedures [2]. Since many drugs are not routinely detected by all immunoassays, contact the laboratory to ensure that the medication you are looking for will be reliably identified by the test ordered. Also be aware of the reporting cut-off concentrations that a particular laboratory uses – the therapeutic doses of some agents might fall below the limit of detectability of UDTs that are designed to deter misuse [62]. An inappropriately negative UDT may also occur secondary to maladaptive behavior, such as bingeing that may lead to running out early of the prescribed controlled substance, which can be addressed in a therapeutic context. Unexpected results should always be discussed with the patient and the testing laboratory.

Problematic patients often want appointments toward the end of office hours, telephone or arrive after office hours or when their primary physician is not available, and may insist on being seen immediately because they are late (for their flight, meeting, child's soccer game) [62]. Aberrant behaviors that suggest substance misuse/addiction include multiple episodes of prescription loss, resistance to changes in therapy, multiple dose escalations or other non-adherence to treatment, and concurrent misuse of alcohol or illicit drugs. However, a study among patients with persistent pain receiving long-term opioid therapy found that monitoring both urine toxicology and behavioral issues captured a greater number of patients with inappropriate drug-taking behavior than either alone [67]. Using UDTs in addition to self-report and monitoring of behavior may provide a more complete diagnostic picture. It is important to be aware that patients who are not addicted to, misusing, or diverting drugs may display the same behaviors; for example, patients whose pain is undertreated (pseudoaddiction) [3].

Patients in recovery from substance misuse disorders are often reluctant to enter into even rational pharmacotherapy for pain management. In these cases, routine UDTs can provide both reassurance and objective evidence to the treatment team and the patient and family of appropriate attention to the increased risks in this patient population [62].

Although only a minority of patients either misuse or become addicted to their prescribed medications, those who do generally have a current or past history of substance misuse or addiction [2]. Therefore, screening for a history of misuse/addiction should be routine before prescribing any controlled substance [62]. This may include a UDT to determine whether the patient is currently taking or has recently taken illicit and/or licit non-prescribed substances. A history of substance misuse does not preclude treatment with a controlled substance, when indicated, but does require a treatment plan with firmly defined boundaries – this may include random UDTs, a treatment agreement, and referral to or continuation with a recovery program [62]. It must be emphasized that the controlled substance is being prescribed to treat the pain syndrome, not for the maintenance or detoxification of a concurrent addictive disorder, which requires a separate registration as a narcotic treatment program. The records must reflect a clear evaluation of the presenting complaint and a clear indication for the medical use of controlled substances. If treatment objectives, such as decreased pain and increased function, are not being achieved despite medication adjustments, a UDT may assist with monitoring patient adherence before making further changes to the treatment plan [62].

Unexpected positive or negative UDT results are useful to support a decision to refer a patient to a specialist experienced in treating patients with co-morbid conditions, such as a pain management specialist who is knowledgeable in addiction medicine [2, 62, 39]. A clearly understood and well-defined description of treatment boundaries, for example, a urine specimen for testing when requested, should be in place when treating patients with controlled substances. The written/oral agreement should outline both the patient's and physician's rights and responsibilities [62, 40, 68].

Frequency of testing should be determined by clinical judgment. For random testing, two to three times per year may be adequate. If the patient is displaying aberrant behavior or third parties, such as family, friends, insurers, or law enforcement, report such behavior, testing may be intensified to as many times as necessary to document that the patient is adhering to the treatment plan [62, 66].

Types of Urine Drug Testing

There are two main types of urine drug testing, which, when used in proper combination, can reduce cost, ensure accuracy, and improve efficiency. The most common immunoassay drug screens, which can be laboratory-based or used at the point of care, are designed to classify substances as either present or absent [59]. The specificity and sensitivity of immunoassays vary depending on the type of assay and on the specific test performed. The primary disadvantage of immunoassays is that the antibodies are seldom specific to a single drug or drug metabolite; therefore, the antibodies may bind with other substances. Positive results based on immunoassays alone are referred to as "presumptive positives" because of factors such as cross-reactivity and different sensitivity and specificity among immunoassays. The results must be confirmed by a more specific method.

Sophisticated laboratory-based techniques, such as gas chromatography/mass spectrometry (GC/MS), are able to identify and confirm the presence of a specific drug and/or its metabolite(s) [59]. Although quantitative results are provided, there is *no* correlation between urine drug concentration and dose taken [61, 66]. This is because there are many factors besides daily dose that determine urinary concentration of drugs and their metabolites. Use a reputable testing laboratory, such as one that is certified by the Department of Health and Human Services (DHHS) or College of American Pathologists (CAP).

Proprietary immunoassays, such as EMIT® II, KIMS®, CEDIA®, DRI®, and AxSYM®, use antibodies to detect the presence of a drug or metabolite in urine [59]. The principal advantage of immunoassays is their ability to simultaneously and rapidly test for drugs in urine. The principal disadvantage is that they vary in the range of compounds detected, some detecting specific drugs, while others recognize only classes of drugs. It is important to know which screen is being used because sensitivity and specificity varies among different testing devices.

An immunoassay's ability to detect drugs varies according to the drug concentration in the urine and the assay's cutoff concentration. Any response above the cut-off is deemed positive and any response below the cut-off is negative [69, 70]. For example, if the cut-off is set at 50 ng/mL, a drug concentration of 49 ng/mL may be reported as negative [62]. Immunoassays are also subject to cross-reactivity; i.e., substances with similar, and sometimes dissimilar, chemical structure may cause a test to falsely appear positive for the target drug.

It is important to note that immunoassays are not static, but are being continually updated by the manufacturer and may even be altered by the testing laboratory itself through, for example, dilution of reagents [63].

Gas chromatography/mass spectrometry (GC/MS; Figure V-8) is the standard method that is used to confirm the presence of a specific drug and/or its metabolite(s) for forensic purposes [59]. However, variation can still exist because of different methods for performing assays, variation in factors affecting assays, potential for

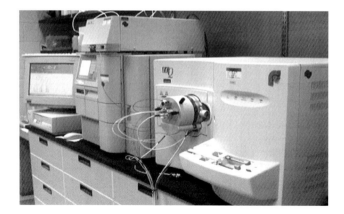

Figure V-8. Laboratory-based procedures using sophisticated equipment are required for chromatographic techniques

carryover from another specimen, and the cutoff concentration chosen [59]. For example, most laboratories have a limit of detection below which they will not report any drug as being present [60].

Clinically, laboratory-based specific drug identification such as GC/MS is needed to confirm the presence of a given drug and/or its metabolite(s); for example, that morphine is the opiate causing the positive immunoassay response, and to identify drugs not included in a given immunoassay; for example, oxycodone, hydromorphone, hydrocodone, and fentanyl [59].

Summary When Using Urine Drug Testing (UDT)

1. Immunoassay screening
   - Laboratory-based or at point of care
   - Classify substances as present or absent
   - Presumptive positives
2. Confirmatory and quantitative laboratory-based specific drug identification by GC/MS standard

INTERPRETATION OF UDT RESULTS

- Immunoassays report each sample as positive or negative for particular drug/class based on predetermined cut-offs
- Positive UDT results reflect recent drug use but cannot determine exposure time, dose, or frequency of use.

Limitations of Urine Drug Testing (UDT)

The term urine drug "screening" is a misnomer
a. All UDTs are not equal
b. There is no "standard" UDT which is suitable for all purposes and settings
c. Indicate whether any substance(s) is(are) suspected or expected
d. For certainty communicate with the testing laboratory
e. In case of positive screen, this has to be validated by GC/MS = gas chromatography/mass spectrometry.
In conclusion, all health care practitioners could improve the detection of addiction disorders:
1. Good pain care requires attention to the assessment of emerging addiction
2. There are reasons for aberrant drug-related behaviors other than addiction
3. Documentation of initial and ongoing findings accompanying continued patient assessment and decision-making process is critical.

Half-Life of Detection and Cut-Offs in Urine Drug Screening

Drug screening tests offer a fast and reliable way to demask a possible drug consumer. Various tests are available as individual tests for 12 drugs and medications as well as different combinations are offered which can be used in diverse circumstances, according to customer needs (Table V-4). They range from quick, competitive, stringent immunoassays to directly qualitative indications of drugs in urine. Depending on the time of abuse there is a large variability in half-life during which the agent can be detected in urine specimen.

The cut-offs presented in the next table are those used for immunoassays in federally mandated urine drug testing programs [59]. The detection time of a drug in urine indicates how long after administration a person excretes the drug and/or its metabolite(s) at a concentration above a specific test cut-off concentration [69, 71]. Although it is governed by several factors, including dose, route of administration, metabolism, urine volume, and pH, the detection time of most drugs in urine is less than 5 days, typically 1–3 days [21, 69, 70]. Long-term use of lipid-soluble drugs, such as marijuana, diazepam, or phencyclidine, may extend the window of detection to as long as a month [59, 21, 69].

At the cut-off value of 1000 ng/mL, urine samples can be positive for amphetamine for up to 5 days after intake [69]. On average, after smoking one marijuana cigarette, tetrahydrocannabinol (THC) may be detectable for 2–4 days in urine; more frequent users can be positive for a month [69]. Street doses of cocaine may be detectable for up to a week [69]. The detection time for opiates is about 1–2 days [65, 69]. Note that a positive "opiate" screen demonstrates the presence of codeine or morphine (a metabolite of heroin) **only**. The duration of detectability of phencyclidine is 8 days, though it may be detectable for up to a month in chronic users [59, 21].

Table V-4. Length of detection of different abused drugs in the urine (PCP = phencyclidine; TCA = tricyclic antidepressants; EDDP = 2-ethylidin-1, 5-dimethyl -3, 3-diphenyl-pyrrolidine)

Amphetamine	1–3 days
Barbiturates	4–8 days; in the case of chronic abuse, several weeks
Benzodiazepines	3 days after therapeutic dosage; up to 4–6 week in the case of long-term usage
Buprenorphine	2–6 days
Cannabis	The half-life is several weeks. Due to its good fat solubility, strong usage of cannabis can be positively detected in urine tests even after 20–30 days.
EDDP (methadone metabolite)	2–7 Days
Cocaine	Half-life ca. 90 min. With a cut-off of 300 ng/ml, detectable after about 2–4 days
Methadone	2–5 days
Opiates/Opioids	2–3 days
PCP	2–3 days
TCA	2–3 days

Table V-5. The cut-off values of different agents used in urine drug screening (EDDP = 2-ethylidin-1, 5-dimethyl -3, 3-diphenyl-pyrrolidine; AMP = amphetamine; MET = methamphetamine)

Drug	Cut-off Value (ng/ml)
AMP300	300
Amphetamines	1000
Barbiturates	300
Benzodiazepines	300
Buprenorphine	20
Cannabinoides	50
EDDP	100
MET300	300
Methadone	300
Methamphetamines	1000
Cocaine	300
Opiates	300
TCA	1000

According to the individual cut-off values, drugs can be detected in urine down to a specific concentration. Anything below the specific cut-off value will not be identified (Table V-5).

Interpretation of Results

The qualitative immunoassay drug panel reports each sample as either positive or negative for a particular drug or drug class, based on predetermined cutoff concentrations [21, 69, 70].

Positive UDT results reflect recent use of the drug, because most substances in urine have detection times of only 1–3 days. Positive results do not provide enough information to determine the exposure time, dose, or frequency of use [69].

Ideally, a UDT would be positive if the patient took the drug (true positive) and negative if the drug was not taken (true negative). However, false-positive or false-negative results can occur for a number of reasons, so it is important to interpret the UDT results carefully [21].

Pitfalls with Urine-Drug-Testing (UDT)

The opiate immunoassay screens were designed to detect heroin use, not adherence to a therapeutic opioid regimen. These immunoassays use monoclonal antibodies to detect morphine and codeine – heroin is rapidly metabolized to 6-monoacetylmorphine (6-MAM), and then to morphine [59].

For patients not prescribed morphine, presence of morphine in urine is often incorrectly assumed to be indicative of heroin use. A morphine-positive UDT may also result from codeine, from morphine use or misuse, and detectable levels are possible from morphine in foodstuffs (e.g., poppy seeds in breads/confectionery) [59, 69, 72]. However, performing opiate immunoassays at the federally mandated level of 2000 ng/mL, which was established in 1998, should eliminate nearly all positive results due to morphine from foodstuffs [59]. Only specific detection of 6-MAM by gas chromatography/mass spectrometry (GC/MS) is proof of heroin intake [59]. In addition, street heroin may be contaminated with codeine [59].

In the clinical setting when monitoring patients' adherence to a treatment plan, it is important that the lower cutoff level of 300 ng/mL be used for both screening and confirmation [62].

The next figure shows some of the pathways by which opioids are metabolized. Heroin is metabolized to 6-monoacetylmorphine (6-MAM) and then to morphine (Figure V-9). Heroin itself is rarely recovered from urine [62]. Codeine is metabolized to morphine, but not vice versa, so both substances may occur in urine following the use of codeine [62]. Hydrocodone can also be produced as a minor metabolite of codeine, and hydrocodone can be metabolized to small quantities of hydromorphone. Clinical experience suggests that morphine may be metabolized to produce small amounts of hydromorphone, possibly through keto-enol tautomerization [62, 73]. Therefore, these pathways may explain the presence of apparently unprescribed drugs. However, at no time should a minor metabolite be in excess of its parent – this would be consistent with use of the second drug [62].

As with any unexpected test results, it is important to clarify the interpretation with someone who is knowledgeable in clinical toxicology.

Also, most semisynthetic and synthetic opioids will not result in morphine or codeine appearing in the urine and are therefore not reliably detected by commonly used opiate immunoassays, even at high concentrations. Nevertheless, cross-reactivity can occur, causing positive results. However, gas chromatography/mass spectrometry (GC/MS) can reliably identify all opioids that are present [59]. If the purpose behind the test is to document the presence of a prescribed medication, such as oxycodone, hydromorphone, or hydrocodone (Table V-6), the laboratory should be informed of this and perform specific-drug identification by GC/MS in addition

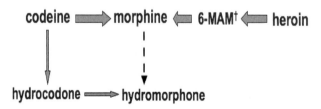

Figure V-9. Not comprehensive pathways, that may explain the presence of apparently unprescribed drugs 6-MAM = 6-monoacetylmorphine, an intermediate metabolite of heroin

Table V-6. Summary of semisynthetic and synthetic opioids not reliably detected by commonly used screens

Natural (from opium)	Semisynthetic (opium-derived)	synthetic (man-made)
• codeine	• hydrocodone	• meperidine
• morphine	• oxycodone	• fentanyl
• thebaine	• hydromorphone	• sufentanil
	• oxymorphone	• propoxyphene
	• buprenorphine	• methadone

to a routine immunoassay screen [62]. It is also recommended that the laboratory be instructed to remove the reporting threshold (cut-off concentration) so that the presence of lower concentrations of the prescribed drug can be documented. This will reduce the risk of missing a drug that is, in fact, present.

Summary of Considerations When Having a Positive Urine Test

1. Codeine is metabolized to morphine, so both substances may occur in urine following codeine use [21, 59, 66].
2. A prescription for codeine may explain the presence of both codeine and morphine in the urine.
3. A prescription for codeine does not usually explain the presence of only morphine (although samples collected 2–3 days after codeine ingestion may contain only morphine). Morphine alone is most consistent with ingestion of morphine or heroin.
4. Codeine alone is possible because a small proportion of patients lack the cytochrome P450 2D6 enzyme necessary to convert codeine to morphine.
5. Prescribed morphine *cannot* account for the presence of codeine. Although codeine is metabolized to morphine, the reverse does *not* occur.

Prescribed codeine may explain the presence of codeine with trace amounts of hydrocodone, which can be produced as a minor metabolite of codeine [73].

Cocaine is a topical anesthetic clinically used in certain trauma, dental, ophthalmoscopic, and otolaryngologic procedures. A patient's urine may test positive for the cocaine metabolite benzoylecgonine after such a procedure for up to 2–3 days. However, a licensed healthcare professional must order its use, which can be checked through medical records or by contacting the treating healthcare professional. There is no structural similarity between other anesthetics that end in "caine" (e.g., procaine, lidocaine) and cocaine or benzoylecgonine; therefore, cross-reaction does not occur, and being exposed to a local anesthetic is *not* an explanation for the presence of benzoylecgonine in the urine.

There have been documented cases of cocaine ingestion by drinking tea made from coca leaves. Although such tea may be available for purchase by unknowing consumers, the product – containing cocaine and/or its related metabolite(s) – is illicit under US federal statutes and regulations, and so is *not* a valid explanation. Patients should be advised not to ingest coca tea.

Clinical interpretation of amphetamine and methamphetamine positive results can be challenging because of prescription use and structural similarities of many prescription and over-the-counter (OTC) products, including certain drugs used in the treatment of Parkinson's disease, diet agents (particularly Mexican diet pills), and decongestants [59, 66]. Knowledge of potential sources of amphetamine or methamphetamine can prevent misinterpretation of results.

Therapeutic uses for amphetamine and methamphetamine include attention deficit disorder, treatment of exogenous obesity, and treatment of narcolepsy and CNS disorders [59]. Examples of prescription medications that contain amphetamine or methamphetamine are Adderall®, Benzedrine®, Dexedrine®, and Desoxyn®.

Immunoassay screening tests cross-react with various amphetamine-related drugs that are not misused, such as dopamine, isoxsuprine (a vasodilator), and ephedrine (an asthma medication). Other amphetamine-like drugs that are sometimes misused and also cross-react are phenmetrazine, phentermine, fenfluramine, and mephentermine [59].

Substances that are known to metabolize to amphetamine or methamphetamine include selegiline (for Parkinson's disease), benzphetamine, clobenzorex, dimethylamphetamine, fenproporex, and mefenorex [59].

Methamphetamine and amphetamine exist as two isomers, which are designated *d*- and *l*-. The *d*-form has a strong stimulant effect on the central nervous system and high abuse potential, while the *l*-form in therapeutic doses has a primarily peripheral action and is found in many OTC preparations [59]. Routine testing, such as immunoassays or gas chromatography/mass spectrometry (GC/MS), does not differentiate between *d*- and *l*-methamphetamine/amphetamine. For example, the OTC Vicks® Inhaler marketed in the US contains desoxyephedrine, the *l*-form of methamphetamine [59]. Patients whose management includes urine drug testing should be advised not to use the Vicks® Inhaler or similar OTC products containing methamphetamine [62].

Specialized tests, such as stereospecific chromatography, can distinguish between the two forms [59]. The separation of the *d*- and *l*-isomers should reveal nearly 100% *l*-methamphetamine following Vicks® Inhaler use. A laboratory quantitative report that indicates there is more than 20% of *d*-methamphetamine present suggests a source of methamphetamine other than the inhaler has been ingested. Illicitly manufactured methamphetamine/amphetamine is a mixture of *d*- and *l*-isomers. However, misuse of even the *l*-form of methamphetamine can have significant central activity and should be addressed clinically with the patient [62].

Several years ago, the nonsteroidal anti-inflammatory drug ibuprofen was found to interfere with the EMIT® immunoassay test and cause false-positive results for

marijuana. However, the problem has been corrected in the currently used EMIT®
II, and ibuprofen no longer causes false positives in initial screening assays [59].

There have been reports of false-positive urine immunoassay test results for THC
in patients receiving proton pump inhibitors, such as pantoprazole [74]. However, a
confirmatory test such as GC/MS will not verify the positive immunoassay result.

Tetrahydrocannabinol (THC), the main ingredient of marijuana, has been
prepared synthetically and marketed under the trade name Marinol® for the control
of nausea and vomiting in cancer patients receiving chemotherapy and as an appetite
stimulant for AIDS patients [59]. More specific testing would be required to distinguish between natural and synthetic THC. Passive smoke inhalation does not explain
positive marijuana results at typical cutoffs (50 ng/mL) [59, 75]. If a positive result
occurs, counsel the patient about the use of marijuana and reinforce the boundaries
set out in the treatment agreement. Repeated positive results for marijuana should
be viewed as evidence of ongoing substance misuse that requires further evaluation
and possible treatment [62].

Although legally obtained hemp food products do not appear to be psychoactive,
there have been concerns that ingestion of these food products, which contain traces
of THC, may cause a positive UDT result for marijuana [59, 76, 77]. However,
multiple studies have found that the THC concentrations typical in hemp seed
products are sufficiently low to prevent a positive immunoassay result [76, 77].
Therefore, consumption of hemp food products generally is *not* a valid explanation
for a urine immunoassay screen positive for marijuana.

False-positive results can be reported because of technician or clerical error.
These results may also occur because of cross-reactivity with other compounds
found in the urine, which may or may not be structurally related; for example, some
quinolone antibiotics, such as levofloxacin and ofloxacin, can potentially cause
false-positive results for opiates in common immunoassays, despite no obvious
structural similarity to morphine or codeine [59, 78, 79]. Fortunately, identifying
specific drugs or metabolites by gas chromatography/mass spectrometry (GC/MS)
is not influenced by cross-reacting compounds.

A UDT result reported as "none detected" may mean any of the following [62]:
1. The patient does not use the drug of interest.
2. The patient has not recently used the drug of interest.
3. The patient excretes the drug and/or its metabolites at a different rate than normal
   (e.g., rapid metabolism, pH effects of urine) [21].
4. The test used was not sufficiently sensitive to detect the drug at the concentration
   present [21]. It is important to know the threshold concentration that your
   laboratory uses when interpreting a report of "none detected." Ask for "no
   threshold" testing to determine if the drug is present at low concentrations.
5. Clerical errors caused a positive UDT result to be reported as negative.

In the case of adherence testing, a negative result may lead to concerns about misuse
(e.g., escalating dose of an opioid leading to running out of the analgesic, bingeing
of prescription medication, diversion of the agent) [62]. The most appropriate use
of a negative result for a prescribed medication is to initiate a dialog with the patient
in order to clarify the result and to preserve the therapeutic alliance.

A false-negative result is technically defined as a negative finding in a sample known to contain the drug of interest [62]. This may occur through technician or clerical error or be due to tampering with the urine sample. Methods employed by a minority of patients who may attempt to influence UDT results include adulteration and substitution of urine, which should be suspected if the characteristics of the urine sample are inconsistent with normal human urine.

Urine creatinine measurement is an inexpensive and well-characterized method to test specimen validity. The pH, temperature, and use of an adulteration panel are also useful [21, 59].

In the second outcome, the immunoassay is negative for opiates, and subsequent gas chromatography/mass spectrometry (GC/MS) failed to detect morphine [62]. Such a negative result suggests that the patient has not recently ingested morphine and may be consistent with diversion or trafficking drugs, but more commonly describes a bingeing pattern of drug use. Further investigation is required; the physician should verify with the laboratory that "none detected" was based on "no threshold" testing. Thereafter an appointment with the patient should be scheduled to discuss proper medication use and explore the possibility of diversion.

In the third outcome, the immunoassay is negative for opiates, but subsequent gas chromatography/mass spectrometry (GC/MS) is positive only for meperidine [62]. This result suggests that the patient is doctor shopping and/or misusing drugs, and requires further investigation to determine whether the patient has a genuine pain syndrome (and whether this behavior might represent a response to undertreatment or pseudoaddiction). Initiate or refer for substance misuse counseling or treatment, as indicated.

In the fourth outcome, the immunoassay is positive for opiates and cocaine [62]. Subsequent gas chromatography/mass spectrometry (GC/MS) confirms the presence of morphine and cocaine. This result suggests that the patient is abusing illicit drugs and may be misusing morphine or abusing heroin. Investigate whether or not the patient does have a pain syndrome, which, if present, will still require treatment, but with tightening of boundaries, counseling, and a referral to a pain specialist or program experienced in the treatment of substance misuse, if necessary.

A note of caution: The routine detection of oxycodone (a semisynthetic opioid) by an opiate immunoassay (designed to detect morphine and codeine) is unreliable [62]. Even large concentrations of oxycodone in the urine may not be detected, although positive results may occur because of cross-reactivity.

To monitor adherence to oxycodone (or other synthetic/semisynthetic opioids), in addition to an immunoassay screen to look for illicit substances, also order gas chromatography/mass spectrometry (GC/MS) without thresholds, which will detect and identify oxycodone, when present [62].

Test Procedure When Using a Multi-Test Card

Two types of test cards are being offered for UDT, both of which differ only in regard to how the specimen is being handled:

1. The dip test – Remove the cap from the test device and hold the absorbent tip into the urine for 10–15 s. There is no protective cap with every single test (Figure V-10).
2. The drop test – Using a pipette 3 drops are dropped into each well (Figure V-10). Read the result after 5–10 min.

Different Multi-Test Cards, either as a dip or a drop-test are available which can be selected in different compositions and combinations for individual drug testing (Figure V-11): Opiates/Opioids, Cocaine, COC 200, Benzodiazepines, Methadone, THC, THC 25, Amphetamines, Barbiturates, TCA Methamphetamine. Buprenorphine, Ecstasy (3,4-Methylendioxy-N-methylamphetamine), AMP 300, MET 300, and EDDP. Since EDDP (2-ethylidine-1, 5-dimethyl-3, 3-diphenyl-pyrrolidine; Figure V-12) is the main metabolite from methadone. By detecting the metabolite

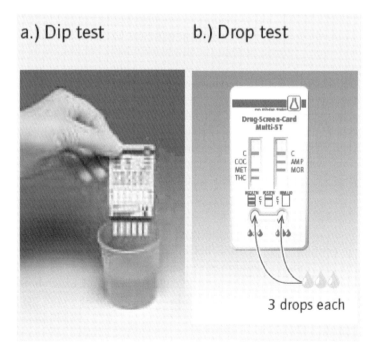

Figure V-10. Different Multi-Test cards using either the dip- or the drop-test method are available for drug analysis of various substances

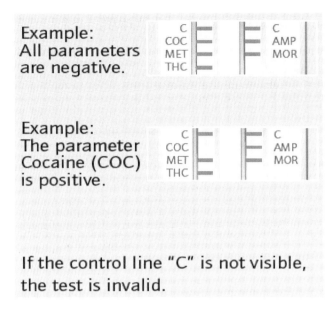

Example:
All parameters
are negative.

Example:
The parameter
Cocaine (COC)
is positive.

If the control line "C" is not visible,
the test is invalid.

Figure V-11. How a Multiple-Test card should be interpreted (AMP = amphetamine; MOR = morphine; COC = cocaine; MET = methamphetamine; THC = tetrahydrocannabinol)

rather than methadone itself, during substitution therapy one has following advantages:

1. Submission of foreign urine with methadone addition is no longer possible. By adding methadone to a negative urine sample, the methadone test will have a positive reading and the patient could make the methadone usage appear believable. Because the EDDP test only reacts highly sensitively to the

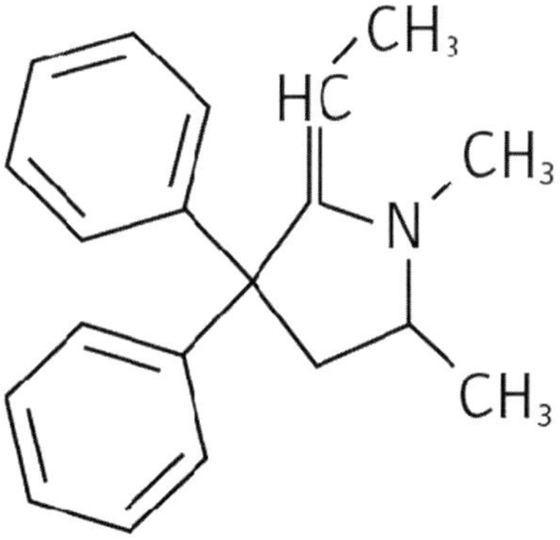

Figure V-12. The compound 2-ethylidin-1, 5-dimethyl-3, 3-diphenylpyrrolidine (EDDP), a metabolite of methadone, which can be detected within a time range of 2–7 days after ingestion

methadone metabolites, any attempt at manipulation remains negative. Those who metabolize quickly will be reliably detected.

2. Some patients metabolize methadone into EDDP very quickly. In such a case, the methadone test still remains negative, because there is no cross-reaction to the EDDP metabolite. With the EDDP test, however, these patients can be reliably identified.

In addition to *Multiple-Test Cards*, single test strips (i.e. sticks; Figure V-13) are also available for the qualitative detection of following abusable substances: Amphetamines, Barbiturates, Benzodiazepines, Buprenorphine, Cannabinoides, Cocaine, EDDP, Methadone, Methamphetamines, Opiates, PCP (phencyclidine), or TCA (tricyclic antidepressants). Having dipped the stick into the urine sample for 5–10 s, results can be viewed after 5–10 min.

Also, a *Cocaine Trace Wipe* is available (Figure V-14), which has been developed in cooperation with Police and Customs Authorities for the determination of cocaine residues on all surfaces such as inside cars, baggage, containers, parcels, textile (jeans etc.). If there are traces of cocaine, there will be a reaction on the tissue (blue color).

Although the specific determination of an antibody only reacts to an antigen, it can occur that a molecule with a very similar structure causes a reaction, leading to false results. Affected patients know this effect and consistently claim that a new medication must be the reason for a positive urine result. A commonly known cross-reactivity is that of codeine to opiates. A patient who takes codeine will test positive for opiates, because the molecules are so similar in structure that the antibodies can't tell the difference. A GC/MS (gas chromatography/mass spectroscopy) confirmation analysis helps in the situation to detect 6-Acetylmorphine as a primary substance, which is a metabolite of heroine, but not of codeine. The results should be available in the lab within 2 working days after receipt of the sample. In the case of a positive result, an approximate quantification will be done. Additionally, the detected illicit substance will be further differentiated, for instance for the type of benzodiazepine. Furthermore, polydrug use, such as LSD and buprenorphine can also be detected.

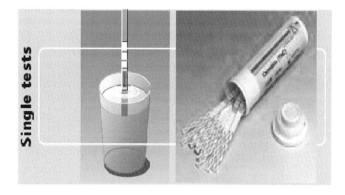

Figure V-13. Single test sticks for qualitative analysis of an abused substance in a urine specimen

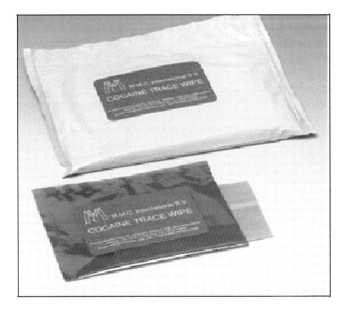

Figure V-14. The Trace Wipe Test for identification of cocaine smuggling or abuse

CONFIRMATION ANALYSIS OF QUICK TESTS

In the case of a positive result, this can only be considered a rough quantification of an abused substance. In the case of amphetamines, barbiturates, benzodiazepines, opiates or tricyclic antidepressants (TCA), the specific substance is only detected qualitatively. Furthermore, the concomitant ingestion of other illicit drugs can be identified. In the case of cross-reactivity, further tests should be conducted in order to clarify the situation. In case of additional drug abuse such as designer drugs, LSD and/or buprenorphine, it is also possible to use gas chromatography or HPLC (high pressure liquid chromatography) for analysis.

Assessing Possible Manipulation of the Urine Sample

The purpose of urine drug testing in clinical practice (Table V-7), where the majority of patients are not going to tamper with their urine sample, is to enhance patient care [62]. However, certain things can be done to improve the reliability of the results. Random collection is preferred, so the patient is not told in advance of the request for the urine sample. This can help to prevent the minority of patients who might tamper with their sample from being prepared with adulterants or substituted specimens.

In all situations, some control of sample integrity is desirable, and it is imperative where the consequences of incorrect results have far-reaching implications [61].

Table V-7. Possible manipulations of urine and how they are detected. Ultimately manipulated urine is unusable. It causes false negative as well as false positive results

Type of manipulation	Substances, methods used	Characteristical changes
Thinning	Can occur in vivo or in vitro	Urine is very light. The temperature is under 32 °C. The specific weight is less than 1.01 g/ml. Creatinine content is less than 30 mg/dl.
Addition of base	Bleaches like acetic acid or Domestos® are added to the sample.	pH value is more than 8. Chloride scent may be present.
Addition of acids	Acids like acetic acid or citric acid are added to the sample.	Marked pH value changes of >8
Addition of other substances	Soap or kitchen salt is added to the sample.	Urine may have flakes. Specific weight is greater than 1.035 g/ml.

Unobserved urine collection is usually acceptable, but observed collection may be necessary in certain situations or with high-risk patients. Ideally, the collection facility should not contain a basin with running water in order to reduce potential for specimen dilution, and blue pigment should be added to the toilet water. An unusually hot or cold specimen, small sample volume, or unusual color should raise concerns. Although urine specimens will cool to room temperature, the temperature of a urine sample within 4 min of voiding should fall within the range of 90 °F–100 °F, which can be checked at the time of collection by a temperature strip built into the urine collection container. Urinary pH should remain within the range of 4.5–8.0, and urinary creatinine concentration should be greater than 20 mg/dL A value less than 20 mg/dL is considered dilute and a value less than 5 mg/dL is not consistent with human urine [71]. Urinary creatinine measurement is an automated, inexpensive, and well-characterized method to test specimen validity. The color of a urine specimen is related to the concentration of its constituents [66]. Urine may be colored as a result of endogenous/exogenous substances derived from food pigments, medications, or disease states that produce excessive analyses. It can appear colorless as a result of excess hydration because of diet, medical condition, or water intake. In the absence of underlying renal pathology, patients who repeatedly provide diluted urine samples should be advised to decrease water intake prior to testing and to provide samples in the early morning. Any results outside of these ranges should be discussed with the patient and/or laboratory, as necessary [62].

The test results indicate whether the urine sample has been chemically manipulated before undergoing the drug test. Thinning of the urine sample is most likely the most frequently used form of urine manipulation. Specific weight and creatinine are significant parameters in case of a suspicious in vivo or in vitro thinning of the urine sample. Selective urine test strips are available, which can assess whether urine has been manipulated. The following parameters are being measured:

pH value – Any adding of acids or basic solution will be identified.

Nitrate – Nitrates in urine with gram-negative bacteria will be converted to nitrates. Nitrates can, if applied, falsify the test results.

Specific weight – A thinning of the urine sample can be identified.

Creatinine – Aside from in-vitro thinning, in-vivo thinning can also be recognized.

Glutaraldehyde – This is found in various disinfection solutions, it can falsify the test and will be detected with the strip. Bleach can affect the results if added to urine.

Pyridine chlorochromate – A chemical that will falsify the test

Screening for Alcohol Abuse

Because concomitant sequelae of alcoholism are often present in addicts an alcohol screen should be done. The Alcohol Screen is a qualitative enzymatic quick test for the detection of alcohol in saliva or urine. The Alcohol Screen is simple and fast and shows a positive result if the level is above 0.1‰ alcohol. The assay detects ethanol at concentrations of 0.1‰ or 10 mg/dL respectively by color change of the test pad to light greenish-grey. The green color intensifies with higher alcohol concentration in the sample. Thus, Alcohol-Screen produces a color change in the presence of alcohol in the specimen ranging from a light green-grey color at 0.1‰ concentrations via middle green at medium concentrations to a dark greenish-grey color at a 3.0‰ alcohol concentration (Figure V-15).

Hair or Saliva for Drug Testing

Urine is currently the most widely used and extensively validated biologic specimen for drug testing [21, 59, 66]. Although alternative technologies using other biologic specimens are marketed for drug testing, information is lacking about false-positive

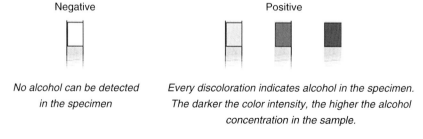

Negative	Positive
No alcohol can be detected in the specimen	Every discoloration indicates alcohol in the specimen. The darker the color intensity, the higher the alcohol concentration in the sample.

Figure V-15. View of the test stick for alcohol and the color, which reflect a positive analysis

Table V-8. Summary of pros ad cons for using saliva and and/or hair for drug testing

Saliva	Hair
Advantages	*Advantage*
• Collection ease	• Long-term measure related to hair length
• Minimal invasiveness	*Disadvantages*
• Close supervision	• Dark hair greater capacity to bind drug
• Limited preanalytical manipulation	• Irregular growth
Disadvantages	• Accessibility
• Shorter retention, lower levels than typically in urine	• Labor-intensive sample preparation

and false-negative results, interferences, and cross-reactivity. At this point, most of these techniques may not be appropriate for use in clinical practice [62].

Factors that influence the selection of a biologic specimen for drug analysis include ease of collection, analytical and testing considerations, and interpretation of results [80, 81]. Advantages of saliva as a test sample include ease of collection, minimal personal invasiveness, collection under close supervision (preventing tampering with the sample), and limited preanalytical manipulation (Table V-8). However, drugs and their metabolites are retained for shorter periods and occur at lower concentrations compared with urine [63, 80–82].

Hair analysis provides a retrospective, long-term measure of drug use that is directly related to the length of hair [66, 81]. Hair analysis is most useful for rapidly excreted drugs like heroin and cocaine, where the likelihood of drug misuse remaining undetected by urine analysis is substantial [66]. However, darkly pigmented hair has a greater capacity to bind a drug than hair that is fair or gray, leading to the claim that hair analysis might have a possible color bias [21, 81]. Other disadvantages of hair analysis include possible irregular growth, accessibility, and labor-intensive sample preparation.

Hair Analysis for the Detection of Abused Drugs and Medications

This analysis is a retrospective method, which uses a gas chromatograph with a mass-specific detector. DIN EN 45001 as well as the 93/42/EWG and 90/385/EWG guidelines should accredit the lab (Table V-9). To complete drug analysis service offerings, hair analysis alongside drug quick tests and confirmation analysis are available. Why is hair analysis a suitable method for long-term detection of abuse? Hair has the advantage of being able to detect the ingestion of drugs and medication over a specific time period. Drugs and medications are stored in the hair follicles and grow along with the hair. Since hair grows approximately 10–15 mm per month, past drug abuse can be determined by examining the respective segment of hair. For the examination, one requires a pen-sized tuft of hair, which was cut directly at the scalp. Individual hairs are not sufficient to run an analysis.

Table V-9. Excess of any of the values below is considered a positive result in hair analysis

Drug	Cut-off value (ng/mg hair)
Amphetamine/Methamphetamine/Ecstasy	1.10
Methadone	1.00
Opiate	1.00
THC (Cannabis)	0.20
Benzoylecgonine (Cocaine)	0.50

Sweat collection using a sweat patch provides a noninvasive, cumulative measure of drug use over a period of days to weeks, which is most appropriate for monitoring drug use in addiction treatment or probation programs [21, 80]. Disadvantages include varying sweat production and risk of accidentally removing or contaminating the collection device [80].

There is reduced possibility that patients can influence test results with blood samples and more accurate determination of drug concentrations could possibly be obtained by a quantitative analysis of drugs in blood [66]. However, blood samples are not amenable to rapid screening procedures (Table V-10), have low drug concentrations, and require invasive collection [21, 66]. Therefore, blood is not recommended for routine testing [21].

The relative detection times of drugs in these biologic specimens are shown in the next figure. Blood and saliva maintain detectable levels of drugs for hours, urine for days, and sweat for weeks with a cumulative device, and hair and nails for several years (Figure V-16).

To summarize, one orders a UDT, takes a detailed history of the medications a patient uses, including prescribed, over-the-counter (OTC), and herbal drugs, with dose and time of last use, and his or her drug misuse/addiction history. And let the laboratory know what you are looking for; i.e., an illicit substance, prescription drug misuse, or presence of a prescribed medication.

Accurate interpretation of UDT results in clinical practice requires information. You should know how the specimen is collected; what prescription, over-the-counter

Table V-10. Summary of pros and cons for using sweat and/or blood for drug testing

Sweat	Blood
Advantage	*Advantage*
• Noninvasive, cumulative measure over days to weeks	• Reduced chance of patients influencing test results
Disadvantages	*Disadvantages*
• Varying sweat production	• Not amenable to rapid screening
• Risk of accidentally removing/contaminating collection device	• Low concentration
	• Invasive collection

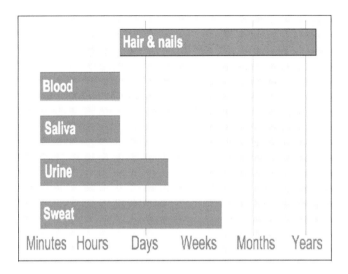

Figure V-16. Differences in detection times of abused drugs in various body fluids Adapted from [83]

(OTC), or herbal drugs the patient is taking; retention times of drugs in urine; alternative medical explanations; metabolism of drugs; scams; and laws, regulations, and guidelines concerning controlled substances. The UDT is an important tool at healthcare professionals' disposal to evaluate patients. Testing cannot, however, substitute for diagnostic skills or an ongoing therapeutic alliance with a patient [62]. It may not be required in every patient, and is insufficient alone in any patient.

The clinical value of a UDT depends on the interactions between the healthcare professional and testing laboratory or manufacturer of a point-of-care test so that the healthcare professional understands the limits of the UDT in terms of what it can and cannot detect, so that appropriate tests are ordered [60]. Healthcare professionals should establish a relationship with the director or certifying scientist from the testing laboratory and consider a medical review officer consult. Medical review officers are licensed physicians who are responsible for receiving laboratory results generated from forensic testing and who have appropriate medical training to interpret and evaluate test results together with medical history and any other relevant biomedical information [62].

In conclusion,

- All clinicians can improve the detection of addiction disorders while prescribing drug medication.
- Good pain care with the use of opioids requires attention to the assessment of emerging addiction.
- There are reasons for aberrant drug-related behaviors other than addiction.
- Documentation of initial and ongoing findings accompanying continued patient assessment & decision-making process is critical.

References

1. National Center on Addiction and Substance Abuse at Columbia University *Missed Opportunity: CASA National Survey of Primary Care Physicians and Patients on Substance Abuse*, 2000: New York.
2. Schnoll, S.H. and J. Finch, *Medical education for pain and addiction: making progress towards answering a need.* J Law Med Ethics, 1994. **22**: pp. 252–256.
3. Weissman, D.E. and J.D. Haddox, *Opioid pseudoaddiction – an iatrogenic syndrome.* Pain, 1989. **36**: pp. 363–366.
4. Savage, S., et al., *A consensus document from the American Academy of Pain Medicine, American Pain Society, American Society of Addiction Medicine. Definitions related to the use of opioids for the treatment of pain*, 2001.
5. Portenoy, R.K. and S.R. Savage, *Clinical realities and economic considerations: special therapeutic issues in intrathecal therapy – tolerance and addiction.* J Pain Symptom Manage, 1997. **14**: pp. S27–S35.
6. Hardman, J.G., L.E. Limbird, and A.G. Gilman, in *Goodman and Gilman's: The Pharmacological Basis of Therapeutics*, L.S. Goodman and A.G. Gilman, Editors, 2001, McGraw Hill: New York.
7. Schnoll, S.H. and M.F. Weaver, *Addiction and pain.* Am J Addict, 2003. **12**(Suppl 2): pp. S27–S35.
8. Camí, J. and M. Farré, *Mechanisms of disease: drug addiction.* N Engl J Med, 2003. **349**: pp. 975–986.
9. Miotto, K., et al., *Diagnosing addictive disease in chronic pain patients.* Psychosomatics, 1996. **37**: pp. 223–235.
10. Cherny, N.I., *Opioid analgesics. Comparative features and prescribing guidelines.* Drugs, 1996. **51**: pp. 714–737.
11. McLellan, A.T., et al., *Drug dependence, a chronic medical illness. Implications for treatment, insurance, and outcomes evaluation.* JAMA, 2000. **284**: pp. 1689–1695.
12. Fernandez, H.H., M.E. Trieschmann, and M.S. Okun, *Rebound psychosis: effect of discontinuation of antipsychotics in Parkinson's disease.* Mov Disord, 2005. **20**: pp. 104–105.
13. Fossmark, R., et al., *Rebound acid hypersecretion after long-term inhibition of gastric acid secretion.* Aliment Pharmacol Ther, 2005. **21**: pp. 149–154.
14. Barkin, R.L. and D. Barkin, *Pharmacologic management of acute and chronic pain: focus on drug interactions and patient-specific pharmacotherapeutic selection.* South Med J, 2001. **94**: pp. 756–770.
15. Vastag, B., *Addiction poorly understood by clinicians. Experts say attitudes, lack of knowledge hinder treatment.* JAMA, 2003. **290**: pp. 1299–1303.
16. Kendler, K.S., et al., *Illicit psychoactive substance use, heavy use, abuse, and dependence in a US population-based sample of male twins.* Arch Gen Psychiat, 2000. **57**: pp. 261–269.
17. Jacob, T., et al., *Genetic and environmental effects on offspring alcoholism. New insights using an offspring-of-twins design.* Arch Gen Psychiat, 2003. **60**: pp. 1265–12721.
18. Kreek, M.J., D.A. Nielson, and K.S. LaForge, *Genes associated with addiction: alcoholism, opiate, and cocaine addiction.* Neuromolecular Med, 2004. **5**: pp. 85–108.
19. Koob, G.F., et al., *Neurobiological mechanisms in the transition from drug use to drug dependence.* Neurosci Biobehav Rev, 2004. **27**: pp. 739–749.

20. Simpson, D., et al., *Screening for drugs of abuse (II): cannabinoids, lysergic acid diethylamide, buprenorphine, methadone, barbiturates, benzodiazepines and other drugs.* Ann Clin Biochem, 1997. **34**: pp. 460–510.

21. Wolff, K., et al., *A review of biological indicators of illicit drug use, practical considerations and clinical usefulness.* Addiction, 1999. **94**: pp. 1279–1298.

22. Girault, J.A. and P. Greengard, *The neurobiology of dopamine signaling.* Arch Neurol, 2004. **61**: pp. 641–644.

23. Prescott, C.A. and K.S. Kendler, *Genetic and environmental contributions to alcohol abuse and dependence in a population-based sample of male twins.* Am J Psychiat, 1999. **156**: pp. 34–40.

24. Enoch, M.A. and D. Goldman, *The genetics of alcoholism and alcohol abuse.* Curr Psychiatry Rep, 2001. **3**: pp. 144–151.

25. Rhee, S.H., et al., *Genetic and environmental influences on substance initiation, use, and problem use in adolescents.* Arch Gen Psychiat, 2003. **60**: pp. 1256–1264.

26. Uhl, G.R. and R.W. Grow, *The burden of complex genetics in brain disorders.* Arch Gen Psychiat, 2004. **61**: pp. 223–229.

27. Toneatto, T., J.C. Negrete, and K. Calderwood, *Diagnostic subgroups within a sample of comorbid substance abusers: correlates and characteristics.* Am J Addict, 2000. **9**: pp. 253–264.

28. Grant, B.F., et al., *Prevalence and co-occurrence of substance use disorders and independent mood and anxiety disorders: results from the National Epidemiologic Survey on Alcohol and Related Conditions.* Arch Gen Psychiat, 2004. **61**: pp. 807–816.

29. Hasin, D., et al., *Effects of major depression on remission and relapse of substance dependence.* Arch Gen Psychiat, 2002. **59**: pp. 375–380.

30. The National Center on Addiction and Substance Abuse at Columbia University. *So Help Me God: Substance Abuse, Religion and Spirituality*, 2001.

31. Schnoll, S.H. and J. Finch, *Medical education for pain and addiction: making progress toward answering a need.* J Law Med Ethics, 1994. **22**: pp. 252–256.

32. Sjøgren, P., et al., *Neuropsychological performance in cancer patients: the role of oral opioids, pain and performance status.* Pain, 2000. **86**: pp. 237–245.

33. Portenoy, R.K. and K.M. Foley, *Chronic use of opioid analgesics in non-malignant pain. Report of 38 cases.* Pain, 1986. **25**: pp. 171–186.

34. Marsden, J., et al., *Psychiatric symptoms among clients seeking treatment for drug dependence.* Br J Psychiat, 2000. **176**: pp. 285–289.

35. American Academy of Pain Medicine and American Pain Society. *The Use of Opioids for the Treatment of Chronic Pain. A Consensus Statement*, 1996.

36. Compton, P., K. Darakjian, and K. Miotto, *Screening for addiction in patients with chronic pain and "problematic" substance use: evaluation of a pilot assessment tool.* J Pain Symptom Manage, 1996. **16**: pp. 355–363.

37. Wilford, B.B., *Abuse of prescription drugs in addiction medicine.* West J Med, 1990. **152** (special issue): pp. 609–612.

38. Portenoy, R.K., *Opioid therapy for chronic nonmalignant pain: a review of the critical issues.* J Pain Symptom Manage, 1996. **11**: pp. 203–217.

39. Federation of State Medical Boards of the United States, I., *Model Policy for the Use of Controlled Substances for the Treatment of Pain.* 2004, A Policy Document of the Federation of State Medical Boards of the United States, Inc.

40. Heit, H.A., *Creating and implementing opioid agreements.* Care Management/Disease Management Digest, 2003. **7**: pp. 2–3.

41. Drug Enforcement Administration. *Physician's Manual: An Informational Outline of the Controlled Substances Act of 1970*, 1990. p. 21.

42. Weaver, M.F., M.A.E. Jarvis, and S.H. Schnoll, *Role of the primary care physician in problems of substance abuse*. Arch Intern Med, 1999. **159**: pp. 913–924.

43. Lambert, L., *Patients in pain need round-the-clock care*. JAMA, 1999. **281**: pp. 689–692.

44. American Pain Society. *Guideline for the Management of Pain in Osteoarthritis, Rheumatoid Arthritis, and Juvenile Chronic Arthritis. Clinical Practice Guideline*, Glenview, IL, 2002.

45. *The Merck Manual of Diagnosis and Therapy*. Vol. 17th edition, 1999.

46. Savage, S.R., *Assessment for addiction in pain-treatment settings*. Clin J Pain, 2002. **18**: pp. S28–S38.

47. Fiellin, D.A., M.C. Reid, and P.G. O'Connor, *Outpatient management of patients with alcohol problems*. Ann Intern Med, 2000. **133**: pp. 85–827.

48. Skinner, H.A., et al., *Identification of alcohol abuse using laboratory tests and a history of trauma*. Ann Intern Med., 1984. **101**: pp. 847–851.

49. Minovitz, O. and M. Driol, *The sexual abuse, eating disorder and addiction (SEA) triad: syndrome or coincidence?* Med Law, 1989. **8**: pp. 59–61.

50. Vastag, B., *What's the connection? No easy answers for people with eating disorders and drug abuse*. JAMA, 2001. **285**: pp. 1006–1007.

51. Ewing, J., *Detecting alcoholism: the CAGE questionnaire*. JAMA, 1984. **252**: pp. 1905–1907.

52. Fiellin, D.A., M.C. Reid, and P.G. O'Connor, *Outpatient management of patients with alcohol problems*. Ann Intern Med, 2000. **133**: pp. 815–827.

53. Bastiaens, L., G. Francis, and K. Lewis, *The RAFFT as a screening tool for adolescent substance use disorders*. Am J Addict, 2000. **9**: pp. 10–16.

54. Knight, J.R., et al., *Validity of the CRAFFT substance abuse screening test among adolescent clinic patients*. Arch Pediatr Adolesc Med, 2002. **156**: pp. 607–614.

55. Sillanaukee, P. and U. Olsson, *Improved diagnostic classification of alcohol abusers by combining carbohydrate-deficient transferrin and gamma-glutamyltransferase*. Clin Chem, 2001. **47**: pp. 681–685.

56. Papoz, L., et al., *Alcohol consumption in a healthy population. Relationship to gamma-glutamyl transferase activity and mean corpuscular volume*. JAMA, 1981. **245**: pp. 1748–1751.

57. Smith, K.E. and N.A. Fenske, *Cutaneous manifestations of alcohol abuse*. J Am Acad Dermatol, 2000. **43**: pp. 1–16.

58. Wiese, J.C., M.G. Shlipak, and W.S. Browner, *The alcohol hangover*. Ann Intern Med, 2000. **132**: pp. 897–902.

59. Shults, T.F., *Medical Review Officer Handbook*. Vol. 8th edition, 2002: Quadrangle Research.

60. Hammett-Stabler, C., A.J. Pesce, and D.J. Cannon, *Urine drug screening in the medical setting*. Clinica Chimica Acta, 2002. **315**: pp. 125–135.

61. Galloway, J.H. and I.D. Marsh, *Detection of drug misuse—an addictive challenge*. J Clin Pathol, 1999. **52**: pp. 713–718.

62. Gourlay, D., H.A. Heit, and Y.H. Caplan, *Urine Drug Testing in Clinical Practice: Dispelling the Myths and Designing Strategies* [monograph]. 2004, Pharma Com Group, Inc: Stamford, CT.

63. Hattab, E.M., et al., *Modification of screening immunoassays to detect sub-threshold concentrations of cocaine, cannabinoids, and opiates in urine: use for detecting maternal and neonatal drug exposure.* Ann Clin Lab Sci, 2000. **30**: pp. 85–91.

64. Passik, S.D., et al., *A chart review of the ordering and documentation of urine toxicology screens in a cancer center: do they influence patient management?* J Pain Symtom Manage, 2000. **19**: pp. 40–44.

65. Perrone, J., et al., *Drug screening versus history in detection of substance use in ED psychiatric patients.* Am J Emerg Med, 2001. **19**: pp. 49–51.

66. Braithwaite, R.A., et al., *Screening for drugs of abuse. I: opiates, amphetamines and cocaine.* Ann Clin Biochem, 1995. **32**: pp. 123–153.

67. Katz, N.P., *Behavioral monitoring and urine toxicology testing in patients on long-term opioid therapy*, in *American Academy of Pain Medicine 17th Annual Meeting*, 2001: Miami Beach, FL.

68. Savage, S., et al., *Public policy statement on the rights and responsibilities of healthcare professionals in the use of opioids for the treatment of pain. A consensus document from the American Academy of Pain Medicine, the American Pain Society, and the American Society of Addiction Medicine*, 2004.

69. Vandevenne, M., H. Vandenbussche, and A. Verstraete, *Detection time of drugs of abuse in urine.* Acta Clinica Belgica, 2000. **55**: pp. 323–333.

70. Casavant, M.J., *Urine drug screening in adolescents.* Pediatr Clin N Am., 2002. **49**: pp. 317–327.

71. Cook, J.D., et al., *The characterization of human urine for specimen validity determination in workplace drug testing: a review.* J Anal Toxicol, 2000. **24**: pp. 579–588.

72. Rohrig, T.P. and C. Moore, *The determination of morphine in urine and oral fluid following ingestions of poppy seeds.* J Anal Toxicol, 2003. **27**: pp. 449–452.

73. Oyler, J.M., et al., *Identification of hydrocodone in human urine following controlled codeine administration.* J Anal Toxicol, 2000. **24**: pp. 530–535.

74. Wyeth-Ayerst, *PROTONIX® (pantoprazile sodium) package insert*, 2004.

75. Casavant, M.J., *Urine drug screening in adolescents.* Pediatr Clin N Am, 2002. **49**: pp. 317–327.

76. Bosy, T.Z. and B.A. Cole, *Consumption and quantitation of Δ9-tetrahydrocannabinol in commercially available hemp seed oil products.* J Anal Toxicol, 2000. **24**: pp. 562–566.

77. Leson, G., et al., *Evaluating the impact of hemp food consumption on workplace drug tests. 2001; 25:691–698.* J Anal Toxicol, 2001. **25**: pp. 691–698.

78. Baden, L.R., et al., *Quinolones and false-positive urine screening for opiates by immunoassay technology.* JAMA, 2001. **286**: pp. 3115–3119.

79. Zacher, J.L. and D.M. Givone, *False-positive urine opiate screening associated with fluoroquinolone use.* Ann Pharmacother, 2004. **38**: pp. 1525–1528.

80. Caplan, Y.H. and B.A. Goldberger, *Alternative specimens for workplace drug testing.* J Anal Toxicol., 2001. **25**: pp. 396–399.

81. Kintz, P. and N. Samyn, *Use of alternative specimens: drugs of abuse in saliva and doping agents in hair.* Ther Drug Monit, 2002. **24**: pp. 239–246.

82. Yacoubian, G.S.J., E.D. Wish, and D.M. Pérez, *A comparison of saliva testing to urinalysis in an arrestee population.* J Psychoactive Drugs, 2001. **33**: pp. 289–294.

Index